# PREFACE

Critical thinking has become imperative in virtually all aspects of life. It is at the heart of the educational reform movement in this country, including nursing education. It is a required outcome criterion for baccalaureate and higher degree nursing faculty who wish to meet the accreditation standards of the National League for Nursing.

Critical thinking is an area of investigation for researchers and of subsequent application for professional practitioners. Interest in critical thinking has swept across the country igniting enthusiasm, scholarly investigation, and curriculum revision. Critical thinking is receiving renewed attention from politicians, philosophers, historians, and ordinary citizens concerned about maintaining our way of life to professional practitioners in all disciplines, including health care. How we think, view ourselves, solve problems, participate in our country's governance, and contribute to society through our professions all determine the quality of our own lives and those around us. Functioning blindly on the orders of someone else is no longer acceptable. Instead, we must be cognitively engaged and participate fully in decision making.

Nursing educators are an increasing presence at conferences on critical thinking, both as speakers and attendees. Many nursing and nonnursing faculty are talking about critical thinking, but few agree on what it is and how it is best applied to nursing practice. There is clear, intense interest in building our knowledge and developing concepts upon which we all can agree. We propose to find and build on areas of agreement in the field of critical thinking as it applies to nursing.

In this book we examine critical thinking as a concept and show how it can be applied to the everyday situations confronting nurses. In every chapter we elaborate on an aspect of critical thinking, explain how to apply it, and provide numerous exercises that lead you through the process itself. We also define concepts, explain how your thinking style affects the kind of thinking you do, and include real life examples and exercises that enable you to apply the process. Not only do we tell you about critical thinking, but we also show you how to do it.

We address the numerous controversial issues about which philosophers contemplate, and with which nurses must deal. We focus on the thinking skills nurses need to deal within the wide array of situations they experience in their daily interactions with clients, families, colleagues, and institutional administrators. We present critical thinking as a set of cognitive skills that health professionals use in all situations. Critical thinking skills are essential to resolving health care situations and to discussing controversial issues in a thoughtful, fair-minded manner. For example, critical thinking skills are necessary for health professionals when they work with clients and families, learn to manage home care, or grapple with caring for a newborn or an aging parent. When a nursing student joins a unit, he or she must engage in critical thinking to negotiate the transition from newcomer to team member. Today health care providers must continually redefine their roles and accommodate new members on their health care team. Critical thinking skills are necessary to participate with administrators in rendering cost-effective care. Critical thinking skills are essential for dealing with controversial and problematic issues: aggressive treatments in the care of the dying client, the ability to come to terms with your own beliefs and values while caring for people such as a young woman undergoing an abortion or a 75-year-old client undergoing a liver transplant, and the redesign of the structure and function of health care delivery in the United States.

Learning to articulate your thinking increases your power to influence others. You are empowered when you confidently state reasoned opinions regarding health care. You increase your chances of being heard when you articulate a logical defense as you communicate effectively about an issue of importance with other nurses, physicians, hospital administrators, legislators, and other significant players in the health care arena. Empowerment changes your position and demeanor. You change the level of respect you command when you articulate clearly about the issue under discussion and how you will be heard on subsequent issues.

Not only should you incorporate critical thinking skills into your own practice, but you also should teach critical thinking skills to clients and families. By helping clients and families work through their health care challenges, you model critical thinking and problem-solving skills, encouraging clients to develop these same skills for themselves. You will find thorough discussion of these issues throughout the book.

Many nursing authors have examined the process of clinical judgment and diagnostic reasoning. Because these topics have been treated by a number of authors, we focus on critical thinking as a broader, more encompassing concept. We believe that critical thinking and clinical judgment are related but different cognitive processes. This conclusion has been posited by both researchers and observers in nursing. Both critical thinking and clinical judgment are important skills for health professionals to cultivate. We believe that the diagnostic focus of clinical judgment makes it more narrow than critical thinking. Further, critical thinking has broad application to all aspects of your personal and professional life.

This textbook emphasizes a holistic view of cognitive processes including many dimensions of critical thinking, as well as other ways of knowing, reasoning, and creative thinking. The perspective of critical thinking as an interaction is followed by treatment of critical thinking as a personal historical development in the individual. Other ways of knowing such as insight and intuition become more important in our world of rapid change and cultural diversity. Examining your own frame of reference and others is followed by information designed to help you refine your thinking. Creative thinking is presented as a phase of all good thinking. Its uses, advantages, and disadvantages are discussed along with methods of promoting it in yourself and others.

Evidence is examined from the perspective of evaluating both quantitative and qualitative research. Learning how to construct your arguments and distinguish between various aspects of the reasoning process is followed by the use of cognitive skills in listening and evaluating the arguments of others. The final chapter emphasizes the use of critical and creative thinking skills to build on the communication process started in the earlier chapters. Persuasion as an important process in nursing and articulating your position to others completes the cycle of communicating with the interacting other.

Each chapter is followed by exercises designed to illustrate points in the chapter, through applications to professional and everyday situations. Readings are included for those whose curiosity is piqued or who wish to do further in-depth exploration of the issues raised in the chapter.

# Critical Thinking
## Applied to Nursing

**Mary A. Miller, RN, PhD**

*Professor of Nursing and Health Care Management*
*Department of Nursing and Health Care Management*
*and*
*Associate Dean*
*School of Professional Studies*
*Metropolitan State College of Denver*
*Denver, Colorado*

**Dorothy E. Babcock, RN, MSN, C**

*Professor of Nursing and Health Care Management*
*Department of Nursing and Health Care Management*
*Metropolitan State College of Denver*
*Denver, Colorado*

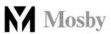 Mosby

St. Louis   Baltimore   Boston   Carlsbad   Chicago   Naples   New York   Philadelphia   Portland
London   Madrid   Mexico City   Singapore   Sydney   Tokyo   Toronto   Wiesbaden

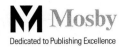
Dedicated to Publishing Excellence

Printed in the United States of America

Mosby–Year Book, Inc.
11830 Westline Industrial Drive
St. Louis, Missouri 63146

**Library of Congress Cataloging-in-Publication Data**

Miller, Mary A. (Mary Alice)
    Critical thinking applied to nursing / Mary A. Miller, Dorothy E.
Babcock.
        p.      cm.
    Includes bibliographical references and index.
    ISBN 0-8151-6962-0 (pbk.)
    1. Nursing--Philosophy.   2. Critical thinking.   I. Babcock,
Dorothy E.   II. Title.
    [DNLM: 1. Thinking.   2. Nursing.   3. Cognition.   WY 100 M649c
1996]
    RT84.5.M54   1996
610.73'01--dc20
DNLM/DLC                                                95-37174

99  /  9 8 7 6 5

*To nurses everywhere
(especially Mary's beloved sister Margaret)
who value critical and creative thinking
and who enrich the lives of others
by their caring ministrations.*

This textbook is for health professionals who are intent on examining their thinking processes and expanding their repertoire of thinking skills. It is an adjunct to textbooks in the basic clinical areas and community health; it provides focus and structure to the discussion of clinical experiences and controversial issues when such discussion moves beyond diagnostic reasoning and into a larger realm, the totality of personal and professional experience.

Throughout the book we have used the word *colleague* to denote nursing students who aspire to professional nursing and practicing clinicians. All of these individuals at their varying levels of expertise and experience are colleagues together. Students should begin at the earliest point possible in their education to see themselves as colleagues with their classmates, instructors, practicing nurses, and other health care professionals and students in the related disciplines. All health care professionals should be challenged to think their best and to keep expanding their thinking abilities. As the roles and responsibilities for administering nursing care shift into pioneering efforts to deliver the safest highest quality nursing care in the most cost-effective manner possible, we will need all the help we can get from experienced and aspiring colleagues wherever we are learning and serving the client. Further, we believe that critical thinking starts in childhood and should be a major outcome of the continuum of education.

At every level of education, instructors must encourage and help students learn to think more critically. We have, therefore, developed an instructor's manual to assist the instructor in making the material herein presented more meaningful to the particular students who confront the instructor. The manual contains both general information on assisting students to learn and guidance for specific chapters. Each chapter in the manual reviews the purpose, expected outcomes, application to the nursing curriculum, and helpful hints about using the exercises at the end of each chapter. Other exercises have been added in the manual. The instructor may select among these according to the students' interests and capabilities.

## Acknowledgments

No book is written in isolation. We want to thank the following colleagues for their invaluable consultation, critique, and effort on our behalf. Darlene Como has encouraged us throughout the development of the manuscript. Mosby reviewers gave us very thoughtful feedback. Lori Allen, a professional editor, provided excellent feedback before reviewers at Shepherd, Inc., scrutinized the manuscript and provided final expert copy editing. Linda Daniel, a nurse educator and doctoral candidate, reviewed the chapters on research. Frederick Doepke and Steve Benson, philosophers and colleagues, reviewed the sections on reasoning and evaluating arguments. Char Spade, Pam Stoeckel, and Mary Johnston, nurse educators in associate degree programs, did a reality check on the relevance of our book to the associate degree curriculum.

Our relatives were equally supportive. Mary's mother, Ida Wall, a retired educator, reviewed and critiqued several chapters, and Dorothy's husband, Clarence Babcock, a retired scientist, reviewed some chapters and changed her scratchings into recognizable drawings. We, of course, take full responsibility for any blunders and mistakes.

# CONTENTS

*Critical Thinking Applied to Nursing*

# A Framework for Critical Thinking in Nursing

## Chapter 1

## OVERVIEW

Learning to think deeply, creatively, and effectively helps you as a nurse to care for your clients and serve as their advocate; it also helps you become more astute in making your own life choices. Thinking critically about your beliefs, circumstances, behavior, and choices will help you develop self-confidence and foster self-actualization, both personally and professionally. This chapter discusses the importance of critical thinking and the reasons nurses should be skilled in its use.

This chapter defines critical thinking, examines factors that influence critical thinking, and identifies and discusses critical thinking skills and attitudes essential for the nurse. The Critical Thinking Interaction Model, which provides a framework for applying critical thinking when working with clients, families, colleagues, and administrators, is introduced. This chapter presents an overview of the components of the model; subsequent chapters develop this model in greater depth.

Finally, each chapter provides exercises that stimulate thinking and apply the content. Chapter 1 introduces you to journal keeping, an exercise that follows every chapter. Chapter 4 explains the value of the journal as a tool to foster critical thinking.

## IMPORTANCE OF CRITICAL THINKING

Why is it important to focus on critical thinking? Why should you think about your thinking? What does critical thinking mean? The answers to these questions depend on your personal and professional values. They also depend on how you perceive your ability to make the choices that shape your personal life and professional practice. To answer these questions, you need to understand why critical thinking is important.

### Learning as a Lifelong Process

Thinking and learning are interrelated, lifelong processes (Chaffee, 1994). To continue to grow you must refine your thinking and become more aware of and more skilled in your cognitive processes. As you add breadth and depth to your reservoir of knowledge, you substantially alter your thinking ability. With practice you broaden your ability to make thoughtful observations and judgments and learn to recognize the influence of your values on your thinking and your behavior. You become more perceptive in identifying assumptions, more articulate in presenting cogent arguments, and more proficient in evaluating the reasoning of others. Although the educational process provides a structured way to teach you to achieve personal and professional cognitive growth, it is not the only way to achieve growth. Learning is a process that, if nurtured, continues over a lifetime.

For example, like all young children, David was egocentric. The world consisted of what he noticed. Anything that he imagined or experienced became his total reality. Later in his childhood, memory, reality testing, and problem solving emerged. During his first camping trip, he heard the adults discussing where to rendezvous. David suggested that they obtain a map at the camp entrance to help them choose a location. It was a good solution.

David's knowledge and experience continued to expand over the years. He learned to apply logic and abstract reasoning to situations he had never encountered and to competently grasp the simultaneous influences of several variables. For example, when he was 16 years old he got a job working in an autobody shop washing and cleaning cars and later was promoted to a painter's helper. He perceived his knowledge base as all-encompassing, but in fact it lacked comprehensiveness. His knowledge and experience were limited in scope and immature. Indeed, he did not know everything. Now that David is an adult, he has acquired more knowledge and experience. As a result, he thinks more effectively and uses better judgment.

As you continue your educational preparation, you will broaden your knowledge and experience. For example, you probably do not know the knowledge base of other health professions. Although you are familiar with the territory of other health professionals, you may not be as adept in thinking and problem solving in their respective fields as they are. The knowledge and experience base of the occupational therapist, medical technologist, and physician are different. These different knowledge bases affect their ability to solve problems in their areas of specialization. Other special knowledge bases include those of professionals such as history professors, lawyers, or plumbers. There is much to know about many things, more than can be known by any one person. Yet, situations occur in which we must interact with others on matters of mutual concern. Focusing on your thinking and expanding your knowledge base will help you interact knowledgeably and effectively with others.

## Professional Growth

When you think critically, you challenge yourself both personally and professionally. Is your usual way of functioning effective? Are you accomplishing your personal and professional goals? Are you getting the results you want? Are you working effectively with others?

As you reflect on your nursing experience, you may find that there are other efficient and cost-effective ways of fulfilling your professional responsibilities. Consider the practice that is becoming routine in some institutions—using fetal monitors on all laboring women (Kenner and MacLaren, 1993). If this is the policy in the hospital where you obtained your obstetric experience, you might believe that fetal monitoring is an essential aspect of nursing care for women in labor. If you were to work at a hospital that applied fetal monitors only to laboring women whose fetal status was unstable, you might think that the hospital was "behind the times" or did not adequately provide for the safety of its clients. If you were to think critically about this issue, you would realize that your first experience in obstetrics shaped your frame of reference and created a personal bias that led you to believe that all laboring women should have fetal monitors attached. Your previous experience influenced you to create this mind-set. What is the reason for using fetal monitors? What value are they under routine conditions? What did hospitals do before this technology was available? Can any harm result from their use? Is there added cost? Asking these questions, seeking supporting evidence, and arriving at a scientifically supported conclusion exemplifies thinking critically.

McCarthy (1992) argues that you should think critically because doing so is efficacious. Efficacious thinking is effective thinking. It is thinking that produces the desired effect, the intended result. The consequences of thinking poorly, or failing to think, are very real. The consequences may affect your life today and impact your future. To think critically is to care about your life and the direction you are moving or wish to move. Critical thinking helps you exert self-direction, power, and control over your life.

## Increase Awareness of Your Attitudes and Values

Focusing on thinking allows you to become more aware of personal attitudes and values and how they affect your perceptions. Often we do not recognize how our own attitudes and values shape the way we perceive situations and how our perceptions affect the way we interact with clients. Perceptions are shaped by each person's own biologic, psychologic, sociologic, cultural, and spiritual influences. Perceptions are shaped by that part of the universe to which we attend. Perceptions are also affected by our attitudes. When we feel confident and self-actualized, we are able to experience our environment more fully. When we feel defensive, we perceive selectively. When we encounter a client whose values vary drastically from our own, we are likely to respond with defensiveness. We may be more comfortable dealing with clients whose values we perceive as being similar to our own.

The inferences we make about the data we perceive influence our response to the situation (Babcock and Miller, 1994). For example, consider your opinion of a woman who has pelvic inflammatory disease (PID), an acute, subacute, recurrent, or chronic infection of the fallopian tubes, ovaries, uterus, and cervix. A common cause is *Neisseria gonorrhoea,* a pathogenic bacterium, but it also may be caused by normally nonpathogenic bacteria in an altered endometrial environment (Nurse's Reference Library, 1981). How does the diagnosis of PID affect the quality of the nursing care you deliver to her? Would it matter to you how she contracted the disease? Would you inquire? Would you assume anything about her at the outset? Is there a difference in your relationship to and perception of a client who is married and develops PID as a complication of childbirth and the client who is single? How do your own values and assumptions influence your nursing care of this woman?

The woman in this example was a young mother who had given birth to her second child 2 weeks earlier and was running a low-grade fever of undetermined origin. A diagnosis was necessary to readmit her to the hospital. The physician hurriedly said PID to accomplish the goal of readmission without actually knowing if the diagnosis was accurate.

## Living in a Complex and Changing Society

Health care delivery in the United States is changing rapidly. As both citizens and health care professionals, we must deal with frequent change and help solve increasingly complex problems. Although our country spends more money on health care than any other nation, many citizens are poorly served or uninsured. Despite skyrocketing costs and technical sophistication, our infant mortality rate is higher than the infant mortality rate in countries that have much smaller health care budgets. The United States' infant mortality rate ranks behind those of Japan, Sweden, Canada, Great Britain, and Australia (Little, 1992). In 1991 health care consumed 13.2% of the U.S.'s gross domestic product and has every prospect of increasing its share (Samuelson, 1993). The U.S. spends one seventh of its national income on health care. This percentage will increase to one fifth early in the next century if present trends continue (Samuelson, 1994). The U.S. government needs to address the health care problems with clear thinking and active participation by both citizens and health care professionals. Critical thinking will help us consider the issues and problems, examine our underlying assumptions, develop creative alternatives, consider the implications, and find effective solutions.

Toffler (1980) correctly stated that we are experiencing the acceleration of change, growing mobility, expanding information exchange, increasingly intelligent environments, and the rising prevalence of consequential thinking. Knowledge and information change rapidly, and their distribution is almost instantaneous as cyberspace becomes the new communications arena. Electronic data bases, newspapers, journals, and books on a broad range of topics are now available. The information superhighway offers health care professionals *Nursing and Health Care* (the official publication of the National League for Nursing) (NLN, 1994) and the *Journal of the American Medical Association* on computer before the hard copy can reach them by mail. With the computer, we can readily access libraries around the world and explore their holdings. Clients can access detailed medical information as quickly as nurses can. Today clients have more extensive knowledge bases and are asking nurses more sophisticated questions.

The technologic environment is transforming our lives. Personal computers are more commonplace than they were 10 years ago. Nurses must possess computer skills to provide competent nursing care. The technologic explosion provides an opportunity for nurses to use their critical thinking skills to create nursing systems that use current technology within an humane and caring environment. Essential to technology is the need to develop decision-making processes for finding ethical solutions that accompany the greater use of technology (Chinn, 1991).

Rapid technologic changes and increased consumer demand for health services affect the nurse's role in health care institutions. Our previous way of defining ourselves is colliding with a paradigm shift. Nurses are moving from the role of primary nurse to the role of case manager along with the many other changes affecting the health care system (Clouten and Weber, 1994). To successfully cope with this shift, you must think in diverse ways, see things from different perspectives, and reconceptualize nursing practice.

To help manage these transitions, talk with your colleagues about your experiences in nursing and discuss the current issues affecting the profession. Consider your classmates, practicing nurses, and all health care professionals as colleagues. As you interact with them, you will grow. As you share with others and expand your own knowledge base, you will develop a vision of how things could be. Your nursing program provides a base of professional experience upon which you can build. With continued research-based practice and interdisciplinary collaboration, you can deepen your ability to think critically, adapt to and help shape the many changes in health care delivery.

## Living in the Evolving World Community

Governments are changing and new ones are appearing. A decade ago, few people believed that the Berlin Wall would crumble, that the Soviet Union would disintegrate, or that black citizens of South Africa would gain the right to vote. The United States has social, political, economic, business, environmental, and scientific problems that need our best thinking and problem-solving approaches if it is to thrive as a nation in the global community. Violations of human rights, human conflict, and ethnic and cultural strife continue to afflict the world. Government leaders need to think from more than one perspective to create a climate respectful for all (Paul, 1992). Developing and refining critical thinking skills are essential to address these issues and create a more humane and healthful world for all.

Interaction with others is the heart of being human. Our world community evolves as people engage each other. Siegel (1980) justified critical thinking as an educational ideal because it requires that we recognize and respect the moral worth of others. The legitimate needs, desires, and interests of others are as worthy as our own. To respect others is to recognize their right to question, challenge, and demand reasons and justifications.

## Multicultural Reality

With increasing immigration and geographic mobility, the population in the United States is changing. Most regions of the country have racially and ethnically diverse populations. In addition to race and ethnicity, diversity encompasses socioeconomic conditions such as education, income classification, and employment. Gender orientation and age are other aspects of diversity. Age cohorts have been labeled generation X, the baby boomers, and senior citizens. Diversity also includes long-standing immigrants (e.g., from South America) and recent immigrants (e.g., from Russia and Afghanistan). Geography creates diversity. Rural communities are distinct from urban ones, and urban communities are distinct from suburbia. Gender orientation and aging cut across race, ethnicity, socioeconomic status, and geography (AAN Expert Panel Report, 1992; Babcock and Miller, 1994; Capers, 1992).

Although members of a race (e.g., Caucasians) share many biologic characteristics, culturally they may be very distinct. The Irish and Germans, for example, are quite different from each other, as are Italians, French, and Russians. Charnes and Moore (1992) identified religious affiliation (e.g., Protestant, Catholic, Islamic, or Jewish) as another basis for diversity among people.

The United States is changing from what was once described as the great melting pot, in which immigrants gave up their own traditions to become Americans, to a "tossed salad," in which new pride and appreciation of the various ethnic groups prevail. More than ever before, ethnic, cultural, and racial groups are celebrating their own heritages, values, and traditions while some are incorporating American values (Tiedt and Tiedt, 1990).

With the increasing cultural and ethnic diversity, we are frequently interacting with people whose thinking, beliefs, values, habits, dress, language, and rules of behavior are different from our own. Leininger (1994) predicts that by 2010, nurses will be interacting with clients and families from virtually every place in the world. As you intermingle in the workplace and in your neighborhood, you may assume that others think and believe as you do without recognizing the cultural differences.

Developing a sensitivity to cultural diversity is an aspect of critical thinking. Sensitivity requires you to move beyond ethnocentricism, which is a concept based on the deep-seated belief that one's own group is superior to all others (Paul, 1990). Recognizing your ethnocentricism and giving empathic thought within the perspective of opposing groups and cultures is Paul's recommendation for overcoming ethnocentricism. Paul criticizes the superficiality of saying others have different beliefs and ways without giving serious consideration to the meaning of these beliefs and ways.

## THINKING

Thinking is essential to living, yet it is a difficult term to define. Thinking is making use of the mind and involves arriving at conclusions, making decisions, drawing inferences, and reflecting. Thinking includes reasoning, recalling and remembering, and encompasses beliefs, opinions, and judgments. It is a creative process of discovery, invention, and conception (Neufeldt, 1991). We do not know how thinking occurs, but consequences of thinking can be observed through human behavior. It is a complex, multifaceted, and dynamic process that involves the creation of mental images (Halpern, 1984). Thinking is the extraordinary process we use to make sense of our world and our lives. It is an active, purposeful, and organized process (Chaffee, 1994). It is a mental activity over which we exercise some control (Ruggiero, 1991).

Directed and nondirected thinking are distinct. Directed thinking is purposeful and goal oriented. Purposeful thinking involves searching for answers and reaching for meaning. For example, when you decide to take a trip to a new area, you may study a map carefully. Nondirected thinking, however, relies on familiar thought patterns. Although it engages the brain, nondirected thinking does not require much conscious thought. Nondirected thinking underlies routine, habitual activities such as getting out of bed, grooming, and driving to work (Halpern, 1984; Ruggiero, 1991). Purposeful thinking is searching for answers and reaching for meaning, whereas habitual thinking is reliance on familiar thought processes. The latter type of thinking obviously engages the brain, but it is done out of habit and does not require much conscious thought. Clearly, purposeful thinking requires considerably more conscious mental effort and involves observing, remembering, imagining, inquiring, interpreting, analyzing, and evaluating.

Other ways to categorize thinking are scientific inquiry, problem solving, decision making, creative thinking, intuitive thinking, and critical thinking. These categories are useful for discussion purposes, but they overlap. Thinking is too complex to be confined by categories. Each of these ways of thinking will be described in the chapters that follow.

## CRITICAL THINKING

Critical thinking is at the heart of the educational reform movement in the United States. Like educators worldwide, American educators are concerned about teaching and refining thinking skills (Chaffee, 1992; Norris, 1985; Paul, 1990; Siegel, 1980; Sternberg and Baron, 1985). The ability to think critically is essential to being a fully functioning individual in our complex society (Glaser, 1985; McPeck, 1990). Parallel to this interest in critical thinking is a similar concern among nursing educators (Beck, Bennett, McLeod, Molyneaux, 1992; Miller and Malcolm, 1990; Nkongho, 1994).

The word *critical* comes from the Greek word *Kritikos*, meaning "critic." To be critical means to question, to make sense of, to analyze. By being critical, you examine your thinking and the thinking of others (Chaffee, 1994). *Critical* is often thought of in a negative, destructive sense; however, using it to describe thinking connotes a positive process in which you challenge your thinking and the thinking of others. Critical thinking helps you arrive at conclusions that have favorable implications for you and those with whom you interact.

Thinking critically is a practical process. Chaffee (1994) defines it as "an active, purposeful, organized cognitive process we use to carefully examine our thinking and the thinking of others, in order to clarify and improve our understanding." (p. 51). Thinking critically involves an integrated set of thinking abilities and attitudes that include the following:

▼ *Thinking actively* by using our intelligence, knowledge, and skills to question, explore, and deal effectively with ourselves, others, and life's situations.

▼ *Carefully exploring situations* by asking and trying to answer relevant questions.

▼ *Thinking for ourselves* by carefully examining various ideas and arriving at our own thoughtful conclusions.

▼ *Viewing situations from different perspectives* to develop an in-depth, comprehensive understanding.

▼ *Discussing ideas in an organized way* to exchange and explore ideas with others (p. 94).

Some use the term *critical thinking* in a vague way to cover a broad range of mental activities, while others see it as a type of thinking that involves specific cognitive skills. Among those who believe critical thinking is mastering specific cognitive skills, there is little consensus on a definition or the inherent nature of these skills. Some people define critical thinking as logic; others define it as solving open-ended problems. Some emphasize the Socratic reasoning processes; others emphasize creativity, which departs from an emphasis on order, structure, and sequence (Klaassens, 1988). Some people believe there is no unitary skill of critical thinking or reasoning and that critical thinking is always relative to particular subject matter (McPeck, 1990, 1981). These proponents believe critical thinking is best taught within subject matter instruction. McPeck states that "there are almost as many different kinds of critical thinking as there are different kinds of things to think about" (p. 10). Others believe that there is a unitary skill of critical thinking and that the current movement to develop courses and programs in general critical thinking is both justified and educationally sound (Adler, 1991; Paul, 1990).

In this book the term *critical thinking* is used to mean purposeful thinking that takes into consideration focus, language, frame of reference, attitudes, assumptions, evidence, reasoning, conclusions, implications, and context when they matter in deciding what to believe or do. In creating this definition, the authors were influenced by a number of writers in the field of critical thinking (Ennis [1985], Browne and Keeley [1994], Ruggiero [1991], Brookfield [1991], Paul [1990], Watson and Glaser [1980]). The relevance of each of these components of critical thinking varies according to the situation.

The Critical Thinking Interaction Model highlights components of critical thinking that may affect your interactions. It is a concrete tool for helping examine any interaction upon which you want to thoughtfully reflect. In this sense it may be used as a problem-solving model. The model is not a linear, step-by-step procedure to follow as you interact with others. Interaction is a dynamic process as indicated by the circles and arrows. The model provides a way to understand yourself and others and all the dynamics that make up interactions from the perspective of critical thinking. Where relevant, each component of the model is discussed in greater depth throughout the text.

## FACTORS INFLUENCING THINKING

Many factors influence thinking, beginning in early childhood. While growing up, children receive different kinds of messages about thinking. Some are positive, such as "You figured that out all by yourself. I'm proud of you!" and "She is a bright one!" Other messages are negative, such as, "If you had a brain you would be dangerous!" and "Others won't like you if you are too smart!" Depending on the nature, consistency, and frequency of these messages and the childrens' reactions to them, children develop varying degrees of confidence in their ability to think clearly.

Many people have a strong influence on your thinking. The closer you are to individuals with whom you choose to associate, the greater their ability to influence your thinking. For example, a spouse may influence your thinking to a greater degree than a neighbor. Your favorite professional role model carries more influence with you than another professional for whom you have less regard.

You are continually bombarded with messages that shape your thinking. Through the media, you receive subtle messages about what the ideal weight is, what you should believe about an issue, and what comforts are essential to living—all messages that in one way or another affect your thinking. During political campaigns you may find it difficult to know the facts about any given issue because proponents of each side want your vote and present messages designed to get it.

The range of factors influencing your thinking is expansive. Consider the influence on your thinking of people such as your teachers, colleagues, friends, employers, religious leaders, politicians, and others. Consider the influence on your thinking of activities such as reading, writing, taking drugs, dancing, drawing, painting, playing video games, playing sports, and listening to music. Consider the influence of culture, socioeconomic status, age, health status, and birth order on your thinking. What can you add to this list?

Paul (1990) identified four factors that influence thinking. First, people think like those around them. It is more comfortable to be with people who think similarly than those who think dissimilarly. For example, we choose friends who hold similar values and beliefs. Second, people may think the way they do because they are rewarded for thinking that way. For example, it may create less interpersonal friction within a family for members to think alike. The same may be true among professional colleagues who are closely associated. Third, people may be afraid to disagree. For example, among friends holding similar religious or political beliefs, an individual may be unwilling to challenge the prevailing beliefs. Fourth, a person's vested interest influences thinking. It may well be in the vested interest for a person to think in a certain way. For example, an employee may get a raise in pay if she does not challenge her boss and does what is asked even though her professional judgment may dictate a different course of action.

How often do you pause to reflect on your thinking? Have you wondered which part of your thinking is uniquely yours and which part results from the influence of your friends? family? various media? How do you separate your thoughts and choices from those of others? Influence is not recognized easily. It requires an awareness of your surroundings and of those factors that most influence your thinking. It requires thoughtful reflection and a deliberate search for reasons to support your views. If you practice these skills, you can strengthen your sense of self and your thinking abilities.

Refining your thinking and learning more about it makes sense if you believe you have some control over your personal and professional life. Although you are influenced by myriad forces that shape your thinking, you still have the power of choice. For example, you can choose to investigate political issues more thoroughly and arrive at your own conclusions. You can examine the living arrangement preferred by an elderly client for yourself rather than assuming the recommendation of another health care professional is best. You also can examine a nursing unit's budget and determine for yourself whether it is economically healthy. You do not have to be a victim of the many influences with which you must contend. If you are aware of these influences and seek reasons to support your own views, you can mitigate their impact on your life and make more informed choices.

## OTHER CONSIDERATIONS

Perfect thinking does not exist. Clarity of thought occurs with experience and with a willingness to verbalize your ideas, thus allowing others to react and challenge them. As you do so, listen to the objections and points of agreement others raise. What are their objections? What convincing points do they make? What reasonable responses can you give to the objections?

By verbalizing and writing down your thoughts, you can better examine your thinking. When you externalize your thinking, you open yourself to alternative explanations, which can come from yourself or the person with whom you are interacting.

Join with others who are discussing interesting topics or generate the discussion yourself. Remember that no one is perfectly logical. Your experiences and thoughts are just as valuable as the experiences and thoughts of others. Some have thought through selected issues more carefully than others, just as some are better informed on certain issues than others. Learning to engage in lively interaction expands your knowledge base and thinking ability. Do not be afraid to challenge others' ideas and thinking. Learn to express your perspective in an objective and forthright manner.

Thinking critically is hard work. You may become so concerned with your thinking that you may grow weary of focusing on it. Thinking about your thinking has a name: it is called metacognition (Ruggiero, 1991). Metacognition means to think about your thinking as you are thinking. It moves beyond those cognitive skills that are directly used in carrying out an intellectual task and involves skills such as planning, monitoring, and revising the progress of the cognitive skills (Norris, 1985). It is important to have confidence in yourself and your ability to reason and to understand the reasoning of others. When you do the very best you can, you build up your confidence and critical thinking skills. When others question your point of view, you can see it as a challenge to your thinking rather than a personal threat. As you refine your reasoning skills, you also become more articulate and more persuasive. Refining your critical thinking skills has lifelong personal and professional benefits.

## CRITICAL THINKING INTERACTION MODEL

We offer a model of critical thinking that has broad application to nursing practice. The Critical Thinking Interaction Model, which conceptualizes the application of critical thinking skills and attitudes to nursing practice, is widely applicable with mentally competent clients in a variety of health care settings. Throughout this text, we construct and discuss the model in stages to illustrate its various components.

### Nurse and Other in Interaction

A nurse in interaction with another person is the essence of nursing practice (Fig. 1-1). Interaction is the heart of the model, illustrated by the two large circles, one representing the nurse and the other representing another person. Nurses interact with a variety of individuals in the health care system and serve in a variety of roles. The

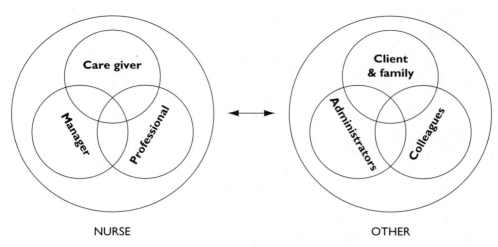

**Fig. 1-1** Nurse-Other Interaction Model.

model focuses on three roles in which nurses engage: care giver, manager, and professional (see circles within the nurse circle). We apply the examples of critical thinking to these roles.

When you function in the role of care giver, you interact with a client and the client's family. In the role of manager, you collaborate with health care colleagues to accomplish goal-oriented activities, such as creating a method to communicate new policies to those who work on a nursing unit. In the role of professional, you focus on activities related to being a member of the nursing profession. Activities might include seeking credentialing or participating on an infection-control committee.

Clients, a client's family, health care colleagues, or institutional administrators are among the most frequent and most significant persons with whom the professional nurse interacts. They are illustrated by the circles within the "Other" circle (Fig. 1-1).

## Individual Characteristics

The central focus of the model is the nurse engaged in communication with another person. Both individuals are complex. Each comes to the interaction with a wide array of life experiences that manifest through the person's frame of reference, attitudes, and assumptions (see smaller circles added to the "Nurse" and "Other" circles in Fig. 1-2). Expressed another way, each person comes to the interaction with a unique blend of biologic, psychologic, sociologic, cultural, and spiritual characteristics that have melded and have become the sum of life experiences for that person.

Biologic characteristics include heredity, gender, age, race, physical capabilities and limitations, and current health status. Psychologic characteristics include motivation, perception, memory, intelligence, learning style, personality, needs,

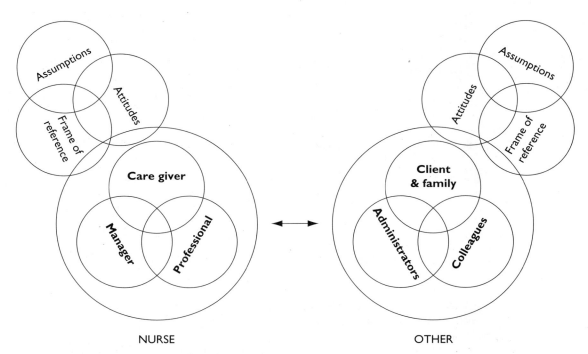

**Fig. 1-2**  Nurse-Other Interaction Model: Individual Characteristics.

emotional reactions, and defense mechanisms. Sociologic characteristics include groups, family, society, social stratification, and education, health, and economic and political systems. Cultural characteristics are the sum total of the way a group of people lives that includes customs, skills, arts, beliefs, attitudes, values, moral principles, habits, dress, language, rules of behavior, diet, health care practices, and attitudes toward economics and politics that are transmitted from one generation to another. Spiritual characteristics include a search for meaning, faith, and beliefs about nontangible realities. Spirituality is a perspective and a belief in a higher power. It includes beliefs about right and wrong, hope, values, divine influence, the soul, and beliefs about what is sacred. The blending of all these characteristics is unique for each person. The result of this blending of characteristics is the unique way each person perceives the world and interacts with others. This blend of characteristics is manifested in the frame of reference through which he or she views every situation, the attitudes the person holds dear, and the assumptions she or he makes, both conscious and unconscious, spoken and unspoken.

If both persons in the interaction have similar characteristics and frames of reference, the interaction will go more smoothly than if they are widely divergent. When these characteristics are very different, the model may be useful in providing perspective for understanding the other person. Awareness of these differences moves the participants beyond egocentric thinking to the consideration of multiple perspectives and frames of reference.

Attitudes also are important in critical thinking. Attitudes are a manner of acting, feeling, or thinking that shows one's dispositions (Neufeldt, 1991). Attitudes create the human climate through which issues and problems are examined. Attitudes of openness, fairmindedness, hunger for truth, and willingness to listen foster critical analysis. Absence of these attitudes diminishes critical thought.

The courage of your own convictions, personal integrity, and intellectual honesty also are important in thinking critically. Other essential attitudes are confidence in multiple ways of knowing, openness to other points of view, willingness to take a position and defend it, and willingness to change one's own opinion based on evidence.

When your critical thinking is slowed down, delayed, or disabled, evaluate your attitude. For example, executives at one large hospital recently received impressive bonuses for merging three large hospitals. When the mergers occurred, nurses at these institutions lost their shift and weekend differential pay and some lost their jobs "to save money." While this was going on, a nurse resigned from one of the merged institutions because she was appalled at the lack of qualified personnel with whom she was expected to work; she did not wish to risk her license. She probably would have difficulty discussing the situation with an administrator and thinking critically. Her anger and righteous indignation would cloud her ability to listen objectively.

## Interaction Event

The interaction event refers to the purposeful and goal-oriented interchange that occurs among the nurse and the client, family, colleague, and administrator. It is the daily communication that is the heart of nursing practice. During the interaction, the nurse and the interacting other focus on significant events or experiences such as client care decisions, professional issues, and nursing unit management. Components of critical thinking that influence the nature and quality of this interaction are focus, language, evidence, and reasoning (Fig. 1-3).

*Focus.*   The interacting participants focus the discussion. Part of focusing is to agree about the central issue and problem, which may involve considerable discussion. The critical thinking skills we associate with focus are distinguishing between the central issue or problem and the peripheral issues or problems, clarifying the central issue or problem, and stating the central issue or problem.

For example, consider the 85-year-old client who is recovering well from hip replacement surgery. The client plans to return to her own home, but you and your colleagues do not believe she has fully considered the assistance she will need once she is discharged. The client believes that she can take care of herself, fears further "confinement," and is annoyed at you for inteferring with her life. She misses her cats and wants to get home to tend to them. She does not believe that she has a care problem because she has several neighbors who will help her. She believes that you, the

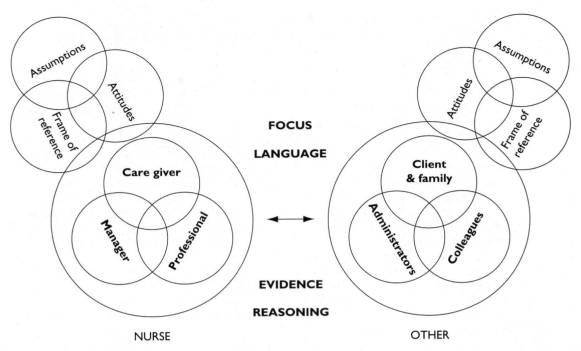

**Fig. 1-3** Nurse-Other Interaction Model: Interaction Event.

physician, and the social worker are her problems. You and your colleagues believe that the client would be better served by staying in a convalescent center for several weeks until satisfactory home care arrangements can be made.

The central issue in this case is the client's actual ability to care for herself in her own home. The client believes that she can care for herself at home and you, the physician, and the social worker do not. Peripheral issues are the client's age; the client's relationship with you, the physician, and the social worker; the care of the client's cats; and the potential support from her neighbors.

Another example in which the interacting participants are colleagues can illustrate the importance of focusing (McGuire-Mahony, 1994). Two colleagues are concerned about a do-not-resuscitate (DNR) order for a client. They both disagree with the order but for different reasons. One believes that the order denigrates the sanctity of life. He believes that nurses should expend their energies to extend life. The other accepts the reality of the DNR order but believes that this client has the potential for many more useful years.

In this example, the central issue is whether or not to resuscitate the client should the need arise. Peripheral issues are the preferences and attitudes of the nurses. The main issue is the desire of the client. As health care professionals, nurses seek to do good for their clients. Although we recognize there is always the potential for harm in all our interventions with clients, our intentions are to produce good outcomes. Further, as moral agents, we accept that all human beings are worthy of respect and that we have an obligation to treat them with dignity. The questions we must ask ourselves in this case are how do we produce good, respect the client, and treat him or her with fairness? Often the issues conflict with each other. For example, if we resuscitate against the client's wishes, we may say we have produced good (the client is alive), but we have ignored the client's wishes. Have we treated our client with dignity and fairness when we reject the client's autonomous decision simply because it is contrary to our personal value? Do we have this right? What is "good" in this situation? Is it to respect the autonomous wishes of a competent adult (even if that results in the client's death), or is it to maintain life independent of the client's perception of the quality of life?

The central issue in this situation is one of respect for the client's rights. Our society recognizes that mentally competent adults have the moral and the legal right to accept or refuse treatment, even if refusal results in harm (or death) to the client. As health care professionals, we seek to help clients and to preserve life. We have difficulty letting clients die when we know we have the ability to keep them alive. By applying critical thinking to client care situations and focusing on the central issue, we can sort out peripheral issues, preferences, and attitudes of each of the participants and resolve the conflict between the colleagues and the client.

***Language.*** Language is a key element in interactions. Our choice of words, intonations, posture, facial expressions, and gestures express our thoughts and feelings. Language allows us to describe how we view the world, what we believe about it, and how we react to it. Engel (1994) observed that "the reality we live in . . . is largely erected by the language with which we describe it to ourselves" (p. 109). Language and words are inseparable. The effectiveness of language depends upon the skill of the user. Many aspects of language affect critical thinking. The critical thinking skills we associate with language are: assessing clarity and precision, defining key words, identifying emotive words, assessing context, and detecting and exploiting labels.

Clarity and precision in language result from clear and precise thinking. Clear language is free of confusion and obfuscation. Precise language is accurate and exact. Jargon, vagueness, and ambiguity are examples of unclear and imprecise language. Jargon is the specialized vocabulary of those in a particular profession or line of work that is not generally understood by people who are not in that profession. Ambiguity refers to a word or phrase that has more than one meaning. Vagueness refers to words that are simply unclear. With ambiguous language, we ponder the speaker's true meaning of the word or phrase. With vague language, we search for any meaning at all or we assume we know the meaning (Engel, 1994).

Vague language is illustrated in the following comment made by a nurse: "The governing boards' decisions to merge the two hospitals was a surprising move to say the least!" Think about the various meanings this statement can have. Does it mean the merger was good? or bad? The speaker's meaning is simply unclear. Ambiguous language is illustrated in the following example: "Noisy children are a real headache. An aspirin will make a headache go away. Therefore, an aspirin will make noisy children go away" (Hughes, 1992, p. 124). In this example, the word *headache* is used to symbolize an annoyance and a physiological reaction.

Another aspect of language is level of diction. The complexity of the terminology used affects how the nurse and interacting other define and understand the terms being used. For example, when a physician tells a client that he or she has basal cell carcinoma and excision will solve the problem, the client may not understand the message as the nurse does. The client may not realize that basal cell carcinoma is an easily curable cancer and may continue to harbor unfounded and unreasonable fears of a recurrence.

The client who states that his stomach aches is another example showing the importance of defining key terms. If taken literally, the nurse may assume the pain is in the epigastric region of the abdomen, but the client may mean the pain is in the lower abdomen. The nurse should ask the client to point to the location of pain. Pointing is the most accurate and fastest way to define the terms in this situation.

Recognizing emotive language is another important aspect of language usage in critical thinking. Emotive language generates strong feelings in listeners. Some examples of emotive language are duty to die, health care reform, gay and lesbian rights, abortion upon demand, right to life, and preserve America first. People tend to stop thinking and listening when these slogans are spoken and react emotionally instead.

**Evidence.**    To decide what to believe or do, you need to formulate good reasons supported by current knowledge and the best available evidence. Evidence is something that tends to prove and provides the grounds for belief (Neufeldt, 1991). Evidence may be derived from personal experiences, from the experiences of others (such as authorities and written documents), from research reports, and from the assessment of clients. Evidence may include facts, figures, and statistical information. The critical thinking skills we associate with evidence are evaluating evidence derived from quantitative and qualitative research, evaluating evidence derived from the assessment of clients, making appropriate inferences based on evidence derived from research and clients, assessing research for its relevance to clinical practice, and participating in systematic and accurate data collection.

To persuade others to your point of view, you must use good reasons supported by evidence. For example, if the nurses wanted a hospital administrator to purchase needed cardiac monitoring equipment, the nurses should provide evidence that continued monitoring of clients' cardiac activity on a step-down unit saves a significant number of lives. The nurses should review the literature to determine if any research has been done in this area. If not, the nurses may want to conduct their own research. They could form a treatment group who would be monitored with cardiac equipment and a control group who would not be monitored. After a period of time, the nurses could determine if a statistically significant difference between the two groups occurred. If the results of the research support the nurses' hypothesis, it would provide strong evidence to support the nurses' position.

If the nurses in this example conduct a well-designed and meticulously implemented research study to compare the differences between the two groups of cardiac clients, and the results show the expected reduction in deaths, their findings will provide a justification for purchasing the cardiac monitoring equipment. Without such a study, the nurses would be basing their request on their opinions about the progress of their clients. The nurses may be highly experienced and well-informed, but without pertinent and accurate data, their argument would be based only on opinions. Professional opinions and seasoned judgments of experienced nurses are very important in clinical practice. Recognizing when opinions are sufficient and when evidence based on research would be better is equally important.

Evidence may be in the form of demographic data, which may be sufficiently persuasive to support an argument. For example, suppose a nurse wanted to persuade the nurse manager to hire bilingual interpreters to be available to all nursing units in a hospital. The nurse should analyze the demographics on the population served by the hospital. If the dominant population served by the hospital were Spanish-speaking, an argument that bilingual interpreters should be hired would be stronger. Demographic data can be a powerful source of evidence.

The client is a rich source of evidence for nurses. The subjective and objective data the nurse gathers during client assessment are other examples of evidence. The nurse makes inferences based upon this evidence and subsequently plans, implements, and evaluates the nursing care.

***Reasoning.***    Another component of the interaction is reasoning. The two kinds of reasoning are deductive and inductive. Reasoning is commonly applied to argument, or thinking that links thoughts together in such a way that reasons provide support for a conclusion. Thus, an argument has two basic elements: a conclusion supported by one or more reasons. Reasoning is also applied to scientific inquiry, problem solving, and the examination of controversial issues.

When we apply reasoning in the Critical Thinking Interaction Model, the interacting participants identify and agree upon an issue. Once agreement is achieved, each participant states the reasons for his or her respective positions. Each participant wishes to be heard, understood, and respected, and may try to persuade the other participants to embrace his or her point of view. For example, nurses in an outpatient surgical setting of a community hospital want to purchase a pulse oximeter to monitor clients in the operating room. One of the early signs for inadequate oxygenation is cyanosis of the nail beds. During surgery the client is draped, so it is impossible to quickly observe the fingers. The pulse oximeter would provide continuous information about the status of the client's oxygenation. The pulse oximeter is a way to determine the oxygen saturation of arterial blood. The nurses ask the hospital administrator to purchase this equipment. The administrator checks on the price of the oximeter, determines the hospital has more urgent expenses, and, in an effort to balance the budget, refuses the request.

What reasons can these nurses generate to persuade the administrator to buy the oximeter? What would happen if the nurses gathered evidence about the number of clients whose inadequate and unrecognized lack of oxygenation resulted in postoperative problems? What would happen if the nurses enlisted the support of the anesthesiologist and the surgeon to tell the administrator that at some time the problem would not be correctable and a client could die? What would happen if the hospital risk management personnel or attorney were reminded that an anesthesia death would quite likely result in a legal action against the institution? Do you think this approach would be more persuasive? Would the administrator rethink his or her position?

Another reason the nurses could use to persuade the hospital administrator to purchase the equipment is the accuracy of the oximeter over the conventional method of checking for cyanosis of the nail beds. Other reasons they could cite are that using an oximeter is less expensive, less traumatic, and less time-consuming than obtaining arterial blood gases.

When you evaluate the quality of your reasons, consider how pertinent they are to the issues you have identified and use only those that are pertinent reasons. Also note the quality of your reasons; some reasons are more compelling than others. In the previous example, reducing risk to the hospital may be a more persuasive reason for the oximeter purchase than the fact that using an oximeter is less time-consuming for staff than obtaining arterial blood gases.

In this example, we have discussed one critical thinking skill we associate with reasoning, that is, distinguishing among issues, reasons, and conclusions. Other important critical thinking skills we associate with reasoning are evaluating deductive and inductive arguments, differentiating between warranted and unwarranted inferences, evaluating pertinence of the reasons, and assessing for errors in reasoning.

## Purposeful Interaction

The final elements of the definition of critical thinking are conclusions, implications, and context when they matter in deciding what to believe or do. Purposeful interaction may lead to conclusions, and each conclusion carries implications for both the nurse and the interacting other. How do conclusions, implications, and context affect critical thinking (Fig. 1-4)?

**Conclusions.**   The interaction between the nurse and the client, family, colleagues, and administrators is goal directed and purposeful. For example, you want to administer safe and effective nursing care to a client, discuss a professional issue with colleagues, or persuade an institutional administrator to consider your point of view. Thus, the movement in the model is toward goal achievement, or deciding what to believe or do. The critical thinking skills we associate with conclusions are supporting conclusions and beliefs with relevant reasons, evaluating deductive and inductive arguments, and evaluating the strength of the evidence supporting conclusions and beliefs.

**Implications.**   Implications are the consequences that result when an issue is resolved, a problem is solved, or a decision is made. Implications extend beyond what is immediately apparent. The critical thinking skills we associate with implications are identifying implications of conclusions and beliefs, evaluating desirability of the implications, and anticipating consequences.

For example, the parents of a 2-year-old child who was born with cerebral palsy and severe seizure disorder made the decision to both stay by the bedside of their child during a prolonged hospitalization. The couple also had a 6-year-old child whom they left in the care of neighbors. The neighbors were good friends, and the parents were confident their child would get good care. As the hospital stay lengthened, the 6-year-old child became withdrawn and began to perform poorly in school. When the parents realized the implications of their decision to remain with their

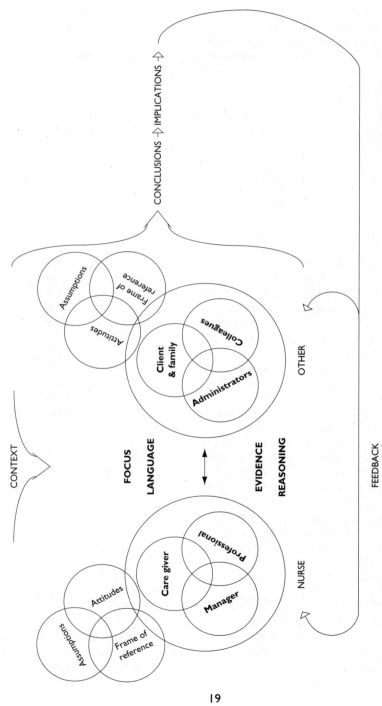

**Fig. 1-4** Critical Thinking Interaction Model.

2-year-old child, they made a change. Thereafter, one parent stayed with the 2-year-old child, while the other stayed with the 6-year-old child. They established a routine for rotating their parental responsibilities.

Reconsider the situation discussed earlier in this chapter about the nurses who requested that the hospital administrator purchase a pulse oximeter for clients undergoing surgery. The implications of not purchasing the pulse oximeter may have resulted in the tragic loss of a client and a possible lawsuit.

Implications exist for every conclusion. Implications can be significant or insignificant, intended or unforeseen, or desirable or undesirable. As a nurse, you should anticipate and predict the consequences. You can minimize uncertainty when you select those outcomes with the most completely known consequences.

When implications become reality, they become feedback to the nurse and the interacting other. Feedback fosters self-correction. When you observe the impact of your choices—those that were effective and ineffective—you open yourself to feedback, which prompts you and the interacting other to do things differently the next time or to continue with an intervention that is working effectively.

***Context.*** Thinking critically includes being sensitive to the context in which thinking occurs. Context in this model refers to the entire situation (universe), background, or environment relevant to a particular interaction. Context includes the societal, institutional, and family circumstances that are relevant to a particular interaction. This sequence moves from the largest context (universe) to the health care system (institution) to the family that is relevant to the immediate client situation.

Context also takes into consideration the background, knowledge, and assumptions of the nurse and the interacting other. Norris (1985) notes that inferences are more likely to be correct when the context relates to personal experience. Collectively, these circumstances and personal backgrounds are the context, or the environment, in which the interaction occurs.

Fig. 1-5 illustrates the interacting influence of several contexts including society, the health care delivery system, a particular community, the family, and the immediate situation. These contexts overlap and may operate simultaneously. They may have more or less impact on any given situation. In each situation, you must assess the context, determine which factors are most influential, and intervene appropriately. As in Fig. 1-4, the exact nature of the context may not be visible, but as in Fig. 1-5, it is very important, and you must determine what the variables are in each situation. When you develop a sensitivity to the surrounding circumstances of a situation, you are contextually aware.

## CRITICAL THINKING INTERACTION MODEL AS A SYSTEM

All components of the Critical Thinking Interaction Model are shown together in Fig. 1-4. The model is based on general systems thinking and includes input, process, output, and feedback. Fig. 1-6 illustrates these aspects of general systems theory. Input refers to the interacting individuals and what they bring to the

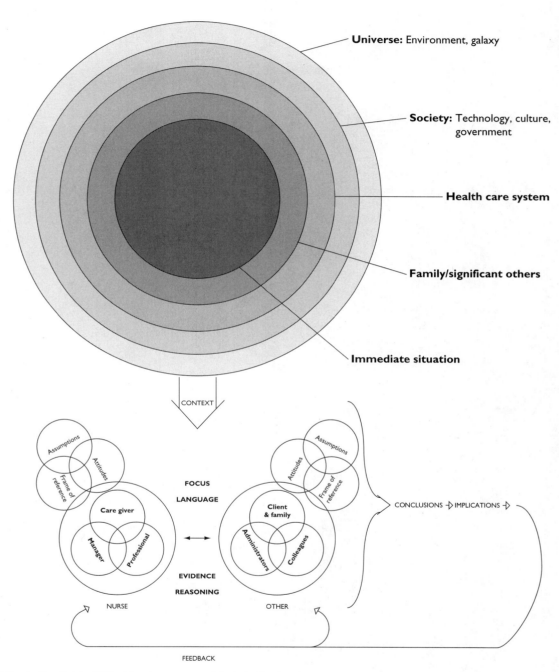

**Fig. I-5**   Critical Thinking Interaction Model:  Context.

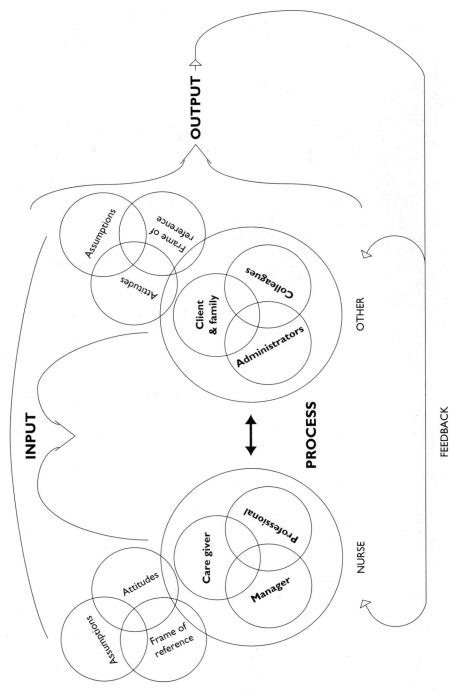

**Fig. 1-6** Critical Thinking Interaction Model: A System.

22

interchange based on their biologic, psychologic, sociologic, cultural, and spiritual experiences. Input includes their frames of reference, attitudes, assumptions, and the context of the interaction. Process is the interaction itself and includes clarification of the issue and problem through focus, use of language, evidence, and reasoning that affect the interaction. Output is the conclusions and the implications resulting from the interactions. Based on the output, feedback is generated. Feedback that is observed and internalized by the nurse and interacting other becomes input into the next interaction.

Learning from your experiences is adapting to feedback. Modifying your thoughts and actions according to the feedback you receive is the basis for personal growth, which comes from continuously adapting to and learning from the surrounding environment. Over time, as your knowledge expands and your experiences multiply, your understanding increases. Understanding forms the foundation for your development as a critical thinker.

Consistent with general system thinking, the model is dynamic with interacting, interdependent components. Each interaction you have is unique and influenced by many factors. The importance of any one component varies from transaction to transaction. For example, culture may be a major factor in one interaction and insignificant in another. Finding agreement on the central issue may be prominent in one interaction and not in another. Because each individual is unique, so also is each interaction.

The model is not meant to be used in a linear fashion. You need not mechanically walk yourself through each skill to believe you have engaged in critical thinking. Instead, let the model lead you to an awareness of the broad aspects of the interactions you are having with clients, families, colleagues, and administrators. When you must focus on an interaction, you have some idea of the areas to explore. And, when appropriate, you can adapt and intervene accordingly.

## CRITICAL THINKING SKILLS AND ATTITUDES APPLIED TO NURSING

Critical thinking skills and attitudes support the Critical Thinking Interaction Model (see the Critical Thinking Skills and Attitudes Applied to Nursing box on p. 24). The essential components in the Critical Thinking Interaction Model are focus, language, assumptions, evidence, reasoning, conclusions, implications, and attitudes.

The items in the box address two broad domains: cognitive skills and affective skills (attitudes). Cognitive skills are the thinking proficiencies associated with the process of knowing in the broadest sense. Examples of cognitive skills include the ability to distinguish the central issue from related but peripheral issues, identify stated and unstated assumptions, distinguish between facts and opinions, and engage in sound reasoning. Refer to the box for a complete list of skills and attitudes that support the Critical Thinking Interaction Model.

Affective skills include attitudes, dispositional traits, and the inclination to act, feel, or think in a given way (Neufeldt, 1991). Attitude is the inclination or tendency to use one's thinking proficiencies. Attitudes are characteristics of a person, not a

**Critical Thinking Skills and Attitudes Applied to Nursing***

**FOCUS**
- ▼ Distinguish between the central issue or problem and the peripheral issues or problems
- ▼ Clarify the central issue or problem
- ▼ State the central issue or problem

**LANGUAGE**
- ▼ Assess clarity and precision
- ▼ Define key words
- ▼ Identify emotive words
- ▼ Assess context
- ▼ Detect and exploit labels

**ASSUMPTIONS**
- ▼ Assess client, family, institutional, and societal contexts
- ▼ Analyze value, descriptive, definitional, and contextual assumptions
- ▼ Assess frame of reference, attitudes, and assumptions
- ▼ Recognize one's own frame of reference, attitudes, and assumptions

**EVIDENCE**
- ▼ Evaluate evidence derived from quantitative and qualitative research
- ▼ Evaluate evidence derived from the assessment of clients
- ▼ Make appropriate inferences based on evidence derived from research and clients
- ▼ Assess research for its relevance to clinical practice
- ▼ Participate in systematic and accurate data collection

**REASONING**
- ▼ Evaluate deductive and inductive arguments
- ▼ Differentiate between warranted and unwarranted inferences
- ▼ Distinguish among issues, reasons, and conclusions
- ▼ Evaluate pertinence of the reasons
- ▼ Assess for errors in reasoning

**CONCLUSIONS**
- ▼ Support conclusions and beliefs with relevant reasons
- ▼ Evaluate deductive and inductive arguments
- ▼ Evaluate the strength of the evidence supporting conclusions and beliefs

**IMPLICATIONS**
- ▼ Identify implications of conclusions and beliefs
- ▼ Evaluate desirability of the implications
- ▼ Anticipate consequences

**Critical Thinking Skills and Attitudes Applied to Nursing—cont'd**

**ATTITUDES**
- ▼ Confidence in multiple ways of knowing
- ▼ Intellectual honesty
- ▼ Openness to other points of view
- ▼ Willingness to take a position and defend it
- ▼ Willingness to change one's own opinion based on evidence

*We acknowledge the influence of many authors in creating this list, particularly Ennis (1985), Browne and Keeley (1994), Chaffee (1994), Ruggiero (1991), Brookfield (1991), LoBiondo-Wood and Haber (1994), Watson and Glaser (1980), and Paul (1990).

feature of thinking itself (McCarthy, 1992). Because nurses are concerned with the application of theory, this discussion of critical thinking focuses on the thinking skills associated with critical thinking and the dispositional traits of the person engaged in thinking. In this context, thinking skills and dispositional traits are equally important aspects of critical thinking. Thinking skills are of little benefit unless they are put to use when appropriate.

Attitudes, dispositions, habits, and character traits are essential to critical thinking. Cognitive skills, such as the ability to evaluate claims based on evidence, are insufficient for being a critical thinker; you must also be disposed to do so. You not only have to be able to engage in principled thinking (i.e., to judge nonarbitrarily, impartially, and objectively), you also have to be willing to conform your judgments to these principles. The critical spirit requires that you be inclined to seek reasons, reject partiality and arbitrariness, and objectively evaluate relevant evidence. You not only have to be able to judge impartially, you also must have a willingness to do so, even when it is not in your self-interest (Siegel, 1980). Both skills and attitudes constitute the "critical spirit" or "critical attitude" that Siegel (1992, 1980) associates with critical thinking.

## WHEN THEY MATTER . . .

What does the phrase "when they matter in deciding what to believe or do" mean? Not every situation requires critical thought (McCarthy, 1992; McPeck, 1990). For example, when you administer nursing care to a client with known health problems and whose current status is uncomplicated by new health problems, your nursing care may be routine and your thinking rational, but critical thought may not be required. If, however, the client's health status has taken a turn for the worse or if a family is facing a new crisis, you may need critical thinking skills as you problem solve. McCarthy (1992) refers to these periodic situations that require critical thought as episodic critical thinking.

Selected critical thinking skills may be needed in different situations. For example, sometimes it will be important to pay attention to values when you become aware that values are affecting the interaction. In other situations the meaning of key terms you use might be more important. For example, you may have one concept of how your client should keep his abdominal wound clean and your client may have quite another. You may define keeping a wound clean as changing the dressing every day, but the client may define it as changing the dressing when it becomes noticeably soiled, which may be after several days.

## SUMMARY

When critical thinking is required, you may need to apply some or all of the many critical thinking skills and attitudes. Learning to think critically is a lifelong process requiring self-awareness, knowledge, and practice. Thinking critically requires a desire and willingness to develop a critical spirit. Each individual is a unique blend of early parental influences mixed with the influence of friends, teachers, employers, government, television, newspapers, and so forth.

When you are confronted with significant issues in your personal and professional life, you must use mental effort to fully consider them and arrive at your own conclusions. Within this context you make choices that may have significant consequences in your life today and in the future. The consequences of thinking and behavior will show you if you were effective or ineffective, successful or unsuccessful. By becoming a better critical thinker, you will learn to make better choices consistently. The Critical Thinking Interaction Model and the Critical Thinking Skills and Attitudes Applied to Nursing provide a structure within which you may conceptualize the interactions you have with clients, families, colleagues, and administrators.

# E X E R C I S E S

## Exercise 1

*Purpose:* *Learn to keep a journal*

### DIRECTIONS

Following each chapter, you will be given an exercise to write about in your journal. We will identify some topics for you to write about, and you also may add your own. We suggest you keep your entries in sequence in a special 2- or 3-ring notebook. After you have read this book and completed the exercises, you can review your notes and reflect on the changes in your thinking over time. Your instructor may require you to turn in certain assignments. These will not be shared with others without your permission. The 2- or 3-ring notebook will allow you to write private thoughts that you do not have to turn in.

To begin your journal, write on the following topics. Write until you feel you have exhausted your thoughts about each question.

1. What does critical thinking mean to me? How is it different from my everyday thinking?

2. Are the critical thinking skills I use in my nursing experiences different from those I use in my everyday life?

3. In Chapter 1 the authors discussed the range of factors that influence my thinking. I considered the influence of people, activities, culture, socioeconomic status, age, health status, and birth order on my thinking. How have these factors influenced me? What other factors can I add to this list?

## Exercise 2

*Purpose:* *Examine factors that influence your thinking and choices*

### DIRECTIONS

Divide into small groups. Discuss the following:

1. What individuals, activities, and other factors have the most influence on your thinking today? Consider government, schools, religions, special interest groups, other social institutions, and the media.

2. Why did you choose to become a nurse and not a physician? An x-ray technologist? A physical therapist? Why do you stay in nursing school?

3. Describe the conditions or circumstances when you do your best thinking. Why is this so?

4. What is your image of a nurse? Describe your ideal nurse. Describe a nurse that you admire who serves as a role model for you.

## Exercise 3

**Purpose:** *Conceptualize your thinking process*

### DIRECTIONS

Figs. 1-7 and 1-8 illustrate how two people conceptualized their thinking. The creator of Fig. 1-7 described his thinking as free associating. He does not organize his thoughts or direct them initially; he chases after his creative, expansive imagination, letting the gestalt emerge when it is ready. Then, he figures out a way to translate his ideas into language others will understand.

The creator of Fig. 1-8 described herself as a linear thinker with dominant driving movement surrounded by ideas that pop into her consciousness. Her ideas are driven by and organized about a central idea or purpose. Within this framework, ideas pop into her mind like fireworks or miniature suns. She notes these ideas briefly and then returns to her central idea or purpose.

Draw a picture of how you think. Then divide into small groups. Describe your drawing to your classmates. How are your drawings similar? Different? What did you learn about how you think? What did you learn about how others think?

## Exercise 4

**Purpose:** *Take a position and support it with reasons*

### DIRECTIONS

Read the following statements. Write a response to each, then form pairs and defend your position.

1. Cardiac resuscitation should not be attempted on anyone who is more than 70 years old.
2. The government should fund abortions for women on welfare who want them.
3. Motorcyclists should be required to wear helmets.
4. People who chronically abuse alcohol should be eligible to receive liver transplants.
5. Physician-assisted suicide should be available for the terminally ill who request it.
6. Intravenous drug users should be given sterile needles.

When you are done, form small groups of like-minded individuals and prepare a group position on any one of the questions. If possible, different groups should take opposite positions on the same issue.

Did your group identify reasons that you had not thought of when you worked alone or in pairs? Share your group's position with the whole class. Which of your group's reasons are the most convincing and which are the least convincing? Why?

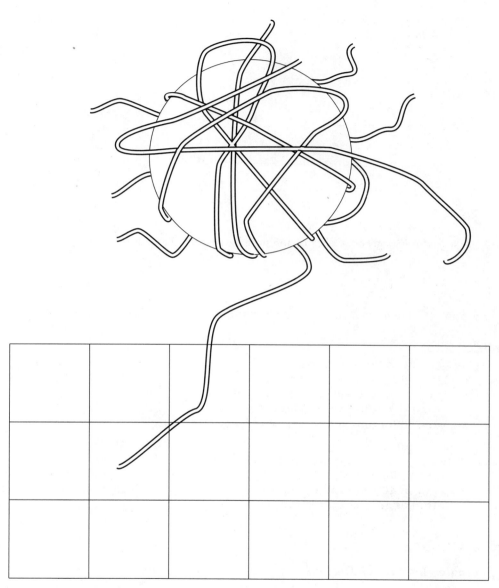

**Fig. 1-7** A way of thinking: Freely associate and then organize.

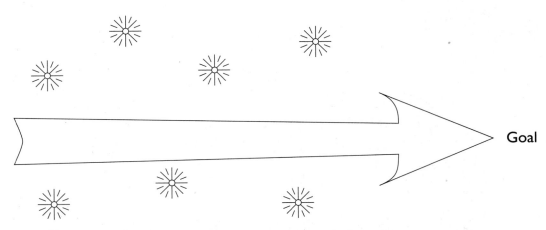

**Fig. I-8**   A way of thinking: Focus on goal and note side issues, digressions.

## Exercise 5

**Purpose:** *Compare and contrast your definition of critical thinking with other definitions*

### DIRECTIONS

Reflect on the various definitions of critical thinking examined in chapter 1 and discussed in class. Compose your own definition of critical thinking. What does it mean to you in your everyday life and in your nursing practice? Then, compare and contrast your definition with at least two other definitions found in the literature. How are your definitions similar? How are they different?

Form small groups. Share your personal definition of critical thinking. How is your definition similar to others in your group? How is it different? Discuss why you defined critical thinking as you did. Were you influenced by the definitions of your classmates or by the authorities referenced in this chapter? If so, how did they influence your thinking?

## Exercise 6

**Purpose:** *Integrate abstract and concrete aspects of thinking*

### DIRECTIONS

Draw a picture or a cartoon of something that occurred to you during or after reading this chapter. Describe it to a classmate(s).

## Exercise 7

**Purpose:** *Examine your support network*

### DIRECTIONS

Think about the people presently in your life. What do you hear them saying to each other or implying about their intelligence and ability? "He (or she) is so intelligent!" "He (or she) doesn't know the left hand from the right!" "That is a great idea!" "That was stupid!" "What a brilliant thought!" "I never looked at it that way." "What a dumb idea!"

Think for a moment to whom you would turn if you wanted to go out and have a good time. Whom would you contact if you wanted sympathy? Whom would you call if you wanted help looking at all the angles of a very sticky issue or problem? Are they the same person? How did you decide?

## Exercise 8

**Purpose:** *Evaluate your critical thinking skills and attitudes and the Critical Thinking Interaction Model*

### DIRECTIONS

1. Examine the list of critical thinking skills and attitudes that support the Critical Thinking Interaction Model and identify those components in which you believe you have some skills and those components in which you need to develop some skills.

2. Evaluate the Critical Thinking Interaction Model. How would you conceptualize the interactions nurses have with others? Reflect on the components in the model that are integral in the interactions between the nurse and others. Would you conceptualize them differently? What parts of the model do you agree with? Would you arrange the model differently? Draw your own picture. What components are not included that you believe should be there? How would you include them in the drawing?

## REFERENCES

AAN Expert Panel Report. (1992). Culturally competent health care. *Nursing Outlook, 40*(6), 277-283.

Adler, J. (1991). Critical thinking, a deflated defense: A critical study of John E. McPeck's *Teaching Critical Thinking: Dialogue and Dialectic. Informal Logic, 13*(2), 61-78.

Babcock, D.E., and Miller, M.A. (1994). *Client education: Theory and practice.* St Louis: Mosby.

Beck, S.E., Bennett, A., McLeod, R., and Molyneaux, D. (1992). Review of research on critical thinking in nursing education. In *Review of Research in Nursing Education, 5,* 1-30.

Brookfield, S.D. (1991). *Developing critical thinkers.* San Francisco: Jossey-Bass.

Browne, M.N., and Keeley, S.M. (1994). *Asking the right questions* (4th ed.). Englewood Cliffs, N.J.: Prentice Hall.

Capers, C.F. (1992). Teaching cultural content: A nursing education imperative. *Holistic Nursing Practice, 6*(3), 19-28.

Chaffee, J. (1994). *Thinking critically* (4th ed.). Boston: Houghton Mifflin.

————. (1992). Teaching critical thinking across the curriculum. In C.A. Barnes (Ed.), *Critical thinking:*

*Educational imperative, new directions for community colleges,* (pp. 25-35). San Francisco: Jossey-Bass.

Charnes, L.S., and Moore, P.S. (1992). Meeting patients' spiritual needs: The Jewish perspective. *Holistic Nursing Practice, 6*(3), 64-72.

Chinn, P.L. (1991). Looking into the crystal ball: Positioning ourselves for the year 2000. *Nursing Outlook, 39*(6), 251-256.

Clouten, K., and Weber, R. (1994). Patient-focused care . . . playing to win. *Nursing Management, 25*(2), 34-36.

Engel, S.M. (1994). *With good reason: An introduction to informal fallacies* (5th ed.). New York: St. Martin's Press.

Ennis R.H. (1985). A logical basis for measuring critical thinking skills. *Educational Leadership, 43,* 44-48.

Glaser, E.M. (Winter, 1985). Critical thinking: Educating for responsible citizenship in a democracy. *Phi Kappa Phi Journal, 65,* 24-27.

Halpern, D.F. (1984). *Thought and knowledge.* Hillsdale, N.J.: Lawrence Erlbaum Associates.

Hughes, W. (1992). *Critical thinking.* Lewiston, N.Y.: Broadview Press.

Kenner, C.A., and MacLaren, A. (1993). *Essentials of maternal and neonatal nursing.* Springhouse, Pa.: Springhouse.

Klaassens, E. (1988). Improving teaching for thinking. *Nurse Educator, 13*(6), 15-19.

Leininger, M. (1994). Transcultural nursing education: A worldwide imperative. *Nursing & Health Care, 15*(5), 254-257.

Little, C. (1992). Health for all by 2000: Where is it now? *Nursing & Health Care, 13*(4): 198-204.

LoBiondo-Wood, G. and Haber, J. (Eds). (1994). Nursing research: Methods, critical appraisal, and utilization (3rd ed.) St Louis: Mosby.

McCarthy, C. (1992). Why be critical? (or rational, or moral?) The justification of critical thinking. *Philosophy of Education, 48*), 60-68.

McGuire-Mahony, K. (personal communication, September 1994).

McPeck, J.E. (1990). Critical thinking and subject specificity: A reply to Ennis. *Educational Researcher, 19*(4), 10-12.

————. (1981). *Critical thinking and education.* New York: St. Martin's Press.

Miller, M.A., and Malcolm, N. (1990). Critical thinking in the nursing curriculum. *Nursing & Health Care, 11*(2), 67-73.

NLN paves a lane on the information superhighway. (1994). *Nursing & Health Care, 15*(5), 265.

Neufeldt, V. (1991). *Webster's new world dictionary* (3rd ed). New York: Webster's New World.

Nkongho, N.O. (1994). Critical thinking: An important outcome of nursing education. *Connections,* Spring. p. 1. New York: National League for Nursing.

Norris, S.P. (1985). Synthesis of research on critical thinking. *Educational Leadership, 42*(8), 40-46.

Nurse's Reference Library. (1981). *Diseases.* Horsham, Pa.: Intermed Communications.

Paul, R. (1992). Why critical thinking? Why now? *Critical Thinking, 1*(1), 3.

————. (1990). *Critical thinking: what every person needs to survive in a rapidly changing world.* Rohnert Park, Calif.: Center for Critical Thinking and Moral Critique.

Ruggiero, V.R. (1991). *The art of thinking* (3rd ed.). New York: Harper Collins.

Samuelson, R.J. (1994, August 15). Will reform bankrupt us? *Newsweek,* pp. 50-54.

————. (1993, October 4). Health care. *Newsweek,* pp. 31-35.

Siegel, H. (1992). On defining "critical thinker" and justifying critical thinking. *Philosophy of Education,* (48), 72-75.

————. (1980). Critical thinking as an educational ideal. *The Educational Forum, 45*(1), 7-23.

Sternberg, R.J., and Baron, J.B. (1985). A statewide approach to measuring critical thinking skills. *Educational Leadership, 43*(2), 40-43.

Tiedt, P.L., and Tiedt, I.M. (1990). *Multicultural teaching.* Boston: Allyn and Bacon.

Toffler, A. (1980). *The third wave.* New York: William Morrow.

Watson, G., and Glaser, E. (1980). *Critical thinking appraisal manual.* New York: Harcourt Brace Jovanovich.

# *Thinking and Learning*

Chapter 2 _____

## OVERVIEW

Before studying content about which to think, you need to understand *how* you think, so you have a foundation for refining your critical thinking abilities. This chapter begins with a discussion about how thinking and moral sense develop from birth to the young adult years. The chapter then discusses several theories about how we learn, including Witkin's field-dependent and independent learning, Kolb's learning cycle and learning styles, Gardner's theory of multiple intelligences, and current thinking about insight and intuition. The chapter applies critical thinking to the role of the nurse. Because more research about how we learn is needed, we should acknowledge and respect other ways of knowing that are not yet well understood.

## THINKING AND LEARNING

In Chapter 1 we discussed learning as a lifelong process and stated that thinking and learning are integrally related. Thinking *is* learning. Thinking is one of the most important aspects of human learning. A broad definition of learning is the acquisition of new knowledge, skills, or attitudes. The focus of this chapter is on the relationship between thinking and learning, that is, how people learn to think and how their thinking affects what they learn.

Mental processes have been the subject of investigation throughout recorded history. Scientific discoveries have complicated the question of what constitutes the mind, thinking, and learning. When you engage in critical thinking, you are thinking about something in a new way (learning) and establishing a new, cognitive structure for arriving at that insight, new knowledge, or conclusion. The path you use to reach that new insight, knowledge, or conclusion then becomes the basis for further critical thinking. When you analyze or synthesize something, you learn. When you rearrange or reorganize knowledge you already have, you learn. When you find it easier to think critically, you learn. Anytime you think, do, or feel something more easily, you learn.

## COGNITIVE AND MORAL DEVELOPMENT: THE EARLY YEARS

Your ability to think critically depends on many factors that encompass the totality of genetic endowment and life experiences.

## Prenatal Influences

Before birth, influences are at work that affect the developing infant's potential cognitive abilities. An individual inherits a mass of gray matter, a nervous system, and other features such as enzymes and genetic glitches from his or her parents. These inheritances may limit or enhance the child's level of wellness. The parents' health habits before conception and the mother's lifestyle during pregnancy all affect the size of the placenta and the amount of nutrients and oxygen the fetus receives. The amount of hormone exposure the fetus experiences will influence masculine or feminine characteristics of brain development. All of these biologic phenomena combined affect the full development of intellectual capacity.

## Infancy

The attitudes of parents, siblings, and other caretakers are affected by the infant's biologic features such as gender, skin color, and size. The baby's nervous system will affect his or her personality, making the baby content, difficult, or uncomfortable with change. An energetic, outgoing baby elicits more feedback from those around than a quiet, reserved child. A smiling, cooing baby elicits responses that are different from those elicited by a crabby, irritable baby. An infant to whom people talk and coo develops the language areas of the brain. An infant becomes noticeably energized when he or she verbalizes and watches an adult attempt to copy his or her sounds. Such responses greatly reinforce efforts to communicate verbally and thus stimulate the language centers in the developing brain. These environmental responses shape the intellectual development of the child, which affects the child's potential to engage in critical thinking.

A family's socioeconomic status and beliefs about lifestyle influence the infant's health and nutrition, which in turn affect intellectual capacity (Pipes and Trahams, 1993). Malnourished children suffer deficits in perceptual performances, memory, verbal ability, and other skills related to critical thinking. A diet too low in fat or lipids—especially in the very young child—can interfere with the manufacture of the myelin sheaths, which are necessary for conduction in the developing nervous system because the brain depends on lipoproteins (such as those found in whole milk) to build these sheaths. Children should receive whole milk until at least the age of two, and at least 2% fat in milk until the age of four (McWilliams, 1993).

A parent who is committed to the intellectual growth of a child will label objects in which the child shows an interest, and name the verb or adjective that describes an obvious experience. For example, a parent who notices the child's listening expression as a plane passes and says "plane" or who says "up" when lifting the child and "soft" when the child feels velvet or cotton batting is promoting the child's intellectual growth. The child who is not given attention or whose interests are not noticed receives less stimulation and fewer messages about his or her importance as a person and the importance of developing his or her intellectual capacities (Tannen, 1990).

## Early Childhood

The family's response to a child's attempt at language gives messages about the importance of the child's thoughts. For example, when one particular 2-year-old child was attempting to speak, the parent deliberately misinterpreted what the child was saying and took great amusement in teasing the child, who walked away frustrated. The parent of another child of the same age responded to the child by stooping to the child's height, listening carefully to the child's efforts, and asking questions in an effort to decipher the child's utterances. Which child was getting the message that thinking was valued?

The socioeconomic level of the child's family and the educational level of the caretakers will influence the type of stimulation the child receives and the way in which the child receives it. For example, mothers with more formal education tend to talk to their children and explain what is happening. Mothers with less education tend to show their children how to do things, and they talk less to their children (Kotliarenco, 1990). Regardless of income level, parenting knowledge is significantly associated with the quality of stimulation (Parks and Smeriglio, 1986).

The extended family also gives messages on the importance of thinking and the child's potential capacity to think critically. A child observes how much importance is given to the opinions and expressed thoughts of the same-sex role models, be they mother, father, sisters, brothers, aunts, uncles, and grandparents. Children learn much about thinking from the words their role models do or do not use to express themselves during the children's formative years. How others respond to the opinions of the child's role models will be equally influential. Young boys and girls receive messages about their ability to think, express emotions, and explore from both the males and females in their family.

The child's culture also will influence the child's perception of the value of thinking critically and the definition of critical thinking. Cultural representatives will teach the child what thoughts are worth pursuing and what topics deserve focus and deep consideration, how much a girl or boy is expected to think, and what the important topics of conversation are.

## Early School Influences

The school-aged child gets messages from his or her family about the purpose of an education and the importance of exhibiting certain behaviors in school. Families that value critical thinking will stimulate it by practicing critical thinking themselves and encouraging it in their children by the way they interact. For example, a respected Jewish scientist was asked about how he learned to think so well. His answer was "My mother was responsible. All of the other Jewish mothers asked their sons, 'What did you learn in school today?' My mother asked me, 'Did you ask a good question?'"

The dominant culture will help to define the child's presence or absence as a significant, thinking individual in society. It also will project expectations on the child as a thinker, an individual capable of thinking, an individual whose opinions should be heard, and an individual who has a right (or lack of right) to critique the opinions of others thoughtfully. Teachers, the books children use, the messages on the walls of their classrooms, and the heros whom they hear about from teachers all give the child an unconscious frame of reference about his or her self-concept as a thinker. For example, a nurse faculty member who is now a doctoral student suffers every time she prepares to make a presentation to her peers and teachers. In her formative years, when this African-American child expressed an interest in becoming a nurse, a number of European-American teachers told her that she might be able to become a nurse's aide or a practical nurse. She clearly got the message that she was not capable of more than that. These old messages continue to plague her as a master's prepared adult, although she now gets respect for her scholarly approach and creative presentations.

Environmental factors and school influences shape the child's perception about the career fields that are viable options for him or her. Research shows that girls in all-girls' academies experience more encouragement to think than girls in coeducational classrooms do. In coeducational schools the average teacher calls on boys four times as often as she or he calls on girls (Holloway, 1993). Changes have been made in the teaching of mathematics. New teaching strategies encourage mathematical talent in females to emerge and remain evident throughout adolescence (Baker and Jones, 1993).

## COGNITIVE AND MORAL DEVELOPMENT: THE YOUNG ADULT YEARS

As children grow into young adults, their cognitive skills continue to develop. Perry (1981) studied the changing ways of seeing the world, knowledge and education, values, and oneself of college-aged students over the span of their baccalaureate education. He identified four major positions in cognitive and ethical development: dualism, multiplicity, relativism, and commitment.

### Dualism

Dualism is thinking in polarized terms such as we versus they, right versus wrong, and good versus bad. A dualistic thinker sees the world as either this or that; nothing exists in between. Dualistic thinkers see themselves in the we, right, and good position. Dualistic thinkers view other people as they, wrong, and bad. This frame of reference sets the stage for frustrating and conflicting relationships with others. Maintaining positive relationships with those who cast you in the they, wrong, or bad role is difficult.

Dualistic thinkers view knowledge as quantitative, or factual. They believe that the way to acquire knowledge is to work hard and memorize facts. They also believe that authorities have the right answers. Dualistic thinkers look to their instructors or supervisors for answers and guidance when it is unnecessary to do so. They may also look to "experts" who are regionally or nationally known, who are published, and who are recognized by respected peers instead of tapping into their own cognitive and creative resources.

Dualistic thinkers are limited in their abilities to act alone or to exert power. The source of action and power is not within; it is without. Dualistic thinkers' source of action and power is in authority, in having the right degree, in getting the right job, in marrying the right spouse, in reaching a given income—always in things or persons outside of themselves.

## Multiplicity

Moving beyond dualism, thinkers progress into multiplicity. Multiplistic thinkers recognize other opinions and values as legitimate in those areas where no one yet knows the right answers. This results in a belief that everyone is entitled to his or her opinions, none of which are necessarily wrong. Multiplistic thinkers do not recognize that some opinions may be better than others or that some may contain more truth than others. They make no distinctions among multiple differing opinions and values.

## Relativism

Relativistic thinkers recognize that some opinions, values, and judgments are based on sources, evidence, logic, systems, and patterns and acknowledge that there is some basis for analysis and comparison. They distinguish between opinions that have little merit and those opinions about which reasonable people will continue to disagree.

Relativistic thinkers realize that teachers want students to think about their own thinking processes. With relativism the concrete, quantitative knowledge of dualism is blended with newly discovered complexity. Relativistic thinkers recognize that there is more than one approach to an issue, more than one factor to consider, and that context is important. Taking a human life is an example of an issue that involves multiple factors and extenuating circumstances. Relativistic thinkers can see differences among a person who kills another in a drive-by incident, a person who kills another to defend his family and himself from an intruder, a child who kills another child in a freak playground accident, a depressed person who commits suicide, and a physician who assists a terminally ill client in suicide at the client's request.

## Commitment

Persons in the commitment position make choices in the face of relativism. They commit themselves to things of importance such as values, politics, careers, and personal relationships. They experience power as coming from within themselves rather than from outside themselves.

## Discussion

Like all linear models depicting a dynamic process, growth is never a straightforward process. Growth can pause or regress—but only temporarily. The larger trend of growth follows a pattern of human maturity. Perry identified these periods as temporizing, escape, and retreat. Temporizing is postponing movement between positions for a year or more. Escape is becoming alienated and abandoning

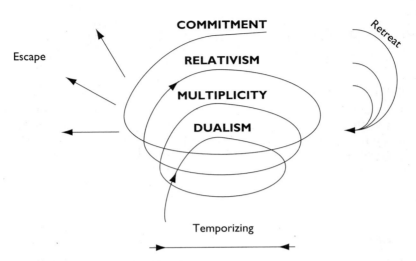

**Fig. 2-1**   Levels of cognitive and ethical development.

Modified from Perry W: Cognitive and ethnic growth: The making of meaning. In Chickering AW, et al. (Eds.), *The modern American college*, San Francisco, 1981, Jossey-Bass.

responsibility. Retreat is avoiding complexity and ambivalence by regressing to dualism. Fig. 2-1 illustrates this dynamic process.

Perry sees growth as nonlinear. He notes that the college student experiences a number of intellectual transitions and plateaus. The spiral connotes growth from one stage to the next. The spiral represents motion, a dynamic process of transition. Students reach plateaus in their intellectual development and have experiences that cause them to digress and then leap to the next level of cognitive development. An individual can take off a year or two to temporize at any level identified by Perry. An individual can retreat from any level and swing back to dualism to find "the answer." An individual can escape the field before coming back and doing the difficult work of growth. Although temporizing, retreating, and escaping have been placed in only one spot on the model, they could be placed anywhere on it.

We believe Perry's concepts fit everyone's adult years. Whenever we run into significant cognitive or ethical challenges, we may escape, retreat, or temporize before doing the difficult work of growth and change.

As you reflect on this model of cognitive and ethical development, you will find it easier to listen to others and assess where they are than to determine where you are in your own thinking. Exercises 2 and 3 at the end of this chapter will help you place your own thinking in Perry's model.

## STYLES OF LEARNING

Recognizing your style of learning is yet another way to understand your thinking. Style of learning refers to a person's preferred way to process information (Garity, 1985), which is also known as cognitive style. Style of learning is the way in which a person acquires knowledge (Kolb, 1981). It is concerned with the form rather than the content of cognitive activity (Witkin, Moore, Goodenough, and Cox, 1977). To help you become aware of your style of learning, study the field-dependence/independence theory (Witkin and Goodenough, 1981), the experiential learning model (Kolb, 1981), and the theory of multiple intelligences (Gardner, 1983).

## Field Dependence and Independence

Field dependence/independence is one dimension of cognitive style and refers to how people take in information, or their mode of perception. The field-dependence/independence dimension is relative and is not intended to cast people into two distinct types of learners. People are relatively field-dependent or field-independent. Each dimension has qualities that are adaptive in particular circumstances. People who possess characteristics of both styles are designated as "mobile" (Witkin and Goodenough, 1981; Witkin, Moore, Goodenough, and Cox, 1977).

People who are relatively field-dependent are more open to external sources of information. They are sensitive to and influenced by their surroundings (their prevailing visual field). People who are relatively field-independent are more autonomous, that is, they rely more on themselves. Field-independent persons experience parts of their visual field as more or less separate from the total surrounding field. Field-dependent persons are more attentive to social cues in the environment and make more use of this information when the situation is ambiguous and when others are seen as likely sources of information for resolving the ambiguity. They are less influenced by others when the opinion of others is unlikely to add to their own effectiveness. They look at others' faces and attend to verbal messages as sources of information about what others are feeling and thinking. They tend to accept the prevailing perceptual frame of reference rather than impose their own upon a situation. They are more social and people oriented, and they prefer close physical proximity to others (Witkin and Goodenough, 1977, 1981; Witkin, Moore, Goodenough, and Cox, 1977).

Field-dependent persons tend to see the whole situation rather than focusing on any one aspect of it. They are inclined to take a spectator role in the learning process and be influenced by authority figures. Field-dependent persons are inclined to conform to group pressure and fulfill maintenance roles such as cooperation, collaboration, and participation. They are more affected by criticism and experience less sense of differentiation from other people (Garity, 1985). When they talk, they refer more to others and less to themselves, whereas field independents make "I" statements such as "I did this" (Claxton and Murrell, 1987; Garity, 1985).

Field-independent persons tend to be less sensitive to the social environment and more impersonal in their orientation. Field-independent persons take an analytic view of a situation and separate aspects of it from the background. They are capable of structuring or restructuring situations on their own. This means that they are able to organize a field that lacks organization or impose a different organization on a field than that which is in place (Witkin and Goodenough, 1981; Witkin, Moore, Goodenough, and Cox, 1977).

Abstract and theoretical concepts are more interesting to field-independent persons. They are task oriented and like to test opinions, ideas, and hypotheses. They are less affected by criticism and are not inclined to conform to group pressure. They are motivated by meeting challenges. They have a strong sense of differentiation from others (Witkin and Goodenough, 1981; Witkin, Moore, Goodenough, and Cox, 1977).

To illustrate what it means to be relatively field-dependent and relatively field-independent, consider how Susan and Rhonda, beginning nursing students, handle a dressing change procedure in the nursing skills laboratory. Both reviewed their notes from the instructor. Rhonda focused on the theory of asepsis and its application to this procedure while Susan discussed the procedure with several other classmates. Susan noticed that some classmates were experiencing mild anxiety, so she offered them encouragement. Susan wanted to observe the procedure before doing it, so she asked Rhonda to perform it first. Rhonda readily accepted the challenge. Rhonda collected the necessary equipment, arranged it on the bedside table, and demonstrated the procedure efficiently. When Susan's turn came, she also demonstrated the procedure efficiently. She spent more time, however, talking with the "client" and explaining the procedure.

Later, when discussing the experience, both Susan and Rhonda made a different suggestion about how the procedure could be done more efficiently and still be equally effective. Their comments generated a lot of discussion. Several classmates disagreed with both suggestions and stated why they disagreed. Susan listened carefully to the comments, decided they had merit, and subsequently revised her suggestion to incorporate her classmates' ideas. Rhonda also listened to the discussion, but she believed her idea had more merit than her classmates' opinions. Rhonda concluded that she was ahead of her time.

In this situation, Susan preferred to observe first, then perform. She assumed maintenance behaviors in the group by being supportive of others. She listened to peer criticism, decided that it had merit, and revised her suggestion for improving the procedure. Contrary to Susan, Rhonda favored a more intellectually independent role in learning. Rhonda was more interested in the technical aspect of the procedure than Susan was. She was less affected by peer pressure and considered others to be less informed than she instead of revising her idea for improving the procedure. Susan is an example of a relatively field-dependent learner; Rhonda is a relatively field-independent learner.

As you reflect on cognitive style, you should think of it as value neutral; that is, one dimension is not preferable to the other. No difference in learning ability, memory, or ability to achieve exists between persons who are relatively field-dependent and relatively field-independent. Field dependence should not be confused with emotional dependence (Witkin and Goodenough, 1977). They are simply different ways of perceiving the prevailing visual field (Witkin, Moore, Goodenough, and Cox, 1977).

## Experiential Learning Model: Learning Cycle

Kolb (1981) proposed an experiential learning model showing learning as a four-stage cycle (Fig. 2-2). Entry into the cycle begins with the concrete experiences after which you move on to the second stage of observations and reflection on their experiences. The third stage deals with abstract concepts and making generalizations.

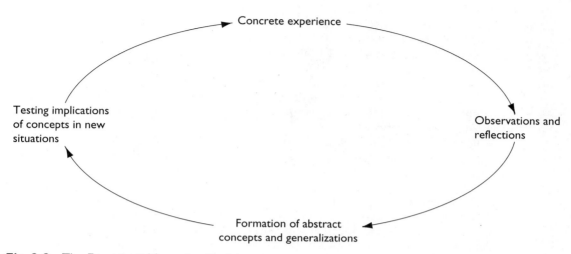

**Fig. 2-2** The Experiential Learning Model.

From Kolb DA: Learning styles and disciplinary differences. In Chickering AW, et al. (Eds.), *The modern American college,* San Francisco, 1981, Jossey-Bass.

Generalizations and principles become the basis for theories that guide further behavior. The fourth stage is characterized by testing implications of new concepts and theories in different and more complex situations. By experimenting and applying new learning, you again engage in concrete experiences. As the cycle continues, you expand your knowledge base as the learning experiences become increasingly complex.

As you reflect on these stages, notice that concrete experience is the polar opposite of abstract concepts and generalizations. Observations and reflections are the polar opposites of testing the implications of concepts in new situations. Learners choose which set of learning abilities to apply in any given situation. Thus, learners move from being actors to observers, and from direct involvement in an experience to general analytic detachment. To take in information and adapt to the environment effectively, learners need all four different sets of abilities: concrete experience, reflective observation, abstract conceptualization, and active experimentation.

Let us look at an example of a learning cycle and apply these learning abilities. Suppose you are working with an Asian client who speaks very little English. The client needs to know that he will be having a diagnostic test the next day and that he will need to collect urine specimens at different intervals during the day. All of your efforts to communicate this message have been unsuccessful. You are aware of your feelings of frustration and suspect the client is also frustrated, although he continues to smile and nod his head frequently, which you interpret to mean he understands. At this moment your instructor comes by and assesses the situation. She tells you that she will try to help, leaves, and returns about an hour later with an interpreter. The interpreter speaks the client's native language and explains your instructions.

Later that evening you reflect on the incident. You think about how frustrated you felt and wonder how your client felt. You fantasized what it would be like to be hospitalized in a country where you did not speak the native language. You reflect on your efforts to communicate by sign language and wonder if your client actually understood because you recall that many Asians are taught to smile and nod to be polite and not to affirm understanding. You think about how easily the interpreter communicated with the client and how, in a brief time, the client understood what he was expected to do. As you reflect on your experience, you remember a similar incident your classmate had and how it was handled by an interpreter who talked with the client by phone.

Both incidents cause you to wonder about the number of ethnically diverse clients served by the hospital and how many other nurses have had experiences similar to yours. You think about the commonalities in these experiences and generalize that all non-English speaking clients would be better served by the hospital if they could communicate effectively with the nurses. You wonder about what could be done to communicate with clients who do not understand or speak English. Then, you have a great idea: The nurses could identify all of the languages and dialects spoken in the community and solicit and train a pool of people willing to serve as interpreters. The master list of interpreters could be kept in a central location, available to the entire hospital staff. As you think about your idea, you also decide that at least three interpreters for each language and dialect would be desirable in case one or two of them were not available when needed. You make a note to run the idea by your instructor tomorrow. In this example, you have been both actor and observer. You have been directly involved and have engaged in reflection and detached analysis.

The following week, you and your instructor meet with the vice president for nursing. She likes your idea and invites you to present it at the next nurse managers' meeting. She also assigns a member of her staff to obtain demographic data on the ethnicity of clients served by the institution and the percentage of those who are non-English speaking. The nurse managers like your idea, and within a month the new pool of interpreters is in place. The nurse managers will evaluate the effectiveness of your idea in 6 months.

The Nursing Application of Kolb's Learning Cycle box on p. 43 places this example in the theoretical framework of Kolb's cycle of learning. You can see how your idea progressed through the various stages of the cycle, beginning with the concrete experience and followed by observation and reflection. You then formed abstract concepts and made generalizations, after which you tested the implications of your concept in a new situation.

***Experiential Learning Model: Learning Styles.***    In his learning cycle, Kolb identified four types of learners: converger, diverger, assimilator, and accommodator. Convergers' dominant learning abilities are abstract conceptualization and active experimentation. Their strengths are in the practical application of ideas. Through hypothetical-deductive reasoning, convergers excel at focusing on specific problems and finding a solution to each question or problem. These individuals prefer dealing with things rather than people—and often specialize in the physical sciences.

Divergers have the opposite strengths of convergers. Their dominant learning abilities are concrete experience and reflective observation. They tend to be people-

## Nursing Application of Kolb's Learning Cycle

**CONCRETE EXPERIENCE**
- ▼ Experiencing nurse/Asian client interaction
- ▼ Noting inability to communicate
- ▼ Feeling frustration
- ▼ Observing that instructor brings interpreter

**OBSERVATION AND REFLECTION**
- ▼ Thinking about the experience that evening
- ▼ Fantasizing self being the client

**FORMATION OF ABSTRACT CONCEPTS GENERALIZATIONS**
- ▼ Wondering about the experience of all non-English speaking clients in this health care institution
- ▼ Proposing a pool of interpreters for non-English speaking clients

**TESTING IMPLICATIONS OF CONCEPTS IN A NEW SITUATION**
- ▼ Meeting with nursing vice president and nurse managers
- ▼ Operationalizing the pool of interpreters
- ▼ Evaluating the effectiveness of the pool

oriented. Their strength lies in generating ideas. Through their imaginative ability, divergers are able to view concrete situations from many perspectives and organize many relationships into a meaningful gestalt (whole). Divergers are often individuals in the humanities and liberal arts.

Assimilators' dominant learning abilities are abstract conceptualization and reflective observation. Their strength is in creating theoretical models. Through inductive reasoning, they assimilate many different observations into an integrated theory. They are more concerned about the logical soundness and precision of a theory than its practical application. They are less people-oriented. The assimilating learning style is more characteristic of people in the basic sciences and mathematics than those in the applied sciences. Assimilators are frequently found in research and planning positions.

Accommodators' strengths are opposite to those of the assimilators. Their dominant learning abilities are concrete experience and active experimentation. Their strength lies in carrying out plans and experiments and becoming involved in new experiences. Accommodators are risk takers who have the ability to adapt to specific immediate circumstances. They tend to solve problems in an intuitive trial-and-error manner, relying heavily on other people for information instead of relying on their own analytical ability. The accommodating learning style is characteristic of persons who frequently hold action-oriented jobs in technical or practical fields. They are comfortable with people but may be perceived as impatient or pushy. The Kolb's Learning Styles box below summarizes these styles.

What would happen if four nurses, each one representing a different learning style, met together for a problem-solving conference? To illustrate how their way of taking in information and processing might differ, let us suppose they are discussing how their health care institution will implement a new nursing care delivery system. Each nurse conceptualizes the situation differently. The converger nurse examines the administration's implementation plan and considers the details of what must be done to make it work on her unit. She thinks about the personnel who will be required and the role and responsibilities of each person. She also thinks about the number and acuity of typical clients cared for on the unit. Her primary concern is how the purposes of the unit will be achieved and how the work will get done.

The diverger nurse sees a larger picture than the converger nurse. In addition to thinking about the impact of the new nursing care delivery system directly on his unit, he also thinks about how it will be implemented on other nursing units, how the change will affect the institution as a whole, and how this might affect the community's perception of nursing care in this institution. He thinks about how the change will affect the nursing and medical staffs and other ancillary help in the institution. He also contemplates the budgetary impact of the change.

The assimilator nurse observes and listens to the other nurses' comments. She has not thought too much about how she is going to implement the new nursing care delivery system on her unit. Instead, she is fascinated with the new nursing delivery

 **Kolb's Learning Styles**

**CONVERGER**
- ▼ Applies ideas in a practical manner
- ▼ Problem solves

**DIVERGER**
- ▼ Uses imagination
- ▼ Sees the larger picture

**ASSIMILATOR**
- ▼ Creates theoretical models
- ▼ Creates logical theories

**ACCOMMODATOR**
- ▼ Carries out plans
- ▼ Likes new experiences
- ▼ Adapts to circumstances

system being created by the institution and contemplates the management process by which it was conceptualized. She has read a lot about various nursing care delivery systems and contributed to the creation of this one. The new delivery system is partially based on a nursing model proposed by a faculty member at a nearby university school of nursing. She compares the new system with what she has read in the literature and mentally blends her own ideas about management with the model. In so doing, she creates her own theory of nursing care delivery and management. She wonders if her own theory incorporates the best of management theory with the model.

The accommodator nurse volunteers her unit for the pilot study. Her Assistant Head Nurse has already focused on an implementation plan and believes he has worked out all of the fine details in preparation for a pilot run on their unit. She tells the staff that such a pilot study is needed to work out any unanticipated problems that may arise before the new nursing delivery system is fully implemented.

As you can see, each nurse has approached the challenge of implementing a new nursing care delivery system from a different perspective. Each has contributed to the richness of the discourse by sharing different views. Each nurse challenged the others to look at the situation from a different perspective.

While these four nurses may experience some minor frustration in understanding each other, this should not in any way detract from the stimulation, enrichment, and challenge that may result by their working together. By recognizing different styles of learning, we learn to appreciate another's point of view rather than discounting it because it is not like our own. Each nurse has a unique contribution to make to the nursing profession.

***Experiential Learning Model: Personal Growth.***    The four learning styles encapsulate a model of personal growth over a lifetime in areas such as decision making, problem solving, and living in general. They eventually become integrated, as illustrated in Fig. 2-3.

Kolb divides personal growth into three broad stages. The first stage, acquisition, occurs from infancy to adolescence. During this time individuals acquire basic learning abilities and information. The sense of self and differentiation from others continues to develop. Thinking is concrete.

The second stage, specialization, occurs from adolescence to mid-career, spanning the time of formal education, career training, work, and personal life. During this stage, individuals are shaped by social, educational, and organizational forces. Individuals become skilled in a particular mode of learning as they strive for competence and mastery over vocational, career, and other life choices.

The third stage, integration, begins after the individual's career peaks and lasts until advanced old age. During this time learning modes that were dormant during the previous stage are reawakened. An individual who was a reflective observer may engage more in active experimentation. An abstract conceptualizer may participate in more concrete experiences. During this stage, individuals may take on new career interests, make lifestyle changes, or become creative in other aspects of work and living. Individuals develop greater competence, complexity, and relativism. Development in and integration of the four learning modes are illustrated by the tapering cone moving toward integration. It is the height of personal development.

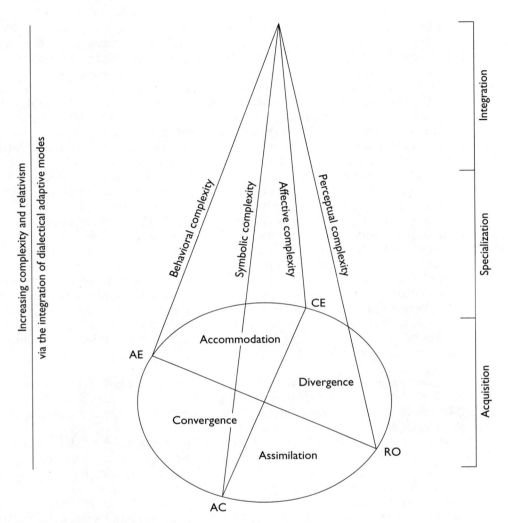

**Fig. 2-3** Kolb's experiential learning theory of growth and development.

From Kolb DA: Learning styles and disciplinary differences. In Chickering AW, et al. (Eds.), *The modern American college,* San Francisco, 1981, Jossey-Bass.

## Multiple Intelligences

Styles of learning based on Gardner's theory of multiple intelligences are yet another way to look at human cognition (Gardner, 1983; Gardner and Hatch, 1990). Gardner eschews the single intelligence quotient (IQ) score as a measure of intelligence in favor of a more comprehensive model. He defined intelligence as "the capacity to solve problems or to fashion products that are valued in one or more cultural settings" (Gardner and Hatch, 1990, p. 5). The term *fashion products* includes things such as writing a symphony, executing a painting, staging a play, building up and managing an organization, and carrying out an experiment.

Gardner described seven intelligences and left open the possibility for others yet unidentified.

**Linguistic Intelligence.**  A person with linguistic intelligence is sensitive to the sounds, rhythms, and meanings of words and possesses a technical facility with words. She or he has a fascination with language and is sensitive to its different functions. Of all the intelligences, linguistic intelligence is the most widely shared among humans. Poets and journalists possess this intelligence.

**Musical Intelligence.**  A person with musical intelligence can produce and appreciate rhythm, pitch, timbre, and the many forms of musical expression. For reasons unknown, this intelligence emerges the earliest in life. Composers and musical artists possess this intelligence.

**Logical-Mathematical Intelligence.**  Persons gifted with logical-mathematical intelligence have the ability to discern logical or numerical patterns and are skilled at handling long chains of reasoning. A passion for abstraction and ideas characterizes this intelligence. Mathematicians and scientists possess this intelligence.

**Spatial Intelligence.**  Spatial intelligence involves the power to create mental images. A person gifted with this intelligence perceives the visual-spatial world easily and can use imagination to transform the scene under observation and re-create past visual experiences at will. Sculptors and navigators are gifted with this intelligence.

**Bodily-Kinesthetic Intelligence.**  Bodily-kinesthetic intelligence is manifested in the person who has the abilities to skillfully use body cues and motions for expression and goal-directed purposes, and for handling objects. Dancers and athletes possess this intelligence.

**Interpersonal Intelligence.**  Interpersonal intelligence is the ability to recognize and make distinctions among the moods, temperaments, motivations, and intentions of other people. Individuals in the helping professions such as therapists and gifted salespersons are examples of this intelligence.

**Intrapersonal Intelligence.**  Intrapersonal intelligence is akin to interpersonal intelligence; however, the focus is inward to one's own feelings and emotions. It is self-knowledge of one's own strengths, weaknesses, desires, and intelligences. It is the ability to discriminate among these and draw upon them as a means of understanding and guiding one's behavior. Persons possessing in-depth self-knowledge illustrate this intelligence.

Some intelligences are relatively independent of one another. A person can excel in one intelligence and not in others; however, few occupations rely entirely on any single intelligence. The intelligences can also be combined in a multiplicity of adaptive ways among individuals of different cultures. Culture is the context in which multiple intelligences reveal themselves and are developed. Gardner noted the educational system in the United States has emphasized two intelligences: linguistic and logical-mathematical. The other intelligences are reinforced in life outside the formal classroom.

Fig. 2-4 illustrates learning styles based on the theory of multiple intelligences. The figure shows the types of learners and what they like to do, what they are good at doing, and how they best learn.

### A Professionally Reinforced Style of Learning

Let us shift our attention to nursing education, the process by which nurses become licensed to practice. What impact does it have on thinking? Kolb (1981) notes that disciplines and professions have characteristic ways of viewing the world, defining and portraying knowledge, inquiring, and solving problems. In many nursing education programs, clients are viewed as living, open systems affected by biologic, psychologic, sociologic, cultural, and spiritual influences in a given environment. Nurse educators define nursing by using various emerging nursing theories, and they portray knowledge by the actions nurses take. Assessment and case studies are common methods of inquiry, and the nursing process is used to solve client care problems.

To be successful in nursing, you must be proficient and comfortable assessing and diagnosing client needs, planning and implementing interventions, and evaluating client outcomes. The nursing process is one way of reasoning by which the nursing profession addresses the very nature of its work, which is caring for clients. To be successful in nursing practice, you must be able to engage in this reasoning process successfully.

If nurses tend to reason in a similar fashion, they are more likely to reinforce each other's thinking rather than to stimulate each other to think or approach problems differently. To move beyond your confines, you may find it stimulating to discuss professional issues and problems with those who can bring a different perspective. You may find opportunities to enjoy this interchange by serving on an interdisciplinary committee at your school or place of employment, attending interdisciplinary conferences, continuing your formal education, participating in community service activities, and participating in local, state, and national political activities. Everyone benefits by this exchange of thoughts and ideas. Getting in a thinking rut or becoming perplexed by a problem or an issue is easy to do. By discussing it with another, you may get a fresh perspective and develop new ideas.

## OTHER WAYS OF KNOWING

Three other ways of knowing are insight, intuition, and awareness of other cultural perspectives. All three are cognitive processes that nurses use in working with clients, families, colleagues, and administrators.

### Insight

Insight is the ability to see and understand clearly the inner nature of things (Neufeldt, 1991). One of the characteristics of insight is that after the insight is gained

# Seven styles of learning

There's no such thing as "generalized intelligence" symbolized by one IQ number, say researchers into intelligence. Rather, people exhibit different types of intelligences.

### Logical/mathematical intelligence

Often called "scientific thinking," this intelligence deals with inductive and deductive thinking/reasoning, numbers and the recognition of abstract patterns.

### Visual/spatial intelligence

This intelligence, which relies on the sense of sight and being able to visualize an object, includes the ability to create internal mental images/pictures.

### Body/kinesthetic intelligence

This intelligence is related to physical movement and the knowings/wisdom of the body, including the brain's motor cortex, which controls bodily motion.

### Verbal/linguistic intelligence

This intelligence, which is related to words and language – written and spoken – dominates most Western educational systems.

### Musical/rhythmic intelligence

This intelligence is based on the recognition of tonal patterns, including various environmental sounds, and on a sensitivity to rhythm and beats.

### Interpersonal intelligence

This intelligence operates primarily through person-to-person relationships and communication.

### Intrapersonal intelligence

This intelligence relates to inner states of being, self-reflection, metacognition (i.e. thinking about thinking) and awareness of spiritual realities.

| Type | Likes to | Is good at | Learns best by |
|---|---|---|---|
| **Linguistic learner** "The word player" | Read, write and tell stories | Memorizing names, places, dates and trivia | Saying, hearing and seeing words |
| **Logical/ mathematical learner** "The questioner" | Do experiments, figure things out, work with numbers, ask questions and explore patterns and relationships. | Math, reasoning, logic and problem solving. | Categorizing, classifying, working with abstract patterns and relationships. |
| **Spatial learner** "The visualizer" | Draw, build, design and create things, daydream, look at pictures and slides, watch movies and play with machines. | Imagining things, sensing changes, mazes and puzzles, reading maps and charts. | Visualizing, dreaming, using the mind's eye and working with colors and pictures. |
| **Musical learner** "The music lover" | Sing, hum tunes, listen to music, play an instrument, respond to music. | Picking up sounds, remembering melodies, noticing pitches and rhythms and keeping time. | Rhythm, melody and music. |
| **Bodily/kinesthetic learner** "The mover" | Move around, touch and talk and use body language. | Physical activities (sports, dance and acting) and crafts. | Touching, moving, interacting with space and processing knowledge through bodily sensations. |
| **Interpersonal learner** "The socializer" | Have lots of friends, talk to people and join groups. | Understanding people, leading others, organizing, communicating, manipulating and mediating contracts. | Sharing, comparing, relating, cooperating and interviewing. |
| **Intrapersonal learner** "The individual" | Work alone, pursue own interests. | Understanding self, focusing inward on feelings and dreams, following instincts, pusuing interests and goals and being original. | Working alone, individualized projects, self-paced instruction and having own space. |

Source: The Instructor, research of Howard Gardner, Harvard University

Jennifer McDonald, Gannett News Service

**Fig. 2-4** Gardner's seven styles of learning.

and expressed, the connection or solution becomes obvious to the inventor and those people who are knowledgeable about the subject matter. What makes the phenomenon "insight" is that it is not obvious before the inventor put the thoughts or parts of the thought together.

The time frame for achieving insight may be months or years. An insight into a field of endeavor does not come by itself, floating through the universe, to some lucky individual. Insight usually occurs to an individual who has been studying intensely, reading, or experimenting with an idea for an extended period of time, such as Kekule, the chemist who initiated the notion of the benzene ring after years of study and contemplation. (Boden, 1991). Insight may be experienced as a gradual dawning of a truth, when various understandings materialize and synthesize. Sometimes it comes in a dramatic flash, as characterized by the "aha" experience, as if the learner suddenly grasps the meaning of a situation at a deeper level of understanding.

Insight is not reached by an orderly progression of logical thought; instead it is reached as a gestalt. All of the pieces of the puzzle (or part of the puzzle) suddenly fall into place. Once the insight is reached, it can be explained using logical thought processes. Although the discovery was there waiting to be discovered, logical thought processes could not find it. Afterwards, logical thought processes can indeed confirm it. Another interesting side effect of an insight is the mind's ability to recall previous observations that had been forgotten, and that now make sense, given the new insight (Poon, Fozard, Cermack, Arenberg, and Thompson, 1980).

People who have experienced insight sometimes describe it as coming "out of nowhere," but they recognize it as soon as it emerges. It is as if some part of an individual's brain has continued the search beyond of the level of conscious awareness, and the individual immediately recognizes the answer to the question when it manifests itself. They also report that their insights come in various forms such as thoughts or pictures. For example, Kekule reported many visions of molecules dancing before his eyes in many shapes on many occasions. One evening as he was dozing, the "snakes" of molecules he often envisioned started chasing after their "tails" and thus the benzene ring was born (Boden, 1991). William Golding, the author of *Lord of the Flies*, reported that he heard dialogue in his head before he added it to his novel. Mozart reported that when he was in a particular state of mind and undisturbed, he experienced a musical work "enlarging itself" inside his head. In his imagination he could hear all the parts of a musical piece all at once, fitting together like a gestalt (Ghiselin, 1952).

People agree more on what insight is than how it is achieved. Some would argue that logical thought processes are indeed occurring and lead to the insight, but they are occurring at a level outside ordinary consciousness, which is called the "submerged chain" theory (deBono, 1970). The thinker experiences the insight as sudden because the thinker can recall only the beginning and end of the chain of thoughts. The other links occurred, but at another level of consciousness. Once the completed end of the chain is experienced (insight), the thinker can work backward and forward to bring the entire chain out into the open to be examined in ordinary light (logic).

Others would argue that the process is more akin to subconscious, covert trial and error. Connections in the subconscious are tried and discarded when they do not satisfy the criteria for the problem. When insight occurs, the thinker recognizes the insight as the answer to the puzzle she or he has been processing and immediately allows the answer to enter the conscious mind.

Some individuals perform particular rituals to increase their chances to gain insight, but insight cannot be achieved on command. Some people work better alone; others discover insights when they discuss their thoughts with interested peers, students, or teachers. The way to a new insight may be through being willing to experience surprise, puzzlement, or even confusion. Being able to tolerate these emotions and stay focused on the uncertainties in the situation may be the key to unlocking the puzzle, which takes intellectual courage, honesty, and curiosity. The thinker must be courageous to stay in a situation that is unclear and be honest enough to admit he or she does not understand it. Given enough time and perseverance, the professional may find a way to reframe the puzzle and solve it. If you can maintain an attitude of humility and curiosity instead of discarding facts that do not fit your theory, you may construct a new theory out of what is before you. As Schon (1983) asserts, when you act on that new theory, you get immediate feedback on its connection with reality.

As technology advances we may soon have a physiological theory that explains the concept of insight. We already know from brain research that the nerve endings in the brain remodel themselves continuously. When a person concentrates on a subject, she or he sends impulses down many nerve fibers. If the person engages in a lot of mental work, the nerve fibers receive much stimulation and remodel themselves according to their stimulation and the reception they are getting from their neuronal neighbors (Raichle, 1994). During these periods of mental searching, new nerve fibers reach out to new neighbors. Perhaps a pathway is finally connected that makes sense to the thinker and an insight emerges. However it is achieved, insight is accepted as thinking that can stand the light of scrutiny, logic, research, and testing. The same criteria cannot be applied so easily to intuition.

## Intuition

Intuition can be defined as knowing something without the conscious use of reasoning. It is immediate comprehension or understanding, or the ability to perceive or know things without conscious reasoning (Neufeldt, 1991). In our speech we display much spontaneous skill and a form of knowing that does not easily lend itself to intellectual reasoning. The skills of speech development are not a result of intellectual reasoning unless we are learning a new language or studying to be speech pathologists.

How do you recognize someone from your own neighborhood in a foreign country? Is it by a reasoning process? Could you describe it? Would you agree that an attempt to describe your process of recognition would be labored and lengthier than your instant recognition of the person? Does that make your recognition of that person less significant or less accurate? If you can accept that such recognition is a common experience for all of us, can you accept the possibility that an experienced nurse forms such patterns of recognition in his or her repertoire of clinical situations? Intuition enhances an individual's ability to solve problems despite relatively small amounts of conscious information. Intuition also has been described as skilled pattern recognition (Benner, 1984), a form of clairvoyance, and a hunch or a gut feeling (Correnti, 1993).

Benner and Tanner (1987) defined intuition as "an understanding without a rationale." Pattern recognition and similarity recognition of fuzzy resemblances are part of the accumulated knowledge that the expert nurse brings to the current client interaction and observation.

One of the striking threads that runs through expert nurses' recollections is their possibility thinking, both for good and ill. Possibility thinking is thoughts that begin with "if . . . then . . . on the other hand. . . ." Possibility thinkers are risk takers; they go with their "gut feelings" and make educated guesses about what is going on or what is likely to happen (Ball and Benner, 1989). The tools they use become extensions of their senses (Schon, 1987). When they look at various chemicals running into the client's veins and the various electronic monitors, they see whether or not the data and connections "look right." They do this while observing whether or not the client's appearance and behavior coincide with the treatments the client is receiving and the client's expected condition at his or her present state of illness. Much of what goes on with a severely ill client lacks precision, because the client's response to the disease process is individual and dynamic (Gruber and Benner, 1989; Stewart and Benner, 1989). The client's unique psychologic, sociologic, cultural, and spiritual responses to his or her illness also affect the physiological processes and psychoneuroimmune responses (McNall and Benner, 1989). The expert nurse knows this at a level of awareness that uses the nurse's own physiological processes and intellect in sensing the client's condition and needs.

Nurses repeatedly report experiences in which they have made lifesaving decisions based on clues they cannot articulate or explain (Benner and Tanner, 1987; Correnti, 1993). The longer they practice, the more confident they are of their intuition. The best proof that intuition is a positive tool is to look at the results. For whatever reasons, they were right; the client was on the verge of deep trouble and their actions were crucial to the client's survival. When asked to justify their actions, they may say, "I don't know; his vital signs were unremarkable and his blood gasses were normal" and continue with a litany of objective data that do not support their intuition. They follow with such statements as "He just didn't look right. I knew something was about to happen and told a colleague to get the crash cart ready and to watch him closely. I called the doctor and said 'You better get over here. I feel uneasy about him'. "When asked how they knew, nurses sometimes describe stories of previous clients who had a few characteristics in common with the current client. They may describe a sketchy pattern on which they have registered, without verbal details. These nurses have information that they have not filtered through the well-known linear logic criteria such as identifying the central issue, recognizing their underlying assumptions, and noticing evidence of bias and emotion. These same nurses state that when they try to be objective, they cannot support their sense of impending doom.

Experienced nurses count their intuition as a valuable part of their clinical judgment, but they do not often talk about it unless they find an open-minded colleague or one who risks reporting similar experiences. Caregivers whom we have interviewed use physical words to describe their intuitive insights such as "gut feeling," "my head spins" (when the client confuses himself or herself instead of facing a problem), "my stomach churns" (when a client is feeling anxious), and "I can feel spikes coming at me" (when confronted with a person who has paranoid schizophrenia).

Sometimes intuitive flashes come with no such physical cues or even significant external cues perceptible to the nurse. For example, a nurse reported, "This man walked into the emergency department with his wife. We were busy. When I asked him what was the problem, he patted himself on the cheek and said 'My face hurts.' I [nurse] said to myself 'This man's having an MI' and had someone put him on a stretcher. He *was* having a myocardial infarction (MI). How did I know? I don't know. A sixth sense? We used to talk about vibrations back in the sixties."

If you consider that intuition is a valuable and worthwhile skill, you may want to ask, "OK, how do I learn intuition? Do I just wait until I have been doing bedside nursing for many years? Will I automatically develop it? How do I know when I am being intuitive and when I am fooling myself or just anxious and panicky?" Use common sense: check out your reactions with a trusted expert. Use your best guess and note what happens.

Correnti (1993) reports that when "nurses at varying levels of experience share their accounts of concepts or knowledge that are difficult to teach or learn, the lessons often have the learning impact of first-hand experience" (p. 93). Further, she notes that certain attributes promote intuitive thinking, such as direct client contact, nursing experience, openness to clients, the desire to tune into them, the ability to tune into them, energy, self-confidence, and a caring nurse-client relationship (Dossey, Keegan, Guzzetta, and Kilkmeier, 1988). Other strategies Correnti suggests that would facilitate nurses' intuitive development include tactics that promote calm and presence such as meditation, mind quieting activities, exercise, progressive relaxation, and journal writing. Skilled pattern recognition (Benner and Tanner, 1987) can be facilitated by sharing case studies, focusing on holistic assessments of situations, and allowing expert nurses to share experiences with less experienced colleagues and students. Schon (1983) characterizes the real world as one of complexity, uncertainty, instability, and uniqueness. He points out that the experienced clinician has a pattern (clear or fuzzy) against which to compare situations. During the process the professional selects and names the variables to be noted. Leners (1992) found that nurses often named "the look" as the main variable they note.

Chinn (1989) points out that nurses feel the need to use all of the ways of knowing at their disposal to know that their care of clients is sufficient. Nurses feel satisfaction when they move beyond the technological care of people, machines, and medicine's illness orientation. Health and wholeness are the goals of nursing care. Caring has again gained acceptability and prominence as a fundamental nursing characteristic (Leininger, 1984). Leners (1992) reports that nurses identified caring as the core of their intuitive ability. "Connected knowing" is the phrase used by Miller and Rew (1989) to describe the nurse's integration of intuitive knowledge with knowledge learned from others.

Nurses who use their intuition do not always find a sympathetic audience; however, this cynicism does not negate that there are ways of knowing about which we do not yet have a satisfactory vocabulary (English, 1993). Our position is that intuition is a legitimate way of knowing. Although nurses may not be able to articulate their thoughts, they should describe them the best they can. The task to explain intuition belongs to nurse researchers, who should interview the intuitive clinician to ferret out the theories, underlying assumptions, and observable clues so that this type of clinical judgment can be communicated to the neophyte. There is no substitute for experience, but perhaps researchers can help neophyte nurses shorten the learning curve of moving from novice to expert (Benner, 1984; Benner and Tanner, 1987).

Hypothesis testing in quantitative research is not the only type of research method available to explain intuition. Bevis (1993) strongly urges nurses to change the research methodology to match the field of investigation. Perhaps ethnographic methods and other forms of qualitative research would be more fruitful methods of investigation as started by Benner (1984), Benner and Tanner (1987), and Correnti (1993).

Of interest is the recognition of intuition as a legitimate and valuable tool in the business community. Barnard (1968) claims that some thinking processes cannot be expressed in the words that are used in reasoning. They are manifest, however, in the thinker's judgment, decisions, and actions. Miller and Rew (1989) assert that holistic knowing means valuing "the whole as more than the sum of its parts, unlike reductionist analysis . . . which relies on breaking things into component parts to understand them" (p. 85).

Like Wolfer (1993), we believe that different kinds of thinking are appropriate under different circumstances. The beginning nurse who is learning the profession may operate differently than the expert. Many learners do better when they are presented with an organized structure at first. After they become familiar with a topic, they may be ready to adapt the structure to suit their own way of conceptualizing. The nursing process is such a structure. The nursing process is akin to scaffolding. When the novice nurse learns to diagnose and treat nursing problems, the nursing process is a scaffold that helps the nurse pay attention to important elements. As the nurse develops expertise, the scaffolding becomes less necessary and may be used as a model or check list for the nurse to make sure she or he has covered all of the important variables. Eventually the nurse functions in a holistic manner, noticing more and taking for granted more routine functions.

Nursing practice should be founded on scientific knowledge, but scientific knowledge remains tentative and should not limit what nurses know and do. Let researchers like Correnti and Benner describe how intuition can be taught. Let the experiments and the attempts to explain intuition continue. Do not refuse to acknowledge talents and patterns of knowing merely because you do not yet have a complete vocabulary to describe what happens or because you do not understand that way of knowing. Expert nurses combine critical thinking and creative thinking in ways that are not always explicable. Individuals who believe that important ways of thinking can be expressed only in the scientific model limit themselves from utilizing other realms of legitimate and valuable knowing, thinking, and communicating.

## Cultural and Interpersonal Sensitivity

All of the cultural relevancies cannot be made explicit, but they are present, affecting the perceptions of the nurse and the client (Giger and Davidhizar, 1995). The nurse who grew up in a multicultural environment is likely to have this awareness at an intuitive level. The nurse who has become aware of this reality through advanced education and practice in transcultural nursing environments will also approach a client or nurse situation with more awareness and notice more clues than a nurse with less transcultural knowledge.

Meaning in such a situation is contributed by both the client and the nurse. The nurse's interpretation of the situation is viewed as only one part of the reality that influences the effectiveness of care and recovery or health promotion. For example, a Vietnamese postpartum woman had to leave her baby in a neonatal intensive care unit instead of taking the baby home with her. The father came by himself as often as he could to visit the baby, but did not bring the mother. When the nurse urged him to bring his wife, he looked very distressed and said she could not come. Her family would not let her. The nurses spent a lot of time trying to convince the father of the importance of bringing the mother in (to promote bonding), although they could see he was distressed by their urgings.

In nursing we need to consider the client and family's ways of knowing as well as our own. To know all of the meanings an event has for another is impossible, but until we stop and listen with an open mind and heart, we cannot learn much. In the previous example, one of the more transculturally minded nurses was able to approach the father differently. She remembered reading that in some oriental cultures the postpartum condition is a "cold condition," and that the mother was at risk for becoming ill if she were exposed to the elements. The nurse assumed that because the baby was not with the mother and was not being cared for by the family, the whole situation might be viewed as more risky by the family. With these assumptions in mind, she approached the father. She told him that he was a good father, coming to see his baby so often, and that she wanted to learn about how the nurses could be more helpful to him and his family. After some time and trust building, the nurse learned that the young mother could not get out of bed because the family feared she would develop a prolapsed uterus. Western logic at this point would not be helpful. She knew enough to guess that power in this family had something to do with the young mother's absence (Marchione and Stearns, 1990).

The nurse reasoned that Vietnamese women had been practicing this method of postpartum care for centuries (as did some American women until after World War II), so she would respect it. Her main concern was to promote bonding with the baby. She then incorporated modern technology that she hoped would appeal to the family: the videocamera and tape recorder. She offered to send the father home with sounds and scenes of himself and the baby together. She requested that the mother record her heart sounds so the nurses could play familiar sounds for the baby. She also asked if the mother and grandmothers would like to record songs for the baby on the tape recorder that the nurses could play to keep the baby company when the father was not there. She asked if amulets would be helpful. She also offered to put an article of the mother's clothing with her scent in the crib, and asked if the father wanted to take home the baby's shirt. When she displayed these creative suggestions for promoting bonding, the father noticeably perked up and added his own recommendations.

In the above example, the nurse did not use her knowledge of "cold conditions" to lock herself into a preconceived way of responding that was proper transcultural nursing. She used what she had studied and read to achieve the proper attitude, one of inquiry and respect for other ways of perceiving the state of new parenthood. She also yielded to the power in the family of this baby. In each situation you must use your ability to tune into the client (Andrews, 1992). When you do this, you can recognize the assumptions and interpretations that must be addressed to facilitate the client's move toward an increased level of wellness.

## TYPES OF CRITICAL THINKING

Understanding how you think is an important aspect of developing critical thinking skills. Paul (1990) described four types of critical thinking: critical thinking, uncritical thinking, sophistic critical thinking, and fair-minded critical thinking (see Paul's Types of Critical Thinking box on p. 57). The types are not discrete, and given the complexity of human behavior, aspects of each may be present in any one individual. For example, in one situation a person may engage in fair-minded critical thinking, and in another situation be uncritical in thought. The ideal is to engage in fair-minded critical thinking most of the time.

Critical thinking describes the process used by a person who is aware of his or her own thought processes and makes an attempt to be more precise, accurate, relevant, consistent, and fair. It is in-depth thinking that is constructively skeptical. The critical thinker is aware of bias, prejudice, and one-sidedness of thought and seeks to remove them. The critical thinker is also aware of what she or he knows and does not know. Paul uses this definition of critical thinking as a point of departure for his other types of thinking.

Uncritical thinking is the least desirable type. It is thinking that is often unclear, imprecise, vague, illogical, unreflective, superficial, inconsistent, inaccurate, and trivial. It is egocentric; that is, everything is viewed in relationship to the self. Uncritical thinking ignores the epistemological demands of good thinking and logical reasoning principles.

Sophistic critical thinking refers to subtly deceptive reasoning. This type of thinking uses logical reasoning principles to serve the vested interests of the thinker. Thus, the sophistic thinker is both egocentric and ethnocentric. This individual is skilled and thinks cleverly, but his or her thinking is not driven by a search for truth and objectivity.

Fair-minded critical thinking is the most desirable type of thinking. This thinking applies logical reasoning principles in situations both when it serves the thinker and when it does not. The fair-minded critical thinker consistently applies principles of logic equally to the self and to others. We all should strive to be fair-minded critical thinkers. The fair-minded critical thinker consistently seeks truth and objectivity.

## RESPECT FOR DIFFERENT WAYS OF THINKING

Novices commonly assume that others think like they do. Accompanying this assumption is an equally problematic one: novices assume that their way of thinking is superior to other ways of thinking. This is especially true for those schooled in Western thought and the sciences. Even when we are aware of different cognitive

**Paul's Types of Critical Thinking**\*

**CRITICAL THINKING**

- ▼ Thinking about your thinking so as to be more clear, precise, accurate, relevant, consistent, and fair
- ▼ Constructively skeptical
- ▼ Identifying and removing bias, prejudice, and one-sidedness of thought
- ▼ Self-directed, in-depth, rational learning
- ▼ Awareness of what you know and do not know

**UNCRITICAL THINKING**

- ▼ Thought captive of one's ego, desires, social conditioning, prejudices, or irrational impressions
- ▼ Egocentric, careless, heedless of assumptions, relevant evidence, implications, or consistency
- ▼ Habitually ignoring eqistemological demands in favor of its egocentric commitments

**SOPHISTIC CRITICAL THINKING (WEAK SENSE CRITICAL THINKING)**

- ▼ Meeting epistemological demands insofar as they square with the vested interests of the thinker
- ▼ Heedless of assumptions, relevance, reasons, evidence, implications, and consistency only insofar as it is in the vested interest of the thinker to do so
- ▼ Skilled thinking that is motivated by vested interest, egocentrism, or ethnocentrism rather than by truth or objective reasonability

**FAIR-MINDED CRITICAL THINKING (STRONG SENSE CRITICAL THINKING)**

- ▼ Meeting epistemological demands regardless of the vested interests or ideological commitments of the thinker
- ▼ Empathy into diverse opposing points of view and devotion to truth as against self-interest
- ▼ Consistent in the application of intellectual standards, holding one's self to the same rigorous standards of evidence and proof to which one holds one's antagonists
- ▼ Entertaining all viewpoints sympathetically and assessing them with the same intellectual standards, without reference to one's own feelings or vested interests, or the feelings or vested interests of one's friends, community, or nation

\*Modified from Paul R: Critical thinking: What every person needs to survive in a rapidly changing world, Rohnert Park, Calif., 1990, Sonoma State University.

patterns related to individual and cultural influences, and have a refined respect for other human beings, we still want others to see things the way we do, or to think as we think. We have difficulty thinking outside of our own frame of reference. And, even if we are able to grasp a frame of reference other than our own, we are likely to continue to believe our way is better.

In nursing we must consider not only our own way of knowing but also the client's and family's way of knowing. This is especially true when working with clients from different cultures. Deliberate energy is required to set aside one's own frame of reference and understand how another person thinks.

To recognize and accept another's frame of reference is one thing; to adopt another's frame of reference or parts of it as your own is quite another. Some immigrant groups have been successful with adopting others' frames of reference with their own. They have kept parts of their own frame of reference (for example, loyalty to family, take care of your own) and accepted parts of the new one (for example, aspire higher, get an education).

Nurses, administrators, and others in health care institutions face multiple economic, social, and political factors that directly impact the institution's viability during this era of rapid change. They must challenge their present thinking, learn to think differently, and reconceptualize their services if they are to compete successfully. This requires critical and creative thought.

## SUMMARY

Cognitive and moral development begin in the earliest years and is shaped by lived experiences and interactions with others. College-aged youth experience characteristic positions in their thinking ranging from either/or thinking (dualism) to commitment to life goals. Style of learning is another way of looking at thought processes. Its focus is on how we process information. Although each of us has a preferred style of learning, we are capable of thinking in any of the styles. Over time we develop a preference for style and consistently favor it when we have new experiences and solve problems. Learning style is shaped by heredity, life experiences, the environment, the nature of nursing practice, and nursing education.

The profession of nursing is exploring the many ways of knowing, including linear, rational processes and intuitive processes. Nursing conceptualizes health as wholeness. Nurses view clients as people needing more than technological care. Medical priorities are not sufficient for creating wholeness and health.

Experienced nurses use the knowledge they glean in many ways. They assess clients in speedy and life preserving ways, even when they cannot explain how they know in objective, scientific language. They can and do convey their knowledge by using other methods of communication such as the metaphor and a description of their lived experiences. Ethnographic and related qualitative research methods may work better for collecting this kind of data. Reasoned hypotheses and measurement, the experimental research design of quantitative research (testing of hypotheses using treatment and control groups), are also legitimate and useful methods for extending the science of nursing. Allen, Benner, and Diekelmann (1986) contend that a pluralistic (multiple ways) method to approach problems rather than a dualistic (either or) or monistic (the one right way to investigate) vision of research will garner us more knowledge. They, along with Bevis (1993), state that human beings, both the nurse and client, must be viewed in their mutually lived experience. Our cultural realities greatly affect how we interact with each other.

# EXERCISES

## Exercise 1

***Purpose:*** *Examine how your thinking and understanding change over time*

### DIRECTIONS

1. Recall your earliest memories of a major holiday such as Christmas, Chanukah, or the New Year. What feelings does it generate? Excitement, trauma, indifference? When and how did your understanding of the holiday begin to change? What does the holiday mean to you today?

2. Recall your earliest thought of wanting to become a nurse. How old were you? What motivated you? What was your first concept of a nurse? What roles and responsibilities did you attribute to nurses? How have your ideas changed as a result of being in a nursing program?

## Exercise 2

***Purpose:*** *Identify elements of Perry's stages of cognition in your own thinking*

### DIRECTIONS

Write a two-page composition discussing one idea you have to improve efficiency and decrease cost at a health care institution about which you are knowledgeable. Discuss the following:

1. How did the situation get this way?

2. Describe your idea.

3. Why has nothing been done before now?

4. What other options might compete with yours?

5. Why should your idea be implemented over others' ideas?

When you are done, trade papers with another student. Examine each other's writing for examples of dualism, multiplicity, relativism, and commitment. Refer to the appropriate figures in this chapter.

# Exercise 3

**Purpose:** *Identify elements of Perry's stages of cognition in your own thinking*

## DIRECTIONS

Write a thoughtful paragraph on one of the following:

1. How did the national deficit become so high?
2. A cure for cancer is available, but the medical community will not let the public know about it.
3. What options do we have to resolve prison overcrowding?
4. Did you vote in the last election? Why or why not?
5. When it comes to improving the health care system, one person's opinion is about as good as another's.

When you are done, exchange papers with another student. Examine each other's writing for examples of dualism, multiplicity, relativism, and commitment.

# Exercise 4

**Purpose:** *Identify elements of Perry's stages of cognition in your own thinking*

## DIRECTIONS

Read the following dialog and answer the questions:

**Sam:**    I support capital punishment and believe it is a deterrent to crime. A society has to establish some limits on what it will tolerate from its citizens. Capital punishment lets everyone know there is a price to be paid for disobeying the law.

**Sally:**    Practically speaking, it's either have capital punishment or have a lawless society. Criminals are released too soon and go back to the streets and hurt other people.

**Joe:**    There are a lot of ways to deter crime besides capital punishment—jail terms, sentences that involve community service, restitution to the victim, and so forth. One way is about as effective as another. We all have the right to our own opinion.

**Jan:**    Surely some of the punishments Joe has identified are more effective than others.

**Zoe:**    My professor is an expert in this area. She can tell you which punishments are most effective.

**Zeb:**    Do you think that the circumstances surrounding a crime should be taken into consideration?

Based on Perry's Scheme of Cognitive and Ethical Development, identify the position each person's statement characterizes. For example, Sam's statement is characteristic of Perry's stage of commitment. How would you classify the others?

# Exercise 5

**Purpose:** *Identify your preferred style of learning*

## DIRECTIONS

1. Take the Kolb Learning Style Inventory, which you must obtain from your instructor.
2. Discuss the results. Do you agree? Disagree? Have you changed over time?

# Exercise 6

**Purpose:** *Examine thinking and learning styles of nurses*

## DIRECTIONS

Debate the following:

Nurses do not reason in a similar fashion. For example, some nurses are artists and others are linear thinkers. Nurses think so differently from each other that they cannot even get together to present a united front to legislators. Nurses give legislators conflicting messages because they cannot agree on a unified message.

# Exercise 7

**Purpose:** *Explore stereotypes*

## DIRECTIONS

1. Separate into pairs. Choose a person who is dissimilar from you. Discuss your mental picture of the following:

   a. A homeless person

   b. A person on welfare

   c. An elderly person living alone

   d. A feminist

   e. A person who is a member of the dominant ethnic group in your community

   What comes to mind when you think of each person listed above? How are your ideas alike? Dissimilar? How comfortable are you discussing your thoughts with someone dissimilar from you? Are there some thoughts you would rather not share? Why?

2. Identify examples that are contrary to the descriptions you shared above or exceptions to your stereotypes. What is your reaction to your partner's examples?

## Exercise 8

**Purpose:** *Distinguish among Paul's types of critical thinking*

### DIRECTIONS

Divide into small groups. Discuss Paul's concepts of critical thinking, uncritical thinking, sophistic critical thinking, and fair-minded critical thinking. State in your own words the central definition of each. How are they different? Alike?

## Exercise 9

**Purpose:** *Reflect on your own thinking and learning style*

### DIRECTIONS

Write about the following in your journal:

1. What were the most significant factors in your upbringing that influenced your learning?
2. How do you learn? What do you do that facilitates your learning?
3. Where would you place your thinking in Perry's model?
4. What do you do best?

## Exercise 10

**Purpose:** *Integrate the rational and creative self*

### DIRECTIONS

After reading this chapter, draw a picture of something that occurred to you.

## REFERENCES

Allen, D., Benner, P., and Diekelmann, N.L. (1986). Three paradigms for nursing research: Methodological implications. In P.L. Chinn (Ed.), *Nursing research methodology: Issues and implementation* (pp. 23-38). Rockville, Md.: Aspen.

Andrews, M.M. (1992). Cultural perspectives on nursing in the 21st century. *Journal of Professional Nursing, 8*(1), 7-15.

Baker, D.P., and Jones, D.P. (1993). Creating gender equality: Cross national gender stratification and mathematical performance. *Sociology of Education 66*(4), 91-103.

Ball, B., and Benner, P. (1989). When the cure is care (simplifying care): Dialogues with excellence. *American Journal of Nursing, 89*(11), 1466-1467.

Barnard, C.I. (1968). *The functions of the executive.* Cambridge, Mass.: Harvard University.

Benner, P. (1984). *From novice to expert.* Menlo Park, Calif.: Addison-Wesley.

Benner, P., and Tanner, C. (1987). Clinical judgement: How expert nurses use intuition. *American Journal of Nursing, 87*(1), 23-31.

Bevis, E.O. (1993, August). Learning to think critically is not a spectator sport. Paper presented at the

Fourth Annual Rocky Mountain Nurse Educators Conference, Copper Mountain Resort, Colo.

Boden, M.A. (1991). *The creative mind*. New York: Basic Books.

Chinn, P.L. (1989). Nursing patterns of knowing and feminist thought. *Nursing & Health Care, 10*(2), 71-75.

Claxton, C.S., and Murrell, P.H. (1987). *Learning styles: Implications for improving educational practices* (ASHE-ERIC Higher Education Report No. 4). Washington, D.C.: Association for the Study of Higher Education.

Correnti, D. (1993). Intuition and nursing practice implications for nurse educators: A review of the literature. *Journal of Advanced Nursing, 18*(3), 91-94.

deBono, E. (1970). *Lateral thinking*. New York: Harper and Row.

Dossey, B.M., Keegan, L., Guzzetta, C.E., and Kilkmeier, L.G. (1988). *Holistic nursing: A handbook for practice*. Rockville, Md.: Aspen.

English, I. (1993). Intuition as a function of the expert nurse: Critiques of Benner's novice to expert model. *Journal of Advanced Nursing, 18*(3), 387-393.

Gardner, H. (1983). *Frames of mind*. New York: Basic Books.

Gardner, H., and Hatch, T. (1990, March). *Multiple intelligences go to school: Educational implications of the theory of multiple intelligences* (Technical Report No. 4), New York: Center for Technology in Education.

Garity, J. (1985). Learning styles basis for creative teaching and learning. *Nurse Educator, 10*(2), 12-16.

Ghiselin, B. (1952). *The creative process*. Berkeley, Calif.: University of California Press.

Giger, J.N., and Davidhizar, R.E. (1995). *Transcultural nursing: Assessment and intervention*. St Louis: Mosby

Gruber, M., and Benner, P. (1989). The power of certainty: A dialogue with excellence. *American Journal of Nursing, 89*(4), 502-503.

Holloway, M. (1993). A lab of her own. *Scientific American, 269*(5), 94-103.

Kolb, D. (1981). Learning styles and disciplinary differences. In Chickerinq, et al. (Eds.), *The modern American college*. San Francisco: Jossey-Bass.

Kotliarenco, N.A. (1990). Mother-child interaction: Impact on children's intellectual competence. *Early Child Development and Care, 58,* 57-70.

Leininger, M. (Ed.). (1984 ). *Care: The essence of nursing and health*. Detroit: Wayne State University Press.

Leners, D.W. (1992). Intuition in nursing practice. *Journal of Holistic Nursing, 10*(2), 137-153.

Marchione, J., and Stearns, S.J. (1990). Ethnic power perspectives for nursing. *Nursing & Health Care, 11*(6), 296-301.

McNall, M.C., and Benner, P. (1989). Healing we cannot explain. *American Journal of Nursing, 89*(9), 1162-1163.

McWilliams, M. (1993). *Nutrition for the growing years* (5th ed.). New York: John Wiley.

Miller, V.G., and Rew, L. (1989). Analysis and intuition: The need for both in nursing education. *Journal of Nursing Education, 28*(2), 84-86.

Neufeldt, V. (1991). *Webster's new world dictionary* (3rd ed.). New York: Webster's New World.

Parks, P.L., and Smeriglio, V.L. (1986). Relationships among parenting knowledge, quality of stimulation in the home and infant development. *Family Relations, 35*(3), 411-416.

Paul, R. (1990). *Critical thinking: What every person needs to survive in a rapidly changing world*. Rohnert Park, Calif.: Sonoma State University.

Perry, W. (1981). Cognitive and ethical growth: The making of meaning. In A. Chickering, *The modern American college*. San Francisco: Jossey-Bass.

Pipes, P.L., and Trahams, C.M. (1993). *Nutrition in infancy* (5th ed.). St Louis: Mosby.

Poon, L.W., Fozard, J.L., Cermack, L.S., Arenberg, D., and Thompson, L.W. (Eds.). (1980). New directions in memory and aging. *Proceedings of the George A. Talland Memorial Conference*. Hillsdale, N.J.: Lawrence Erlbaum Associates.

Raichle, M.E. (1994). Visualizing the mind. *Scientific American, 270*(4), 58-64.

Schon, D.A. (1987). *Educating the reflective practitioner*. San Francisco: Jossey-Bass.

———. (1983). *The reflective practitioner: How professionals think in action*. New York: Basic Books.

Stewart, P.B., and Benner, P. (1989). A moment of truth: Dialogues with excellence. *American Journal of Nursing, 89*(11), 1467-1468.

Tannen, D. (1990). *You just don't understand: Women and men in conversation*. New York: William Morrow.

Witkin, H.A., and Goodenough, D.R. (1981). *Cognitive styles: Essence and origins*. New York: International Universities Press.

———. (1977). Field dependence and interpersonal behavior. *Psychological Bulletin, 84*(4), 661-689.

Witkin, H.A., Moore, C.A., Goodenough, D.R., and Cox, P.W. (1977). Field-dependent and field-independent cognitive styles and their educational implications. *Review of Educational Research, 47*(1), 1-64.

Wolfer, J. (1993). Aspects of "reality" and ways of knowing in nursing: In search of an integrating paradigm. *IMAGE: Journal of Nursing Scholarship, 25*(2), 141-146.

# Examining Frame of Reference, Attitudes, and Assumptions

Chapter 3

## OVERVIEW

Chapter 3 focuses on frame of reference, attitudes, and assumptions as they relate to critical thinking. Frame of reference, attitudes, and assumptions are unique characteristics that individuals bring to interactions. These characteristics affect what is said, how it is said, what is heard, how it is interpreted, and how each participant evaluates the interaction.

Frame of reference is the lens through which the world is viewed. It is the unique sum total of each person's lived experiences. Attitudes are personal dispositions, which are fundamental to the development of critical thinking skills. Both frame of reference and attitudes contribute to the formation of assumptions, which are unquestioned givens that we take for granted and about which we are frequently unaware. A close examination of these human qualities helps us understand the interactions the nurse may have with clients, families, colleagues, and administrators and helps us to assess the effectiveness of interactions.

## FRAME OF REFERENCE

Frame of reference is the unique patterning of perceptions and attitudes by which people view themselves and the world and evaluate events (Rathus, 1990). It is the lens through which each person filters reality and creates a point of view of the world. Frame of reference is developed based on a person's lived experiences and a distinctive blend of biologic, psychologic, sociologic, cultural, and spiritual factors shaped over time. Frame of reference is dynamic and changes with new learning.

Each person's frame of reference is unique. Similar life experiences may result in agreement on certain issues or aspects of living, but the totality of each person's view of the world is different. Each person has experienced, reacted, interpreted, and evaluated life in a way that no one else has, even siblings raised in the same family.

Frame of reference is a phrase that has been used in psychotherapy for many years (Elder, 1978). Reframing, a psychotherapeutic strategy, encourages the client to go through a traumatic experience from a different viewpoint to experience some healing. Reparenting is another technique in which the client recalls needs from his or her childhood that were responded to inappropriately, perhaps with violence, neglect, or distraction. In therapy, the client addresses those needs from the vantage point of an adult with a different frame of reference who has acquired many more coping resources.

Students commonly experience changing frames of reference because they are exposed to other points of view. One of the tasks of educators is to offer students alternative frames of reference through which to view a particular set of facts. For example, a beginning nursing student who lived in one community all of his life gained new knowledge about people from cultures that were different from his own through his educational coursework and clinical experiences. These experiences were entirely new to him. Some of what he learned conflicted with what he thought people from other cultures would be like. As a result of exposure to another culture, the nursing student changed his frame of reference.

## Perception

Perception is the process of actively selecting, organizing, and interpreting what is experienced by the senses (i.e., sight, hearing, smell, touch, and taste). The senses allow us to become aware of the world outside ourselves. Using our senses and active, purposeful, and organized thinking brings about an understanding of our lived experiences. Thinking is the process by which we make sense of information, work toward our goals, solve problems, and understand other people (Chaffee, 1994).

Perception is an active, creative process that involves three activities: (1) selecting sensations, (2) organizing them into a design or pattern, and (3) interpreting the information. Data are taken in through the senses, coded into the language of the nervous system, and then organized into a meaningful design or pattern. We then interpret these designs or patterns and give them meaning derived from our unique personal experiences (Chaffee, 1994; Smith, 1993).

Selecting perceptions means that we accept certain data and filter out other information based on our personal experience, needs, and interests. For example, when you are hungry you are more aware of the sensory data derived from your sense of smell as you take in the aromas from a nearby restaurant. Mothers with small babies are more attentive to auditory sensory data and selectively listen for their baby's cries amidst general environmental noises. Experienced nursing students make the distinction between a firm and cystic breast mass by attending to sensory data derived from touch.

Organizing perceptions means that the sensory data taken in forms a meaningful design or pattern. The brain is more than a repository for random meaningless bits of sensory information such as patches of color, isolated sounds and aromas, different textures, and haphazard tastes. The brain instantly organizes these data so that we perceive a unified and meaningful whole. We see colorful flowers and trees, hear the sounds of music, smell aromas, and enjoy the taste of our favorite foods (Chaffee, 1994).

Interpreting perceptions means that we assign meaning to the sensory data organized in the brain. The data becomes something we recognize such as a person, a thermometer, or a color. It also may be clusters of data that indicate a health problem. For an example of the perception process, consider the situation in which the night nurse reported that a client who had surgery the previous evening was increasingly restless. While making her rounds, the day nurse closely examined the client, noting a large amount of bright red blood. She changed his dressing, examined the incision, and took his vital signs. She concluded that his bleeding was excessive and he was showing signs of early shock. Based on her assessment, she promptly notified the physician. In this example, the day nurse *selectively attended* to the night nurses' report about the client. As she examined him, she used her senses to observe him and hear how he felt. Her brain *organized* this information into a recognizable pattern of bleeding and abnormal vital signs. She then *interpreted* this information to mean that the client was hemorrhaging and in the early stages of shock.

Perceptions are very individual and may differ quite radically, even when two or more people view the same event. Perception is different from reality. With perception, the mind takes in more than just the physical characteristics of the stimuli. Perceptions are influenced by our expectations, emotions, and needs (Smith, 1993). For example, often health care providers write "the patient looks older (or younger) than his stated age" on a client's chart. What does this tell you about the client's appearance? Does the age of the observer make a difference in this instance? Will a 25-year-old observer judge a client's appearance differently than a 50-year-old observer?

Ideal body weight is another example of how perceptions are individual. Young women with eating problems typically perceive themselves as overweight, although other observers would say they are thin or even emaciated (Williamson, Kelley, Davis, Ruggiero, and Blouin, 1985). Their actual weight can be determined objectively by using weighing scales and making a comparison to a standard weight-to-height chart. However, this factual information may have little to do with how a young woman sees herself. Individual perception of ideal body weight is influenced by early messages about weight from family and friends, advertisements, movies, television, and magazines.

## Context of Perceptions

Context, or the overall situation in which something occurs, influences how we interpret our perceptions (Chaffee, 1994). For example, when a client reports that his skin is itching, does it make a difference to know he just received an injection of penicillin or to know he has chronic eczema? When a client reports shortness of breath, does it make a difference to know she is 25 and just walked 2 miles on a treadmill or to know she is 60 and in the critical care unit with a diagnosis of pulmonary edema? An experienced nurse psychotherapist felt secure and confident dealing with clients in crisis in her usual setting, a neighborhood mental health clinic. When she substituted for her colleagues in the city-operated hospital emergency room, she felt all thumbs!

Consider the situation of Mae. As a young woman in her twenties, she often misplaced things such as her car keys. At 80 years old, Mae is a very active, vivacious woman who still misplaces things but now she quietly worries that she may be developing Alzheimer's disease. Her children are also more aware of her habit of misplacing things than they were in their formative years.

## Assess Client, Family, Institution, and Societal Contexts

One of the critical thinking skills expected of nurses is to assess the client, family, institutional, and societal contexts. Doing so assists the nurse to gain a better understanding of the interacting other and to select effective nursing interventions. Exercise 3 at the end of this chapter is designed to guide you in assessing how a client perceives his or her world. Each client develops perceptions based on lived experiences, family interactions, community characteristics in which he or she lived and now lives, and the social institutions with which he or she is now associated (as appropriate) such as employment, education, and social groups. As a nurse you will learn to sort through the information and distinguish that which has a significant bearing on the client's present situation and to which you must attend.

For an example of assessing a client's needs, consider Mr. Grady, a 50-year-old client who was hospitalized every fall for several years because of asthma, a condition that was under control the remainder of the year. He lived in a small community, and the nurses were aware of his life circumstances. He was employed at a large electronic manufacturing firm, and the firm's busiest season was during the fall months. He also was primarily responsible for maintaining a home life for his three teenage children. His wife had a chronic illness and was confined to bedrest much of the day. Knowing Mr. Grady's circumstances, the nurses did not limit their nursing care to the treatment of Mr. Grady's asthma. The nurses focused on the underlying depression he was experiencing due to the multiple problems in his life. They assessed his present coping status, how he was solving problems, and how he was dealing with his children. Then, working with Mr. Grady's perceived needs, they taught him new coping and parenting strategies appropriate to the stress he was having. By assessing this client's context, the nurses were able to intervene and alter his frame of reference by teaching him new coping and parenting strategies.

## Imperfections of Perception

Perceptions are often incomplete, inaccurate, and subjective and may be a source of bias and distortion. Bias is a mental leaning or partiality, and distortion means a twisting, or a misrepresentation or misstatement. Perceptions are influenced by a multitude of factors. To avoid distortion, you can externalize your perceptions by asking questions about what you perceive and compare your observations with those of others. When you do this, you allow yourself to move outside of your own frame of reference and accept the thinking of others. Through open dialogue you can learn if you missed something that someone else picked up or interpreted an event in a different way than you did. Open dialogue helps you clarify and validate your own perceptions (Chaffee, 1994). By comparing and contrasting your observations, you learn to see things from different perspectives or from different frames of reference.

Being aware of your frame of reference and how it shapes your thinking and subsequent behavior is important. Being aware that you view the world through subjective lenses and entering into dialogue with others about your perceptions may help you to clarify your perceptions and understand the unique way in which you and others view the world.

## ATTITUDES

Attitudes are manifested in a manner of acting, feeling, or thinking that shows a person's disposition, opinion, or mental set (Neufeldt, 1991). The ABC model of attitudes is widely accepted by social psychologists. *A* refers to affect (emotions and feelings), *B* to behavior (predispositions to act), and *C* to cognitions (beliefs and ideas). Attitudes are beliefs or opinions that have a positive or negative evaluation of something (an object, person or event) and that predispose us to act in a certain way. For example, based on their personal beliefs, people have positive or negative attitudes toward people who are different from themselves. The difference could be attributed to ethnicity, race, group membership, religion, or politics and causes them to behave in a given way (Plotnik, 1993; Rathus, 1990).

Attitudes serve several functions, two of which are a utilitarian function and a value-expressive function (Plotnik, 1993). As a utilitarian function, attitudes serve as guidelines for interpreting and categorizing objects and events and deciding whether to approach or avoid them. For example, if you have a positive attitude toward the elderly, you are likely to see their individuality and plan their care accordingly. If you are afraid of young men who appear to be gang members, you will try to avoid them. As a value-expressive function, attitudes help us define and stand up for beliefs and values that we consider central to ourselves. For example, if you value reason and clear thinking, you are less likely to get into a shouting match when discussing a problematic issue with others.

### Attitudes and Critical Thinking

Attitudes and dispositions are important aspects of being a critical thinker. Being reflective, open-minded, curious, persevering, precise, and tolerant of ambiguity; maintaining an internal locus of control; and having high self-esteem are commonly cited attitudes and dispositions that accompany good thinking (Baron, 1987). Paul (1990) refers to attitudes and dispositions as traits of mind, such as intellectual humility, intellectual courage, intellectual perseverance, intellectual integrity, and confidence in reason.

Ennis (1991, 1987) created a list of essential critical thinking dispositions (see Ennis' Critical Thinking Dispositions box on p. 69). He based it on his definition of critical thinking as reasonable reflective thinking that is focused on deciding what to believe or do.

### Critical Thinking Attitudes Applied to Nursing

The Critical Thinking Attitudes Applied to Nursing box on p. 69 lists important critical thinking attitudes for nurses. The attitudes support the Critical Thinking

## Ennis' Critical Thinking Dispositions*

1. Seek a clear statement of the thesis or question
2. Seek reasons
3. Try to be well informed
4. Use and mention credible sources
5. Take into account the total situation
6. Try to remain relevant to the main point
7. Keep in mind the original and/or basic concern
8. Look for alternatives
9. Be open-minded
    a. Consider seriously others' points of view than one's own (dialogical thinking)
    b. Reason from premises with which one disagrees without letting the disagreement interfere with one's reasoning (suppositional thinking)
    c. Withhold judgment when the evidence and reasons are insufficient
10. Take a position (and change a position) when the evidence and reasons are sufficient to do so
11. Seek as much precision as the subject permits
12. Deal in an orderly manner with the parts of a complex whole
13. Use one's critical thinking abilities
14. Be sensitive to the feelings, level of knowledge, and degree of sophistication of others

*From Baron and Sternberg: Teaching thinking skills: Theory and practice, New York, 1987, W. H. Freeman and Co.

## Critical Thinking Attitudes Applied to Nursing

▼ Confidence in multiple ways of knowing
▼ Intellectual honesty
▼ Openness to other points of view
▼ Willingness to take a position and defend it
▼ Willingness to change one's opinion based on evidence

Interaction Model and are essential for the nurse when working with clients and families, colleagues, and administrators. The attitudes are interrelated and interdependent.

***Confidence in Multiple Ways of Knowing.***   The first attitude, confidence in multiple ways of knowing, is supported by emerging theories that value the intuitive and the rational modes of thought. This attitude recognizes the multiple ways of knowing that the nurse and the interacting other (clients, families, colleagues, and administrators) may have as legitimate. The nurse with this attitude listens to others, attempts to understand them, and takes their concerns seriously.

***Intellectual Honesty.*** Intellectual honesty means to represent reality (events and people) as truthfully and objectively as possible, or to be fair, straightforward, and free from deceit. Intellectual honesty underlies all of the other attitudes. To be intellectually honest means that you challenge yourself to see things fairly, regardless of whether or not you agree. It may mean that you entertain multiple points of view. It may mean to acknowledge those moments when you cannot find a theory to fit your observations—when what you see does not fit within the framework of what you were taught. As a critical thinker you will act on the evidence that you see and your own experience regardless of whether or not you can explain it in a rational sense.

***Openness to Other Points of View.*** Openness to other points of view is an attitude that connotes a willingness to examine the thinking of others. A nurse is not required to embrace all points of view, but only be willing to listen and attempt to understand them. In so doing, the nurse acknowledges her or his own egocentricism and ethnocentricism and how they affect his or her perception and attitudes.

This attitude recognizes the limitations of one's frame of reference and indicates an openness to other points of view. It is a personal acknowledgement that one's own way of thinking is not the only or even the best possible way to think.

***Willingness to Take a Position and Defend It.*** Underlying willingness to take a position and defend it is courage, the courage to defend your convictions as important. As a critical thinker, the nurse must be willing to deal with important issues and believe that she or he has something important to contribute as an individual and collectively as a member of the profession. To be an effective health care provider, a nurse will demonstrate this attitude by his or her willingness to take a position and defend it when necessary.

***Willingness to Change One's Own Opinion Based on Evidence.*** Willingness to change one's own opinion based on evidence assumes intellectual honesty on the part of the nurse and connotes flexibility of thought. This attitude assumes that opinions are somewhat fluid. It does not mean that the nurse is persuaded by any case that appears strong and is eloquently presented if that case does not stand up under close scrutiny. It does not mean an openness to anything that sounds "good." It does mean that, when provided with sufficiently persuasive and compelling evidence, the nurse is willing to change his or her opinion.

## ASSUMPTIONS

An assumption is something we take for granted, or something we believe to be a fact but which may or may not be true (Neufeldt, 1991). "Assumptions are the seemingly self-evident rules about reality that we use to help us seek explanations, make judgments, or decide on various actions. They are the unquestioned givens that, to us, have the status of self-evident truths" (Brookfield, 1991, p. 44). When assumptions have become fully internalized, we perceive them to be common sense.

Assumptions are unstated yet, if known, they would help to clarify why we believe or act as we do. Assumptions influence our beliefs and subsequently direct our behavior; however, we seldom recognize them.

We make assumptions about virtually every aspect of life. Our assumptions affect our relationships with clients, families, colleagues, and administrators. Assumptions may be related to ethnic and socioeconomic background, educational preparation, or perceived social status. For example, we often make assumptions about the needs of physically disabled clients, mentally ill clients, and wealthy clients.

Assumptions are difficult to recognize in our daily interactions; however, they are essential to daily living. Some assumptions serve us well, while others may interfere with our ability to function effectively. For example, when you get up in the morning, you assume that the sun will come up, that there will be hot running water for hygiene, and that you will make it safely to your destination. As you arrive for class, you assume that it will meet in the usual location, that the instructor will be present, and that the topic to be discussed matches that assigned. In the clinical area you may assume the best way to take care of a client is the way you have always done it, that the client needs and appreciates your services, and that your instructor, nurse manager, and physician know what is best for the client.

We perceive our assumptions as fully justified and use them as a framework within which to operate. In fact, they are essential. You would be exhausted if you had to concern yourself with many of these assumptions on a daily basis. However, not all assumptions are completely justified. How many times have you been in the uncomfortable position of operating on an assumption only to find out that it was incorrect? Perhaps you erroneously assumed there would not be a quiz in class because the instructor had just given one in the previous class. Or perhaps your instructor, nurse manager, and physician assumed they knew what intervention was best for the client only to find the client rejecting it and seeking another treatment. Or perhaps you ordered orange juice for a client's breakfast because it is your preferred breakfast drink and you erroneously assumed it would also be the client's choice. Or perhaps you observed a change in your client's condition and incorrectly assumed that your instructor and nurse manager were also aware of it. Or perhaps you assumed your female client desired privacy during a medical procedure only to learn that in her culture, the husband never leaves his wife unattended during any procedure.

Experience tempers our assumptions. We make different assumptions at various stages in our lives based on our accumulation of knowledge and experience. For example, some beginning nursing students assume that biologic factors such as bacteria and viruses, fat accumulation in blood vessels, and uncontrolled cell division (tumors) are the primary basis for illness. With more information and experience, these nurses will learn that many illnesses have strong psychological, social, and environmental components, and they will revise their assumptions accordingly.

The Critical Thinking Skills Applied to Nursing: Assumptions box on p. 72 lists the critical thinking skills we associate with assumptions. The first critical thinking skill (assess client, family, institutional, and societal contexts) was discussed in a previous section.

**Critical Thinking Skills Applied to Nursing: Assumptions**

▼ Assess client, family, institutional, and societal contexts
▼ Analyze value, descriptive, definitional, and contextual assumptions
▼ Assess frame of reference, attitudes, and assumptions
▼ Recognize one's own frame of reference, attitudes, and assumptions

## Analyze Value, Descriptive, Definitional, and Contextual Assumptions

Assessing the value, descriptive, definitional, and contextual assumptions of both the nurse and the interacting other is an important critical thinking skill when solving problems or discussing issues of significance. By doing so, the nurse and the interacting other can establish a common frame of reference for their discussion.

***Value and Descriptive Assumptions.*** Our values affect how we see the world and the assumptions we make about it. Browne and Keeley (1994) identify two types of assumptions, value and descriptive. Value assumptions are prescriptive; they are beliefs about how the world *should* be. Descriptive assumptions are beliefs about the way the world *was, is,* or *will* be.

Values are "ideas that someone thinks are worthwhile" (Browne and Keeley, 1994 p. 49). Value assumptions are beliefs about which values are important. The more value we assign to an idea, the more influence it has on our choices and behavior. For example, if you place a high value on human life, you are likely to oppose war, capital punishment, and mercy killing as solutions to human problems. If you value quality of life, you are likely to attend to a client's circumstances, support systems, and lived experiences.

Values are also standards of conduct that we endorse and expect others to meet (Browne and Keeley, 1994). For example, nurses place a high value on caring, truthfulness, responsibility, and accountability. They expect ethical behavior from their colleagues and assume that the motivation for all nursing acts is the desire to do good for others. Since many nurses hold these values in common, it is not so much the value itself but the intensity with which nurses hold this value and the priority to which they assign it that is important. It is here that nurses may experience value conflicts with their colleagues. For an example of a nursing value conflict, consider the client who had surgery and radiation treatments for primary liver cancer a year earlier and was readmitted with widespread metastasis in the peritoneum, the serous membrane lining the abdominopelvic walls and covering the viscera. The physicians discussed the client's prognosis (5 to 6 months at best) and the current treatment options (surgery and chemotherapy). The client requested aggressive treatment, and his wife was reluctantly supportive. She was aware of the difficult time he had earlier and the reality of his current prognosis. The nurses were divided on whether the client should undergo further treatment. Some of the nurses wondered if the pain and stress of surgery and subsequent chemotherapy were worth it and would detract significantly from the quality of the client's remaining life. Other nurses believed the client should take every treatment option in the hope that it would prolong his life until a cure could be found. In this situation, all the nurses valued caring, supporting life, and doing good for others; however, they were in conflict over what constituted reasonable treatment efforts given the context and circumstances surrounding this client.

When we associate with people whose values are like our own, we gain support and reinforce each other. When our values are in conflict with others, we may experience confusion and misunderstandings. At these times we should examine our assumptions and ask about the assumptions of the interacting other. By examining our assumptions, we develop a better understanding of other points of view and a greater appreciation for those with whom we interact.

***Definitional Assumptions.***   Language and assumptions are related. Your understanding of an issue or your reasoning about it may be based on an unstated definition of a key term that you assume others share. Browne and Keeley (1986) call this a definitional assumption. For example, two students were engaged in a lively discussion about the effectiveness of psychotherapy before they realized that they defined psychotherapy differently. Each assumed the other defined it the same. One person defined psychotherapy as deliberate, intelligent and careful listening, and well-timed confrontation. The other person assumed it meant doing nothing for or with the client, expecting that the client would identify his or her own problem, discover its meaning, and find a way to resolve it. Notice that both students assumed that psychotherapy is defined in terms of therapist's behaviors.

Another way of looking at psychotherapy is from the reference point of the client. One client defined psychotherapy as lying on a couch and free associating several times a week for several years while another believed it to be intensive Gestalt work with self-disclosure in a group for a year. Yet another client defined it as a weekend marathon designed to produce a dramatic personal shift. Before any meaningful discussion can occur, the students should compare their definitions of the word psychotherapy.

Making definitional assumptions is very common. Consider the following statements:

▼ Should the medically indigent receive full health care benefits?
▼ Are the numbers of physically disabled individuals increasing?
▼ Do ethnically diverse clients receive adequate health care?
▼ Do most elderly require nursing home care?

What key words in each statement need to be defined before you engage in further discussion? To whom does the "medically indigent" refer? How would you define "full health care benefits?" Continue this line of questioning as you think about the other statements. A critical thinker identifies key terms, questions their meanings, and does not base a discussion on an assumed definition.

***Contextual Assumptions.*** Assumptions are related to context. In the Critical Thinking Interaction Model, context refers to the client, family, institutional, and societal environment, or the total situation surrounding a particular person or event. Contextual assumptions are assumptions that we make about the environment or surrounding situation. For example, we may assume that a client is supported by a loving family but learn later that he is divorced and living alone. We may assume a family has sufficient food, clothing, and shelter to meet their needs and later learn the breadwinner is no longer employed, leaving the family temporarily dependent on the generosity of friends and neighbors.

A common assumption nurses make is that mistakes are always bad, costly, and to be avoided if possible. This assumption is justified in the context of working with sick clients, but how appropriate is it in other contexts, such as in managing a nursing unit or solving unit problems? In the latter instances, an appropriate strategy would be to try out different approaches before settling on one that is right for the particular unit and its unique circumstances. Successfully managing a nursing unit depends on a number of variables such as the leader's preferred leadership style, the experience and educational background of the staff, and the nature of the situation. What works well in one situation may not work in others. To determine what works best, nurses need a willingness to experiment, to engage in trial and error, and to risk new behaviors, especially during periods of transition when the future is unclear and parts of the health care system are changing (Miller and Malcolm, 1990).

## Common Assumptions

Assumptions form around individual rights and obligations, duties, appropriate behaviors, beliefs, norms, values, myths, hierarchies, and expectations (Brookfield, 1991). The boxes on pp. 75 and 76 list some common assumptions nurses make in relationship to clients, colleagues, and administrators. The box on p. 77 contains some assumptions nurses commonly make about themselves. Review these assumptions and discuss them. How alike and how different are they from your own assumptions? How similar and dissimilar are they to your colleagues' assumptions? If you are unsure, ask them. In your opinion, are some of the assumptions well-founded? In error?

## Challenging Assumptions

Identifying and challenging our assumptions are both central to understanding our thinking and learning to think critically (Brookfield, 1991). To be a critical thinker you must be willing to set aside some previously unquestioned assumptions and to absorb the meaning of a new experience. This requires reflection and analysis.

When you experience cognitive dissonance, or the unpleasant psychological tension that results when you notice an inconsistency between what you thought was true and what you actually find is true based on your experience, then question your assumptions. When you question your assumptions, you begin to form new theories and explanations that are consistent with your actual experience. Through reflection

**Common Assumptions Nurses Make about Clients and Families**

**NURSES**

- ▼ know what is best for clients
- ▼ are obligated to care for clients in a sensitive and competent manner
- ▼ are responsible for maintaining smooth interpersonal relationships with clients and their families

**CLIENTS**

- ▼ have the right to quality care
- ▼ are obligated to comply with nurses' requests
- ▼ should be told the truth about their diagnosis and prognosis
- ▼ have the right to know their treatment options
- ▼ have the right to ask questions and to make informed decisions
- ▼ should behave like "patients"
- ▼ tell the truth about health matters affecting them
- ▼ value healthful behaviors as much as nurses do
- ▼ will comply with the nurses' health teaching
- ▼ do things in their best interest to maintain their health
- ▼ understand how their body works
- ▼ understand technical health care jargon
- ▼ want to get well
- ▼ will stop doing things not in their best interest

**FAMILIES**

- ▼ are loving, supportive units
- ▼ are willing and able to help the client after discharge

and analysis you will find theories and explanations that work in particular situations, arrive at explanations as to why they work, and develop a readiness to change your ways of working based on changing circumstances (Brookfield, 1991).

As you become aware of your assumptions, you may question the validity of some of them. To challenge your assumptions is to bring into question the very foundation upon which you have built your frame of reference (your view of the world). Challenging your assumptions can be unsettling and anxiety provoking, and it also carries a certain degree of risk. When you have no meaningful explanation for your experiences, you may find yourself temporarily feeling ungrounded. You may feel that your very being is threatened. You may question what you believe to be true about the world in which you live. Like many people, you probably prefer answers to ambiguity (Brookfield, 1991). Challenging the assumptions of others is something that must be done with great care and respect.

### Common Assumptions Nurses Make about Colleagues

**COLLEAGUES**
- ▼ should notice when a nurse needs help and offer it
- ▼ who look and talk alike have the same values
- ▼ who are ethnically diverse are alike and share the same values
- ▼ who are ethnically diverse hold the cultural values recorded in the literature
- ▼ value the same health behaviors to the same degree
- ▼ share the same definition of health
- ▼ put their client's needs above their own needs
- ▼ always report accurate data
- ▼ solve problems in a similar manner

### Common Assumptions Nurses Make about Administrators

**ADMINISTRATORS**
- ▼ have the best interests of nurses and clients at heart
- ▼ care more for profit than they do for nurses or clients
- ▼ are more concerned about public relations and their reputations in the community than with client care
- ▼ are helpful in a crisis
- ▼ are in control of the institution
- ▼ know what they are doing
- ▼ know how to manage a budget
- ▼ expect nurses to defer to them

## ASSESS FRAME OF REFERENCE, ATTITUDES, AND ASSUMPTIONS

How can you identify the frame of reference, attitudes, and assumptions under which you and others are operating? It is not always easy, but as with many aspects of critical thinking, it is worth the effort.

### Enter Another's Frame of Reference

When you care about another person, you try to understand what life is like from his or her perspective. Because each person has a unique frame of reference, you need to listen to what a person says and how he or she interprets the world. Try to enter

**Common Assumptions Nurses Make about Themselves**

**NURSES**

▼ do good and help others to the best of their abilities
▼ are the "good guys"
▼ should be able to work alone and not ask for help
▼ are responsible for everything that happens to the client
▼ should put others' needs before their own
▼ should "fix" what is "broken"
▼ who are capable of doing something must do it
▼ must meet everyone's needs
▼ must be prompt and clean
▼ must defer to physicians and administrators
▼ are responsible if something goes wrong
▼ choose nursing as a career for the same reasons
▼ solve nursing problems in a similar manner
▼ care more about the psychosocial aspects of clients than physicians do

sympathetically into his or her experience to capture a feeling of what life must be like for him or her. Try to listen with an open mind and heart.

By listening carefully, you are more likely to hear the subtle differences in how an illness or injury experience is affecting a client. Avoid making superficially reassuring statements such as "Everything will be alright," when that may not be the case. Instead, ask "What was that like for you?" or "How are you and your family adjusting to the illness?" or "Tell me more about what this means to you." Such statements are open-ended and invite the client to set the direction for the interaction.

## Discuss Discrepancies and Inconsistencies with Others

As you become aware of discrepancies and inconsistencies between what you assumed to be so and what your actual experience is, share these with your instructors, colleagues, and mentors. By discussing your perceptions and insights with others, you reduce any self-doubt that you might feel. Discussing your perception and insights will not immediately resolve the discrepancies and inconsistencies, but it will alleviate the feeling that you are alone and that no one else has ever made your observations or had your insights. When you share and discuss your observations with others, they can reflect back what they hear you say. When you realize that others have had similar observations and insights, you will be in a better position to reflect and analyze their meaning (Brookfield, 1991).

### Examine a Person's Background

Consider a person's background and how it may influence her or his thinking (Browne and Keeley, 1994). What frame of reference, attitudes, and assumptions might the person have based on that background? Consider such things as approximate age, ethnicity, gender, socioeconomic status, educational background, and professional experience. Ask yourself why a person would want to take this position. What vested interest would a person want to protect? Do the outcomes promoted by the person appear favorable to him or her? Try to think like a person with that background might think.

The purpose of this recommendation is not to encourage you to make unfounded assumptions about others but to analyze the thinking of others more fully. A great diversity of thought among members of a profession and among those in a given age group exists. A person's background does not give you the whole story about his or her motivation. Neither does it mean that a person's motivation is always self-serving.

### Recognize One's Own Frame of Reference, Attitudes, and Assumptions

As you become aware of the concepts of frame of reference, attitudes, and assumptions, you can consider them as you interact with clients, families, colleagues, and administrators. In developing this awareness you will also develop the ability to recognize the effect of these in shaping your own thinking. You can use the same strategies we previously discussed to develop an awareness of your own frame of reference, attitudes, and assumptions.

## EXPANDING YOUR THINKING

Some people think infrequently and at a superficial level. Some people think periodically when they are faced with new challenges that do not fit solutions they already know. Others develop a passion for thinking throughout their life and continuously strive to think better and deeper. Fig. 3-1 illustrates these levels of cognitive expansion.

Scientists can observe cognitive activity. Sophisticated technological advances such as electroencephalogram (EEG), x-ray computed tomography (CCT), positron emission tomography (PET), and magnetic resonance imaging (MRI) allow scientists to actually monitor the normal human brain in action. When this technology is combined with powerful computers, scientists can detect circumstances under which the brain "lights up" through the measurement of electrical activity, changes in blood flow, and accumulations of oxygen (Fischback, 1992). These techniques allow scientists to note that even the simplest mental task is accomplished by the action of networks of many communicating areas of the brain. When certain circuits are repeatedly stimulated, the brain changes the way it organizes itself to increase the functional efficiency of doing the task. This type of reorganization is evident within 15 minutes of practice (Raichle, 1994).

Some ways to achieve cognitive growth are to think about something important more often, think critically about more things more often, or think about something you never thought about before. Another way to achieve cognitive growth is to explore others' points of view by reading and listening. Reading the editorial page of

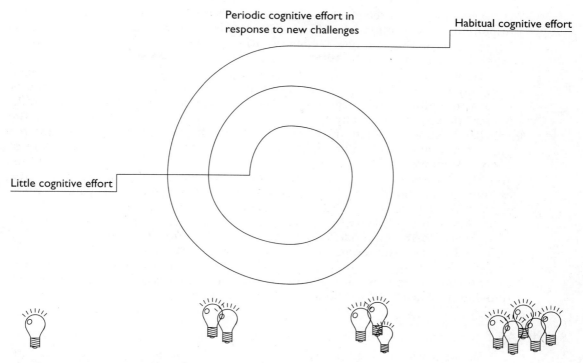

**Fig. 3-1**    Levels of cognitive expansion.

your local newspaper or publications such as *Forbes* and *Newsweek* is a way of exercising your brain regularly about current issues. You will be in touch with a larger community, not just nursing and health care. Reading professional publications such as the *American Nurse* and the *American Journal of Nursing* keeps you informed about current issues in nursing and health care. Attending inservice education meetings and workshops and conversing with respected colleagues also will provide opportunities for cognitive growth.

Sometimes you may simply need comic relief. Seek out a friend who is good at seeing the funny side, clowning, and making jokes. When you need to complain and moan, find a sympathetic ear or a friend who will commiserate with you. You need this kind of periodic catharsis. When you feel the need to solve a problem or feed your brain with more substance, seek out someone who listens to you, challenges your perceptions and assumptions, and is knowledgeable about your area of concern. As you develop professionally and become empowered, you will find yourself spending more time in the latter activity because you have confidence in your mental efforts. You will realize that you can put your thinking into action and have a positive impact on the situation. Fig. 3-1 illustrates this cognitive expansion.

Expanding yourself includes experimenting with new roles and ways of responding. Good role models are excellent sources of inspiration and provide an opportunity to visualize new behaviors. You can gain much from observing how others think and behave.

Thinking critically is emancipating and allows you to explore multiple points of view and ways of behaving. As a critical thinker you are not afraid to take a stand or make a commitment, although you maybe criticized. You are able to make commitments, but only after critically examining the available evidence. You are aware of the socializing influence of family, community, education, religion, media, race, and the profession itself. You are informed about issues and wrestle with the pros and cons of various positions. You are able to take a position and support it with good reasons. You think through the implications and consequences of your positions. You examine assumptions and reject stereotypes. You have confidence in your ability to reason. You analyze your positions thoroughly and own your commitments fully.

When you expand yourself, you encourage your clients and colleagues to expand themselves. When you model critical thinking and elicit it from others by the questions you ask and the rewards you provide, you receive thoughtful responses from others more often. By stimulating others to think critically along with you, you expand your vision of what is possible, generate better decisions, and create an environment in which critical thinking occurs more often.

## SUMMARY

Each participant in an interaction is a composite of many influences including biologic, psychologic, sociologic, cultural, and spiritual factors. This composite results in a unique frame of reference or point of view that directly affects all interactions with others. As you enter sympathetically into another person's frame of reference, you refine your ability to grasp and understand what life is like for that person. As you do so, you develop the ability to perceive more accurately, to reason more thoughtfully, and to understand more fully the thinking of others.

Attitudes are *attributes* of the thinker, not the thinking process itself. Attitudes may foster or hinder the development of our ability to think critically. Attitudes such as confidence in multiple ways of knowing, intellectual honesty, openness to other points of view, willingness to take a position and defend it, and willingness to change one's own opinion based on evidence are essential to developing the critical spirit.

Assumptions, those hidden, unquestioned givens that hold the status of self-evident truths, affect our interactions with others. They influence how we enter, structure, and engage in interactions with others. We make assumptions about values (i.e., what the world should be like), about the definition of words, and about what we believe the world was, is, or will be like.

When you reflect on your interactions and how they have been influenced by frame of reference, attitudes, and assumptions, you are engaged in critical thinking. As you learn to ask more questions, you discover new information and develop new insights. By analyzing your experiences and your thinking, you are able to consider new, more effective ways of thinking and behaving.

# EXERCISES

## Exercise 1

**Purpose:** *Explore other frames of reference*

### DIRECTIONS

1. Get in touch with your sibling(s) or childhood friend(s). Talk together until you can agree on an event that you all recall from your childhood. Separately, write about the event in as vivid detail as you can remember. Ferret out any assumptions you can detect that influenced your perceptions. Draw out the conclusions that you made and the decisions that flowed from your conclusion.

2. Discuss your accounts together. How alike (different) are your points of view? Were your assumptions the same? What conclusions and decisions were drawn by your sibling(s) or friend(s)?

## Exercise 2

**Purpose:** *Explore other frames of reference*

### DIRECTIONS

1. Compile a list of controversial issues that concern members of your class.

2. Select one issue about which you personally have strong feelings. On one sheet of paper, list the reasons why you believe as you do.

3. When you have finished writing, divide into small groups of individuals who are concerned about the same issue. Report the reasons why you believe as you do. Group members should analyze and evaluate the reasons.

4. After everyone has reported, write a cogent position in defense of a point of view opposite your own. Create the best, most logical, and most persuasive reasons you can.

5. When you have finished writing, return to your same group. Report on the new defense you have prepared. Group members should analyze and evaluate your reasons and how fairly you have represented another point of view.

## Exercise 3

**Purpose:** *Explore the frame of reference of a client, colleague, or administrator*

### DIRECTIONS

Interview a client (and the family if possible), colleague, or administrator whose race or ethnic background is different from your own. Use the following interview guide and add other questions as appropriate.

### Biologic assessment

1. How is your general health?
2. What are your personal health goals?
3. What activities do you engage in to stay healthy?
4. Have these activities made a difference in your health?
5. What was your childhood like?

### Psychologic assessment

1. How do you define good health?
2. How do you handle stress?
3. What do you do with your free time?
4. What relationships are important to you?
5. How do you maintain those relationships?

### Sociologic assessment

1. Describe your family and other social groups to which you belong. What importance do they have in your life?
2. What is your educational level? How do you feel about your education (formal and informal)?
3. What is your impression of this health care agency and its health care providers?
4. What are your beliefs about work? What role does employment have in your life?
5. How do you feel about democracy and capitalism in this country?

### Cultural assessment

1. Describe any health beliefs and practices in which you engage.
2. Describe your beliefs about health and the cause of illness.
3. What dietary practices are important to you, particularly as they affect your present health status?
4. Describe your family structure, its communication patterns, and how decisions are made.
5. Describe the meaning and importance of time in your life. Are you present or future oriented?

### Spiritual assessment

1. What is the meaning of life for you?
2. Do you believe in a higher being? If yes, describe your beliefs.

3. What nontangible realities do you believe in?

4. Describe the meaningful rights and wrongs to which you adhere.

5. What influence do sacred things or matters of religion have for you?

When you have completed your interview, write a paragraph summarizing the person's frame of reference in each assessment category (biologic, psychologic, sociologic, cultural, and spiritual).

Discuss the following questions: Did you assume you should ask all of the questions as given? Did you modify any of them to suit your interviewee? Report on changes you made in the interview questions to make them more intelligible to your interviewee. What questions did not fit? Why? What are your hunches about this?

Compare the person's frame of reference with your own. Take turns sharing your findings with your classmates. Discuss what this exercise taught you about the importance of seeing life from another point of view.

## Exercise 4

**Purpose:** *Explore different frames of reference*

### DIRECTIONS

Divide in groups of four (if more, change the directions in "1" accordingly).

1. *Person 1:* Tell a vignette that involves a nurse and at least 3 other people who are not nurses.

2. *Person 2:* Retell the vignette from the frame of reference of a member of the client's family.

3. *Person 3:* Retell the vignette from the frame of reference of a colleague.

4. *Person 4:* Retell the vignette from the frame of reference of an administrator.

## Exercise 5

**Purpose:** *Become more aware of the perceptions you receive through your senses*

### DIRECTIONS

Perform a physical assessment on a client. Use the four chief methods of physical examination: inspection, palpation, percussion, and auscultation. Organize your perceptions in a meaningful way and arrive at a conclusion about the health status of the client by interpreting your findings.

1. Discuss how you used your senses (sight, hearing, smell, and touch) to collect data. What visual observations did you make? What information about the different body systems did you obtain through palpation? percussion? auscultation?

2. Discuss your interpretation of the above information. What is the significance of your findings?

3. Compare your interpretation of the findings with those found in the client's chart and with those made by the unit nurses and your instructor. How closely aligned are the various interpretations?

# Exercise 6

**Purpose:** *Compare and contrast different perceptions of a single scene*

## DIRECTIONS

Examine the photograph in Fig. 3-2 then discuss the following:

1. Describe your perceptions and interpretation of the photograph. What is going on? What does it mean?

2. Compare and contrast your responses with those of your classmates.

3. How are your perceptions and interpretation affected by your descriptive assumptions (i.e, what you believe life was, is, or will be like)?

4. How are your perceptions and interpretation affected by your value assumptions (i.e., what you believe life should be like)?

# Exercise 7

**Purpose:** *Identify your disposition to think critically*

## DIRECTIONS

Take "The California Critical Thinking Dispositions Inventory" (CCTDI) developed by Facione and Facione (1992). Your instructor will need to obtain the Inventory for you. The CCTDI contains Likert-style questions on seven scales: truthseeking, open-mindedness, analyticity, systematicity, critical thinking self-confidence, inquisitiveness, and maturity. What did you learn about your dispositions to think critically based on this inventory? What dispositions would you like to change? What dispositions would you like to develop in greater depth?

# Exercise 8

**Purpose:** *Explore your assumptions about clients, colleagues, and administrators*

## DIRECTIONS

1. Review the assumptions in the boxes on pp. 75, 76, and 77. Form small groups and discuss how similar and dissimilar they are to yours. What assumptions would you add to or delete from the list?

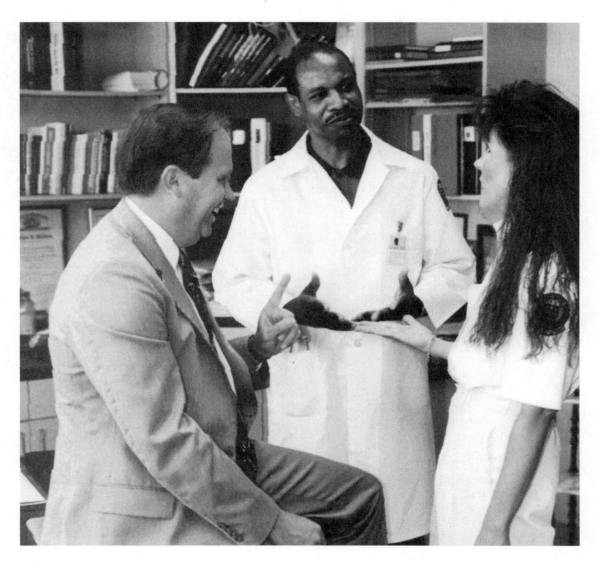

**Fig. 3-2** Photograph for Exercise 6.

From Wise Y: *Leading and managing in nursing,* St Louis, 1995, Mosby.

2. Create a list of your assumptions about nurses, clients, families, colleagues, and administrators. Consider the following areas around which assumptions form: individual rights and obligations, duties, appropriate behaviors, beliefs, norms, values, myths, hierarchies, and expectations.

3. Interview two individuals in each category (nurses, clients, families, colleagues, and administrators), one whom you believe to be like you and one whom you believe is different from you. Ask questions that will prompt them to reveal those aspects about themselves upon which you based your assumptions.

4. Rejoin your small groups and discuss your findings. Were your initial assumptions accurate? What did you learn about each person? Did this experience change your thinking? In what way?

## Exercise 9

**Purpose:** *Identify the values embodied in a written document*

### DIRECTIONS

Read the *American Nurses' Association Code for Nurses* found in your library. What values can you identify? Compare your list with your classmates. How are their lists similar or dissimilar from yours? Were the values you identified what you expected from the code? What new insights about nurses have you gained based on this exercise?

## Exercise 10

**Purpose:** *Examine the consequences of faulty assumptions*

### DIRECTIONS

Read the following incident:

Ivan and Brent had a great time decorating the getaway car for the wedding of Ivan's sister to her new husband. They painted "just married" in large letters on the back window, tied balloons to the radio antenna, and tied a trail of aluminum cans to the back car bumper. At the appropriate moment, the newlyweds got in the back seat of the car. With Ivan at the wheel and Brent videotaping the happy couple, the foursome sped away for the 2-hour drive to the airport where the couple would catch a flight to their honeymoon destination. As they drove along, few people in other cars noticed them.

During the return trip, however, Ivan and Brent had an entirely different experience. They generated a great deal of attention as many people in other cars looked at them. Some of the looks they received appeared hostile. Occasionally drivers would honk at them. At first Ivan and Brent were at a loss to explain the attention they were receiving. Suddenly it dawned on them that people in the other cars were assuming they were newlyweds in a homosexual union. As they drove along, the attention did not abate, and they decided to have some fun by playing the role of lovers. Brent slid closer to Ivan and put his arm around his shoulder. Occasionally they put their heads together in an affectionate pose. To them it was humorous, and they played up to the attention they were receiving.

Discuss the following questions:

1. What value, descriptive, and definitional assumptions were present?

2. How many observers do you think would have tried to validate their assumptions with Ivan and Brent had they the opportunity to do so?

3. Do you think Ivan and Brent jeopardized their safety in this situation?

# Exercise 11

**Purposes:** *Illustrate how assumptions affect the nurse-client interaction*
*Illuminate conflict between assumptions and reality*

## DIRECTIONS

Reflect on the experiences you have had with clients whose race or ethnicity is different from your own. Identify one experience you would call satisfying and one that you would call frustrating. For each experience, discuss the following:

1. Describe the circumstances (context) in which the experience occurred.

2. Who was involved in the situation? What role did each person play?

3. What occurred that caused you to feel the way you did?

4. What was your role in the situation? How did it contribute to your feelings?

5. What was it about this situation that brought about your feelings of satisfaction/ frustration.

6. What was the outcome or consequences of the situation?

7. After you have completed the assignment, reflect on the differences. Why, in your opinion, do you suspect one experience was more satisfying than the other? What does it mean to you?

# Exercise 12

**Purpose:** *Examine how well-intentioned information contributes to the creation of faulty assumptions*

## DIRECTIONS

1. Role-play the following situation:

Ms. France, age 65, is awaiting health education about complications surrounding her diabetes mellitus. Before you see the client, you talk with another nurse who knows the client from previous admissions. She tells you that the client is not very bright and is not interested in changing her health behavior. Ms. France is in the clinic awaiting you. Role-play your first encounter with her.

2. Now, assume that the nurse tells you that the client is brilliant, alert, and strongly motivated to change her behavior. Role-play your first encounter with the client.

## Exercise 13

**Purpose:** *Reflect on your assumptions over time*

### DIRECTIONS

Write in your journal about the assumptions you make before giving care to one of your assigned clients. Record your assumptions and then judge how accurate they were after you complete your care assignment. Continue this activity each week until the end of the quarter or semester. Review your journal at quarter or semester's end. What did you learn from this intensive focus on assumptions? Did your process of forming assumptions change? In what way? Did you learn to withhold judgment until you had further information? Did you become more tolerant of ambiguity?

## Exercise 14

**Purpose:** *Record your thoughts and insights*

### DIRECTIONS

Write in your journal about the following questions:

1. What are some of your assumptions about nurses, clients, families, colleagues, and administrators?
2. Put yourself in each of these roles. What assumptions do you think they make about nurses?
3. Where does making assumptions cross the line into making stereotypes?
4. Identify people whom you consider intelligent, thoughtful, reasonable, and articulate. What behaviors do they display that indicate to you that they are good thinkers?

## REFERENCES

Baron, J.B. (1987). Evaluating thinking skills in the classroom. In J.B. Baron and R.J. Sternberg (Eds.), *Teaching thinking skills: Theory and practice* (pp. 221-247). New York: W.H. Freeman.

Brookfield, S.D. (1991). *Developing critical thinkers*. San Francisco: Jossey-Bass.

Browne, M.N., and Keeley, S.M. (1994). *Asking the right questions* (4th ed.). Englewood Cliffs, N.J.: Prentice Hall.

————. (1986). *Asking the right questions* (2nd ed.). Englewood Cliffs, N.J.: Prentice Hall.

Chaffee, J. (1994). *Thinking critically* (4th ed.). Boston: Houghton Mifflin.

Elder, J. (1978). *Transactional analysis in health care*. Menlo Park, Calif.: Addison-Wesley.

Ennis, R.H. (1991). Critical thinking: A streamlined conception. *Teaching Philosophy, 14*(1), 5-24.

————. (1987). A taxonomy of critical thinking dispositions and abilities. In J.B. Baron and R.J. Sternberg (Eds.), *Teaching thinking skills: Theory and practice* (pp. 9-26). New York: W.H. Freeman.

Facione, P.A., and Facione, N.C. (1992). *The California Critical Thinking Dispositions Inventory (CCTDI); and the CCTDI test manual.* Millbrae, Calif.: California Academic Press. (217 La Cruz Ave., Millbrae, Calif. 94030).

Fischback, G.D. (1992). Mind and brain. *Scientific American, 167*(3), 110-117.

Miller, M.A., and Malcolm, N. (1990). Critical thinking in the nursing curriculum. *Nursing & Health Care, 11*(2), 66-73.

Neufeldt, V. (Ed.). (1991). *Webster's new world dictionary* (3rd ed.). New York: Webster's New World.

Paul, R. (1990). *Critical thinking: What every person needs to survive in a rapidly changing world.* Rhonert Park, Calif.: Sonoma State University.

Plotnik, R. (1993). *Introduction to psychology* (3rd ed.). Pacific Grove, Calif.: Brooks/Cole.

Raichle, M.E. (1994). Visualizing the mind. *Scientific American, 270*(4), 58-64.

Rathus, S.A. (1990). *Psychology* (4th ed.). Fort Worth, Tex.: Holt, Rinehart and Winston.

Smith, R.E. (1993). *Psychology.* St. Paul: West Publishing Company.

Williamson, D.A., Kelley, M.L., Davis, C.J., Ruggiero, L., and Blouin, D.S. (1985). Psychopathology of eating disorders: A controlled comparison of bulimic, obese, and normal subjects. *Journal of Consulting and Clinical Psychology, 53*(2), 161-166.

# Refining Thinking

## Chapter 4

## OVERVIEW

Chapter 4 focuses on factors that help to refine thinking. Making a distinction between a person and the idea that person presents and making a distinction between thinking by choice and thinking by habit are necessary to refine thinking. When we make these distinctions, we achieve a higher level of thinking that considers the multiple subtleties inherent in everyday interactions.

Ignorance is a very human quality. In this chapter, we discuss various kinds of ignorance such as beliefs, cultural biases, and lack of insight. We can appreciate the subtleties of these distinctions through reflection, which is the ability to recall and contemplate the meaning of an experience or event.

Reflection, the soul of critical thinking, serves as a rudder to our thoughts and consequently to our behavior. Through reflection we find meaning and purpose in life. To make critical distinctions, to reflect, and to have an awareness of our ignorance deepen our thinking.

This chapter concludes with a discussion on how language structures, defines, and externalizes our frame of reference. Clear language reflects clear thinking; vague language reflects vague thinking. When we refine our language and choose our words to express our thoughts accurately and clearly, we simultaneously clarify our thinking.

## IMPORTANT DISTINCTIONS

When working with clients, families, colleagues, and administrators, you need to make some important distinctions between people and their ideas, taste and judgment, fact and interpretation, and an idea's validity and the quality of its expression (Ruggiero, 1991). You must also make a distinction between truth and beliefs, stereotype and individuality, people's differing frames of reference, and thinking by habit and thinking by choice.

### Person and the Idea

Personal opinions of a speaker affect perceptions of an idea's credibility. How often have you noticed an idea being discredited because the person who expressed it was disliked? Have you ever noticed an idea being received more favorably because the person who expressed it was liked? Have you ever ignored an idea because you did not have confidence in or respect for the speaker?

Who would you expect to command the most credibility: a physician, a nurse, or a client with a long-term disability or illness? To expect the physician to be more informed on issues of medical diagnosis and treatment and the nurse to be the expert on issues of nursing diagnosis and care is reasonable. However, many clients with a long-term disability or illness are highly informed about their diagnosis and treatment. They may be better informed about current research and treatment methods than either the physician or the nurse. We are conditioned to believe that the physician and nurse are the experts; however, this is not always true.

Does an idea to improve hospital efficiency have more credibility when it is expressed by a hospital administrator than when it is expressed by a nurse's aide? When an idea has the weight of organizational authority, it takes on an added dimension of influence that it does not have when spoken by someone with less organizational authority.

We make a distinction between the person and the idea the person communicates. Learn to evaluate an idea on its own merits rather than the merits of the person who is expressing it. An unpleasant, disliked person can still make truthful statements and articulate valid reasoning.

Become aware of your feelings about others and how you react to their ideas and verbalizations. Learn to focus on the merits of the idea instead of the person. Remember that no one person has a corner on good ideas. Excellent ideas can come from disliked individuals, and poor ideas can come from favored people.

## Taste and Judgment

Taste and judgment both are broad types of opinion. Many people believe that everyone has a right to his or her own opinion without providing justification. Many people believe that their opinions are right simply because they hold them, or because they are more experienced, older, more educated, and so forth. Although this is true in matters of taste, it is not true in matters of judgment.

Taste is a matter of personal preference that requires no defense. Taste describes an internal state, something you like or dislike. For example, you may prefer long skirt lengths, a catheterization tray made by a certain manufacturer, and working the evening shift. Others may or may not agree with your tastes; however you need not defend your tastes.

Opinions dealing with matters of judgment are different and *do* require a thoughtful defense. "Expressions of judgment are assertions about the truth of things or about the wisdom of a course of action" (Ruggiero, 1991, p. 28). For example, a claim that long skirt lengths are a deterrent to assaults on women requires justification. Is the statement true? Why does the speaker believe it is true? On what evidence does the speaker base such a claim? Is it a wise statement for women to heed?

Suppose a colleague states that brand XYZ catheterization tray is less likely to become contaminated than brand ABC. This is a judgment that requires justification. Is it true? Why is the person making such a claim? What are his or her reasons?

## Fact and Interpretation

"A fact is something known with certainty, something either objectively verifiable or demonstrable. An interpretation is an explanation of meaning or significance" (Ruggiero, 1991, pp. 56-57). An example of a statement of fact is "Between 1965 and 1991, health spending rose from 5.9% to 13.2% of the gross domestic product in this country" (Samuelson, 1993). This statement of fact is based on selected governmental documents. The general interpretation of this finding is that health spending is excessive and therefore, undesirable. Another interpretation is that health care costs are out of control. Yet another interpretation is that the United States is finally realigning its priorities and contributing more of its resources to health care. Which interpretation do you choose?

Before you choose an interpretation, you should reflect on the cause of the increase in health spending. Could it be due to the longer life span of people in this country? Is it due to the increased numbers of people living below the poverty line who receive Medicaid funds? Is it due to the expansion of high-tech medicine? Are health care providers too greedy? Are fraudulent claims out of control? Is the health care insurance industry too profit-oriented? Is it due to the increasing numbers and amounts of malpractice awards? Is it a combination of all of these? Is any one factor more of a contributor than others? These numerous questions illustrate the importance of considering all the facts before making a final interpretation.

## An Idea's Validity and the Quality of Its Expression

How a speaker expresses an idea influences the idea's validity. Some speakers are more articulate than others. Some speakers are able to express their ideas with conviction and enthusiasm; they readily persuade others to their point of view and inspire followers.

Other speakers may have great ideas, but they lack the ability to express them effectively and persuasively. They may lack enthusiasm, speak in a monotone, or misuse language. They generally fail to reach their listeners.

In either instance, the validity or truthfulness of an idea is unrelated to the speaker's ability to express it. When you listen to a speaker, distinguish between *what* the speaker is saying and *how* she or he is saying it. Evaluate the idea on its own merit. Evaluate the presentation skills of the speaker as a separate issue.

## Truth and Beliefs

What is truth, and how is it different from beliefs? Truth is that which conforms to fact or agrees with reality. Truth is accurate, right, correct, and in accord with experience. It is an established or verified fact or principle (Neufeldt, 1991). Examples of true statements include the following: the United States is on the continent of North America; two plus two equals four; and the earth spins on its axis and revolves around the sun. Truth may mean vision or insight ("All men are created equal"), or it may refer to the end product of an analytical appraisal by the human mind (matter can neither be created nor destroyed).

Conducting research is one particular approach to seeking truth. Scientists seek to verify the authenticity of ideas and theories by employing a systematic reasoning process known as the scientific method. The scientific method consists of five steps: (1) identifying an event to be investigated, (2) gathering information about the event, (3) developing a theory or hypothesis to explain the event, (4) testing the theory or hypothesis through experimentation, and (5) evaluating the theory or hypothesis (Chaffee, 1994).

In contrast, a belief is a conviction or acceptance that certain things are true or real (Neufeldt, 1991). Beliefs may or may not be true. For example, at one time scientists believed the earth was flat, that disease was caused by "bad" body humors, and that getting cold and wet led to upper respiratory tract infections.

Beliefs are influenced by culture. For example, consider the medical physician who tried to help an Asian-American man understand why he should stop using opium. The physician tried reasoning, using factual information derived from Western biomedical research, but got nowhere. The physician called in the local healer from the man's cultural center. The healer was successful after only one session with the addict. When asked about the healer's successful intervention, she said she told the man that a dragon would devour him if he did not stop using opium. The dragon was threatening to the man because the man believed in dragons. This approach was more effective than the message of the Western physician to whom magical dragons mean nothing. Beliefs are a function of our frame of reference, and the man's frame of reference included a belief in dragons.

Truth, then, "is the reality of the matter, as distinguished from what people wish were so, believe to be so, or assert to be so" (Ruggiero, 1991, p. 21). Ruggiero recommends reserving the word *truth* for situations in which we know the final answer and using the words *belief, theory,* and *present understanding* more often.

## Stereotype and Individuality

To rely on familiar stereotypes is easy. When you think of clients from a specific ethnic group, you might think in terms of stereotypical characteristics based on your background—where you were raised, what your family taught you, and how you learned to view other people. You should attempt to view clients as individuals raised in families and to learn the particular beliefs, thoughts, and needs of each individual client.

Consider the example of the monolingual Hispanic woman from Chile who was hospitalized in the United States. The nurses were concerned about her because she was not eating well. Communication was a problem; the client did not speak English, and the nurses did not speak Spanish. The nurses assumed the client would eat better if she were served Mexican foods such as burritos, tacos, beans, and tortillas. They made a special effort to order these foods but found that their efforts were ineffective and unappreciated. The client picked at the food, leaving much of it uneaten. After several days the nurses were able to locate an interpreter who spoke the woman's particular dialect. Through the interpreter, the nurses learned that the client lived near the Chilean sea shore and ate primarily fish and other types of seafood. She was unaccustomed to eating the Mexican foods the nurses offered her.

In this example, the nurses unwittingly operated from a commonly held stereotype about Hispanic clients and assumed that people who share a common culture also share food preferences, beliefs, values, and habits. They created a dietary treatment based on this unquestioned stereotype.

## One's Own Frame of Reference and Other Frames of Reference

To get outside of ourselves and see life from another perspective is difficult for all of us. To recognize when your frame of reference is a factor in gaining a better understanding of another person is another important distinction to make. Frame of reference is the window through which a person views the world, or what a person believes life was, is, and will be like based on the sum total of life experiences.

As we go about our daily routines, we listen to information that we understand and with which we agree; we need only to assimilate the information. We have difficulty listening to information that requires us to change our way of thinking. To illustrate this concept, refer to the nurses' experience with the Chilean client. If the client had relished the Mexican foods, she would have validated the nurses' frame of reference; her enjoyment of the food would have been exactly what they expected, and the experience would have merely confirmed what they already believed. When the client indicated a preference for fish and other seafoods, the nurses had to change their way of thinking about Hispanic clients. They had to incorporate a new and more complicated reality into their frames of reference. Seeing only your own frame of reference is egocentric. Learning to recognize other frames of reference is part of learning to think critically and allows you to recognize that everything you have been taught is not the only truth there is.

## Thinking by Habit and Thinking by Choice

When we think by habit, we agree with the thinking of others—possibly because we were trained this way or perhaps because the issue is simply unimportant to us. Thinking by habit has been described as "being on automatic pilot." Habitual thinking requires less intellectual work. We tend to use habitual thinking until something happens to make us aware that our thinking no longer works. We then realize that we need to give the issue or problem our full conscious attention.

Thinking choice requires time to reflect on an issue. Thinking may be stimulated by discussions with others or by reading about an issue. In whatever manner it occurs, thinking by choice is a conscious decision to examine an issue fully.

Consider the example of Hedrina who was in group counseling with a psychiatric nurse. Hedrina and her husband Otis lived in close proximity to his family. For years Otis's family treated him as if he were an oddball, incompetent, and undeserving of respect. Through counseling, Hedrina came to realize she was unwittingly treating Otis in the same way that his family was treating him. She realized she was being influenced by his family. Because she loved her husband and wanted to respect him, the next time a family member made a disparaging remark about Otis, she objected to it and offered her opinion. Soon she was in conflict with his entire family. It was not long until Hedrina and Otis decided it would be in their best interest to establish themselves in a new community, one that was a considerable distance from his family.

In this example, Hedrina made a distinction between thinking by habit and thinking by choice. When confronted with a problem, she chose to critically examine her feelings about her spouse and the importance of their marital relationship. Realizing the impact of her unthinking behavior on Otis, she changed her thinking and her behavior. She was thinking by choice.

History is replete with individuals who have gone against the tide of conventional thinking, or thinking by habit. Margaret Sanger, who started Planned Parenthood, is an example of such a figure. In her time, the primary role of women was to bear children. She vigorously fought for women's right to control their reproduction, and introduced the diaphragm as a method of birth control. She challenged the thinking of society during her time, endured the contempt of many, and even served time in jail. She eventually prevailed.

## REFLECTION

### Definitions

Reflection has many meanings. Dewey (1916) described it as the process of inquiry or the results of inquiry. Reflection is the fixing of the mind on some subject, serious thought, contemplation, the result of such thought, or an idea or conclusion, especially if expressed in words (Neufeldt, 1991). In the context of this book, reflection is a mental activity during which we recall and contemplate an event. We give careful thought to and seek to discover the meaning and purpose of that event. The event may be a transaction between the person reflecting and another person, or it may be something the person reflecting saw, felt, heard, or read. Reflection is a form of self examination and self analysis. We may reflect in solitude or with others.

Reflection connotes quieting the mind to focus on a subject and taking the time to think about it in an unhurried manner. You may set aside time for reflection in the easy chair, just before sleep, or while gazing into a fire or a beautiful sunset. Reflection may also come unbidden when you allow time for it to happen. It may even start when you are in the midst of another activity. Many people who do rhythmic athletic activity such as swimming laps, walking long distances, and running, say that they do their best thinking while thus engaged. Rhythmic activity promotes the trancelike, focused state that is conducive to reflection.

Some situations may be more amenable to reflection than others. When it suits us, we take the time to review the events—perhaps through several perspectives—and consider what truth, meaning, or other kinds of learning we can derive from the experience.

Reflection allows you to process each event and attempt to consider it from all possible angles. You may wish to contemplate such questions as: What led up to the event? What possible causes precipitated it? What exactly did the other person mean by that statement? What evidence did the other person present for that point of view? Was the evidence the other presented relevant? Did the descriptions of the event offered by the other person match or conflict with your own observations?

You can also review your own thoughts and actions: Did I say what I really meant? How did I back up my position? Did I use reasons that the other person could relate to? Did I make my premises clear? Did we agree on basic premises? Did we disagree? What merit has the other person's ideas? Was I uncomfortable because there was something wrong with the event or the other person's use of logic and I cannot put my finger on it? Did the other person's statement threaten my position? Would I have to give up my position if I believed him or her? What will the cost of giving up my position be? What will I gain? How else can this event be explained?

## Ways to Reflect

Engaging in the activity of reflection is very individualized. All people deal with new knowledge by associating it with something familiar. This basic principle of learning, however, is handled by individuals in very different ways. Some individuals immediately make pictures of the new information. For example, one Hispanic woman told her mentor "Slow down! When you talk, I get all of these pictures in my head!" Others prefer quiet contemplation of the concepts they encounter. Still others who are more outwardly active learners reflect upon new knowledge by discussing it with someone else. For example, one student drove her roommate crazy by discussing each book she read as if she was giving the author a personal critique.

Many creative artists, writers, and scientists have described gaining their best insights while reflecting upon their experiences and thoughts in solitude. For example, one nurse said, "I find I need a quiet time to reflect. When circumstances require me to sit still (as in a lecture), I find I can reflect. Sometimes answers will come. I will be listening to others and suddenly this problem I have been stewing on emerges along with some insights."

Another nurse described two very different circumstances under which she reflected. One situation presented a painful conflict that caused her to raise her defenses. She experienced a block. She found it impossible to reflect deeply, even though she knew that the situation had to be processed and dealt with. She realized that attempting to overcome the block was futile at that moment. She did not experience denial, which occurs when a person refuses to deal with an issue worthy of contemplation; she was experiencing problems of timing. Later, after she had enough time and distance, she reflected on the issue. "When I am ready, then I can reflect on it, whatever the troubling event was." At other times, this same person cannot settle down for the night until she processes the event: "I cannot do anything else until I settle it."

Another nurse said that he can wind himself up in knots and keep himself up all night ruminating about a conflict or troubling event and exhaust himself. His solution is to do whatever is necessary to lay it aside and get a good night's sleep. When he awakens the next day, refreshed, he often has the solution. "I do not know how it works, but it does!"

Thinking individuals have different ways of coping with transactions and events that call for reflection. We vary in the timing of reflection and the methods we use to reflect depending on our role models, brain chemistry, personalities, state of energy, the circumstance under which we encounter a situation, and the way we react to it. You should attempt to notice what circumstances promote *your* ability to reflect, and use that inner wisdom in your own behalf.

Reflecting in the company of another person or a few trusted individuals is productive for some people. This type of activity may promote reflection for a person who has trouble thinking about a particular issue. Reflecting with peers is crucial to the development of moral judgment. The process of stating our beliefs and discussing it with others helps us to move and evolve effectively.

*Debriefing* is the word used to describe directed reflections after an important event by an individual or by a team such as the nurses and physicians involved in responding to a COR-O (emergency cardiopulmonary resuscitation) or in psychiatric teams after a group or family therapy session. The team members reflect together on what transpired, what interventions seemed to work and why; other concerns of psychiatric teams would be what various transactions meant, what information the clients revealed about themselves, what insights were demonstrated by clients and therapists, and what was "really going on" when specific overt actions occurred.

Reflection can serve as an antidote to boredom. Some nurses who work in acute care settings return to school to get out of a rut. As exciting as acute care is, some nurses have expressed boredom with the situation. As they become more expert in caring for critically ill clients, they no longer find it challenging.

By reflecting, you can raise to the surface and analyze the tacit understandings of your routine activities. Often these reflections occur at quiet moments while studying, or during discussions with peers. Reflection may happen right during the situation itself (Schon, 1983). A nurse said very excitedly, "I can see right before me the theory I was reading!"

## Reflection and Action

One of the strong messages that Dewey (1933) relayed is his attitude toward action. Thinking well is only half the story. He asserts that the worth of reflection is evident in the actions that result from it. If you succeed, you should reflect on why you succeeded. What dimensions do you believe were crucial to your success? If you did not succeed, you should reflect on why you failed. What dimensions did you overlook? What suspicions did you neglect or discount that were very important? Did your reflection lead to a modification? Did you consider scrapping the whole method and adopting a different approach?

The Denver International Airport's baggage system is an example of a dilemma in which a method was discarded in favor of a new one. In the spring of 1994 the Denver International Airport was scheduled to open with a state-of-the-art baggage system. The only problem was that the system did not work. All summer the city council, various airlines and other interested parties argued about who was responsible for the fiasco, and debated whether to scrap the whole method and start over or continue with the present method and add a backup system. In the fall, United Airlines assumed responsibility for the baggage system and stated that they would redesign it more simply (Weber, 1994).

Reflection often leads to synthesis. Synthesis occurs whenever we carry over any meaning from one object to another that had previously seemed to be of a different kind (Dewey, 1933). Organizing your information from this point of view consists of three steps: (1) reviewing the facts and ideas you gain through researching your subject, (2) noting the facts that you see for yourself, and (3) relating them to each other on a new basis, namely the hypothesis you make or the tentative conclusion that you draw. Reflection is mental work, and most people usually do not do it unless they find themselves dealing with a puzzling, thoughtful, or unsettling situation.

The opposite of reflection is to deny feelings, thoughts, and observations. People selectively attend to only those situations in which they feel confident and in control. Another option is to deny the significance of the situation, or to deny that anything can or should be done about it (Laing, 1994). In other words, people are more apt to practice reflection if they have developed the attitude of emotional and intellectual honesty. One way to combat the temptation to ignore an issue is to develop an attitude of curiosity. Being able to tolerate surprise, puzzlement, or even confusion may be the key to unlocking the puzzle; this requires courage and honesty.

## Journal Keeping

In addition to reflecting in solitude or in the company of trusted others, some people find it easier to reflect and write their thoughts. Keeping a journal can develop and strengthen the ability to engage in reflection (Bradley-Springer, 1993). By writing about your thoughts in a journal, you can reflect upon any event at your own pace. A journal is an excellent tool for enhancing critical and creative thinking.

Good thinking takes time and discipline. First thoughts and the words chosen to express those thoughts, however, may not arrive in good order. All thoughts are valuable and a journal is a great way to capture these raw thoughts and then refine them over time. In our economy-minded era, the idea of "conversing" with each other at leisure, or even getting others to listen to an idea fully, seems like a luxury. Making others wait while you struggle with a thought or try to convey your thoughts can seem disrespectful to others who desire to "get on with" the topic at hand.

When you write in a journal, you may take your time describing your observations, and use as many words as needed to convey the entire picture you are contemplating. You may use the journal to speculate and to wonder aloud about other directions and paths. If your thoughts are captured in a journal, they are not lost. You may retrieve them whenever you choose. The advantage of journal keeping is that it allows you to think about ideas without fear of being ridiculed. You can record "half-baked" ideas with the security that they will not affect others' opinions. Journal keeping also allows you the opportunity to revise ideas while becoming more knowledgeable, thinking more intently, or observing more closely.

In addition to being a valuable tool to promote your own emotional growth, problem solving skills, and ability to think critically, journal keeping can have positive physiological effects. Adams (1990) reported that spending just 15 minutes a day for four consecutive days writing about emotionally sensitive issues can increase immune system functioning, lower blood pressure, and improve your physiological response to stress.

## PROBING OUR IGNORANCE

The purpose of most formal schooling in the United States is to transmit knowledge about specific subject matter from those who know (teachers and books) to those who do not (students). Educators examine human experience and understanding through the frames of reference of the historian, psychologist, linguist, mathematician, chemist, and other content specialists. Most educators focus on known content such as facts, principles, and concepts without a concomitant focus on what is unknown. Nursing educators have followed a similar pattern in nursing curricula, focusing on nursing content that is believed or known to be true. Little attention is given to those areas in which little or no information is available, areas about which we are ignorant. For example, we know the pathophysiology of many diseases such as diabetes mellitus and cancer but we do not know why the pancreas fails to meet the body's demand for insulin or why cell division goes awry.

There is much about nursing, clients, and relationships that we think we know but do not know, do not know and know that we do not know, or do not know and are not aware that we do not know. By acknowledging our ignorance, we gain a greater awareness of the limitations in our present knowledge and the vast expanse of knowledge about which we know little or nothing. Marlys Witte, a physician educator, calls these gaps the "black holes" of knowledge. She encourages medical students to develop an awareness of these black holes in two ways: by taking them on "wondering rounds" during which they discuss the biological, clinical, social, and ethical questions raised by the clients' conditions; and by conducting "pondering sessions" in which students freely ponder a variety of topics (Blum, 1993).

When we acknowledge our ignorance and reflect on it without embarrassment, we nurture that most wondrous of human qualities, curiosity. Curiosity is a desire to learn and an eagerness to know—an inquisitiveness manifest by asking questions and seeking more information. Critical thinking and curiosity are compatible companions. Through scientific inquiry, we structure and formalize our curiosity as we seek to validate our present knowledge and discover new knowledge.

Having knowledge gaps should not interfere with thinking critically. You should not expect more from critical thinking and the Critical Thinking Interaction Model than either can deliver. Critical thinking may not necessarily lead you to a truth or a final answer; some things you will never know. Critical thinking will, however, help you to think deeply and thoroughly and develop confidence in your ability to reason, which will inspire you to continue learning throughout your lifetime.

# USE OF LANGUAGE

Language is the tool we use to communicate the essential components of critical thinking: focus, frame of reference, attitudes, assumptions, evidence, reasoning, conclusions, implications, and context. Language allows us to understand and communicate issues and problems, ascertain assumptions, evaluate evidence and reasoning, anticipate implications, and assess context. Through language we also communicate information, express feelings, and evoke emotions in others (Engel, 1994). To put it more simply, the main function of language is to communicate (Kim, 1994).

All words are symbols of something else; that is, they represent something. For example, *syringe, catheter, liver,* and *heart* are symbols of equipment and organs with which we are familiar. Without this symbolization, words would be meaningless. For example, what do *zephonie, triameride,* and *besordt* mean? Nothing comes to mind because those words do not arouse images or emotions. Words are abstract items; they symbolize or represent concrete things (Engel, 1994).

Thinking and language are distinct but closely related processes. The ability to use language is closely associated to the ability to think meaningfully. When we speak or write, we use language to express our thinking. When we listen or read, we use language to understand the thinking of others (Chaffee, 1994). In dialogue, our goal is to communicate our thoughts and feelings accurately. When others understand the message as we intend it, we have successfully communicated. To achieve this level of communication, we must use language precisely and clearly, the two keys to effective thinking and communicating. When language is sloppy (vague, indistinct, imprecise, foolish, and inaccurate), it reflects similar thinking. When language is clear and precise, thinking is also clear and precise (specific, distinct, significant, and accurate). Thinking and language are interactive processes, each continually influencing the other. As we improve our skill in one process, we will improve our skill in the other (Chaffee, 1994; Halpern, 1984).

Words frame how we view a topic. Malone (1994) comments on the changing language we use to describe ill people. For example, 20 years ago ill people were consistently called "patients," which connotes a care giving relationship that has existed between nurses and ill people throughout nursing's history. Today patients are known as "clients" because nurses recognize that not all patients are ill, injured, or hospitalized. This change in terminology occurred as a result of changing patterns of health care giving and nursing roles. Terminology continues to evolve. Within the past 5 to 6 years, clients have been called "consumers," nursing care became a "product," and health care became a "business." Recent terminology describes clients as "guests" and nurses as "hostesses."

Malone argues that the language we use suggests a relationship between nurses and people who need care. Nurse-patient, nurse-client, nurse-consumer, and hostess-guest create images of different kinds of relationships. Nurses should be mindful of how language can alter this relationship and use language that connotes the desired relationship.

The critical thinking skills we associate with language are found in the Critical Thinking Skills Applied to Nursing: Language box on p. 101.

## Critical Thinking Skills Applied to Nursing: Language

▼   Assess clarity and precision
▼   Define key words
▼   Identify emotive words
▼   Assess context
▼   Detect and exploit labels

## Assess Clarity and Precision

Clarity and precision in language result from clear and precise thinking. Clear and precise language is especially important to communicate and record nursing observations, construct arguments, and persuade others. Jargon, vagueness, ambiguity, and style are four aspects of language related to clarity and precision.

***Jargon.***    Jargon consists of words, expressions, and technical terms that are used and understood by a particular group of people but not by the general public (Chaffee, 1994). Medical terminology is an example of jargon. For example, a nurse may ask a client if she has *voided*. Many clients do not know that voiding is the same as urinating. Later this nurse encouraged the client to ambulate, and the client was baffled again. She had no idea what the word *ambulate* meant. Fortunately the nurse went through the activity of getting the client up. "Why not just tell me to walk? Why use big words for everyday words?" she asked. Without realizing it, the nurse used language that had meaning for her but little meaning for the client.

Many commonplace Latin abbreviations used in health care are informative to health care providers but may be meaningless to clients. For example, NPO (nothing by mouth), per os (by mouth), tid (three times a day), and qd (every day) are not generally understood by clients. As a nurse, you must remember not to use jargon that clients may not understand. Jargon can interfere in communicating important heath information to clients.

***Vagueness.***    A word or phrase is vague when the meaning is unclear and imprecise, or when you search for any meaning and find none (Engel, 1994). A vague word "lacks a clear and distinct meaning" (Chaffee, 1994, p. 330). Some examples of vague language includes the following:

▼   Draconian cost containment measures impact health care delivery.
▼   What a resuscitation effort!
▼   Nurses should get involved.

Each statement is imprecise and will need further clarification to make its meaning understood. What does "draconian" mean in the first example? What does "cost containment" mean? What impact (positive or negative) does "cost containment" have on "health care delivery"? In the second statement, "resuscitation effort" is unclear. Does it mean the client was successfully revived? Does it mean that the resuscitation procedure was perfectly executed by the staff? The third statement that nurses should "get involved" is also meaningless. What does involvement mean? How involved is involved? What will nurses be doing if they are "involved"?

Many words health care providers use daily lack a clear and precise meaning. Consider words such as young, old, underweight, overweight, health, illness, normal, abnormal, high, low, dependent, independent, mature, and immature. You may have a vague understanding of what these words mean, but as a critical thinker you use precise terminology, particularly when charting, reasoning, and persuading others. In charting, for example, to record a client's skin as "normal" is vague and insufficient. To note color, moisture, temperature, texture, condition of hair and nails, and the presence of lesions is precise. If lesions are present, noting their size, color, shape, type (morphology), grouping (configuration), location, and tenderness is more precise.

To clarify vague language, Chaffee (1994) recommends that we ask who, what, where, when, how, and why. Consider this statement:

Health care should be both universal and accessible so that everyone can receive the needed health care and engage in activities to prevent illness and maintain health. It may increase costs in the short run, but it would decrease costs in the long run.

To apply Chaffee's questions, ask:

**Who:** To whom does "everyone" refer and what does "universal" mean? Does it include citizens and noncitizens? Does it mean that preexisting conditions are no longer a factor in determining insurance coverage?

**What:** What is the central point? What is the context? Is it an idle statement by an errant politician, or the position of a professional organization? What does "accessible" mean? Does it mean available to everyone regardless of race, age, health status, citizenship, and socioeconomic background?

**Where:** Where should health care be universal and accessible? Throughout the United States? In just those states that elect to participate?

**When:** When should health care become universal and accessible? Immediately? In 5 or 10 years?

**How:** How should health care become universal and accessible? By a phased-in process? By mandating individual, state, and business participation? By voluntary individual, state, and business participation? By increasing taxes on individuals, business, or property?

**Why:** Why should health care become universal and accessible? Only to reduce costs? Are there other reasons?

Clarifying these vague terms will affect the position you take on this issue. For example, if taxes were significantly increased to make health care "universal" and "accessible," you might oppose the issue, whereas you might support it if it requires no such increase.

***Ambiguity.***　　Many words have more than one meaning. A word or statement is ambiguous when it has more than one meaning and that meaning is not made clear by the context in which it is used (Moore and Parker, 1992). If the meaning remains indeterminate when placed in context, then the word(s) are ambiguous (Engel, 1994). Consider this statement by a nurse: "How is Mrs. Rose doing this morning? The night nurse reported that she complained of abdominal pain and had her call light on a lot. The doctors cannot find any cause and think that her problem is psychosomatic. She complains so much!"

Which word is ambiguous? How is the word *complain* used? Its first use refers to the client's report of abdominal pain. The second use refers to the nurse's reaction to Mrs. Rose's behavior, but we are left to wonder what the nurse really means by her statement. Does she mean that Mrs. Rose consistently reports her abdominal pain, or that Mrs. Rose continuously expresses her displeasure and annoyance?

Being aware of ambiguity is important, especially in group meetings when new ideas are discussed and in interpersonal communications when one person tries to persuade another to accept a particular point of view. How can you locate ambiguities? Browne and Keeley (1994) recommend that you begin by examining key words for alternative meanings. Identify the key words to define in "Everyone should have equal access to health care." The words *everyone, equal access,* and *health care* are all potentially ambiguous.

Abstract words tend to be more ambiguous than are concrete words. Abstract refers to thoughts that are apart from any particular instances or material objects. Abstract thoughts are more difficult to understand because they are general in nature. Concrete refers to things that have a material presence that can be perceived by the senses (Neufeldt, 1991). A distinction between the abstract and concrete is illustrated in the mental status examination to assess a client's higher order cognitive skills. A client is asked to explain the meaning of a proverb such as "People who live in glass houses should not throw stones." An abstract answer to the proverb would be a statement such as "Vulnerable people should not criticize others." A concrete answer would be "People should not throw rocks because rocks can shatter glass."

Next you must determine whether your understanding of the key words matches those of the speaker or writer. To do this you must avoid assuming that the word has an obvious definition and that your understanding matches the speaker or writer's meaning. Does the definition of the ambiguous word remain constant throughout the discussion? Could it have another meaning and still make sense in the discussion? For example, does "everyone" include legal and illegal immigrants too? Does "equal access to health care" mean that every medical treatment should be available to "everyone" regardless of age, physical condition, and ability to pay? The more abstract the key words, the greater the likelihood they will be misunderstood. Ask for clarification when you identify ambiguous words. For example, you can ask a speaker to "clarify what you mean by 'equal access.'"

You must also consider context. What is the context of the possible ambiguity? Does context affect the meaning? For example, how does context affect your understanding of the statement, "Everyone should have equal access to health care"? What does the statement mean to you? Ask what it means to your peers. Would it mean something different to wealthy people living in Oregon than it would to poor people living in Alabama? Would it mean something different to Canadian versus American citizens? To people living in Rwanda or Bosnia? Following these suggestions will help you identify significant ambiguities in discussions and arguments.

**Style.**    Style, or the unique manner in which a person communicates, is an important aspect of clear communication. A person's choice of words and how they are arranged and expressed create an overall effect. The level of language used, point of view, purpose, and tone are a part of style (Wassman and Rinsky, 1993). Consider how you speak to your children and family, clients, colleagues, and administrators. Does it change with your audience? In what way does your style change?

Good style means communicating clearly, simply, appropriately, and concisely (Engel, 1994). Good style can be achieved by paying attention to four rules (Mirin, 1981). First, avoid unnecessary words. Use short sentences rather than long ones. Avoid redundant words and sentences. If the information is complex, attempt to communicate it as simply as you can and still transmit the desired meaning. Second, use familiar, simple words and phrases. Avoid using complex words when simple words will suffice. When conversing with clients, use words that are appropriate. Translate medical jargon into suitable language that takes client characteristics into consideration (Babcock and Miller, 1994). Third, use explicit, clear-cut words rather than abstract words. Abstract words are subject to multiple meanings and therefore are easily misinterpreted. Finally, choose words that reflect your meaning accurately. Think about what you want to communicate and select your words accordingly.

## Define Key Words

When we communicate we may assume that others understand the message as we intended it, or that the words we use have the same meaning for the listener as they do for us. For example, Ralph had a benign tumor in his large bowel that was surgically removed. The physician clearly told him the tumor was benign, but Ralph did not define "benign" in the same way as the physician. A benign tumor is one that is not malignant (cancerous). Ralph assumed that all tumors were cancerous and that his definition of "benign" was correct.

Some words require defining on a larger scale. Recall the difficulty our society had in arriving at an acceptable definition of the word *death*. Is it the cessation of life as indicated by the absence of a heartbeat and respiration? Is it the total absence of brain activity? Our society still grapples with a definition of when life begins.

How key words are defined determines how acceptable the reasoning is. Defining key words is an important skill in the precise use of language. Definitions may be either reportive or stipulative (Engel, 1994). A reportive definition is one that is used in a certain way by a specific group. For example, word definitions are commonly attributed to *Webster's Dictionary.* In health care, practitioners use definitions from expert sources such as the National Institutes of Health and the U. S. Centers for Disease Control and Prevention.

A stipulative definition is one that a speaker or writer intends to use in a certain way. For example, nurse researchers must define the meaning of terms used in the conduct of research. The definition of critical thinking in this book is a stipulative definition. When defining key words, always state the source of the definition.

The importance of defining key terms has everyday application for nurses. For example, a nurse visited a postpartum client in her home. The client had a mild vaginal drainage, and the nurse instructed the client to use a vinegar and water douche daily. When the nurse returned 2 weeks later and inquired about the effectiveness of the douches, the client replied that she douched only the first day. She stopped because she could not stand the taste of the vinegar and water mixture. In this example, the nurse failed to verify that the client understood the key term, douche.

Culture may affect the meaning of words. For example, in Western medicine, hypertension is defined as blood pressure in excess of 130 over 85 (Johannsen, 1993). Some blacks may confuse it with nervousness and stress and "high blood," a natural folk illness. "High blood" may mean that there is an excessive amount of blood in the body or that the blood has shifted its location such as when they believe an increased flow to the brain has occurred. Both of these events are related to diet and emotions and may result in a stroke (Snow, 1983, 1991). Similar misunderstandings were found among Mexican Americans of whom only 28% knew the correct definition of hypertension (Ailinger, 1982). Incorrect definitions included bad circulation, rapid heart rate, tension or nervousness, and feeling hot.

## Identify Emotive Words

Word meanings have two dimensions: denotation and connotation (Wassman and Rinsky, 1993). Denotation is a word's literal meaning, its dictionary definition, dissociated from any emotional association. For example, the dictionary defines *patient* as someone who is undergoing treatment for a disease whereas a *client* is a person for whom a professional person is acting. A *customer* is someone who buys or patronizes an establishment regularly. Each definition refers to someone who receives services, but the mental image of each is different.

Connotation of a word goes beyond the dictionary definition of a word and suggests ideas, associations, and implications. Connotations can be positive or negative. They evoke an emotional response, stir up feelings, and create a visual image. For example, the *dull, malnourished* patient was undergoing treatment for a *debilitating* disease. The *astute* client contracted with the home health care agency for *superior* services. The *faithful* customer finally became weary of *substandard* and *inattentive* services and decided to take his business elsewhere. Within the context of these sentences, patient, client, and customer evoked mental images that include much more than the literal definitions.

Words may have a powerful emotive force (Moore and Parker, 1992). Consider the emotive force of the following words: benign, overweight, indigent, smoker, mental illness, geriatrics, baby, and birth control. What images come to mind when you read each word? Compare your images with those of your colleagues. Are they similar? Different? Are your emotional reactions positive, negative, or indifferent?

Emotive words may indicate the user's personal opinion or evaluation (Chaffee, 1994). Note how a person describes another person, subject, or situation. What words does that person choose? What does it reveal about that person's frame of reference and attitude toward another person, subject, or situation? The key to assessing the appropriateness of a given use of language is establishing its intention (Engel, 1994). Is the intention to inform, to express emotion, or to move us to action? Is it all of these? After you establish intention, assess whether the language is consistent with that intention.

Emotive language has a legitimate place in our language. It adds a descriptive dimension that enriches our understanding of life and the human condition. Although emotive language is discouraged in the study of argument, it does have importance. The emotive force of written or spoken words is not related to the logical validity of an argument (Engel, 1994).

Many students with whom we work tell us that they wish they could show less emotion when they express their opinions and could state better, clearer reasons for their positions on issues and problems. They state that they get emotional, which interferes with their ability to persuade others. To improve this situation, we offer the following suggestions. First, reflect on the issue or problem. What do you believe about it? What is your position? Next, consider your intention and goal(s) in interacting with another person(s) about it. Do you wish to inform? Express your emotion? Persuade others to believe as you do? Persuade others to take action?

The next step is to create strategies for your goal(s). What will be most effective? What reasons will be most effective? How will you verbalize your position? Take timing into consideration when you plan your strategies. When is the best time to present your position? Choose a time when the other person is available and can listen without interruption.

Then, practice your presentation. If you feel very strongly about the issue or problem, practice presenting your case in calm language and demeanor. Practice until you get it right. Role-play it with a trusted colleague who will respond as you anticipate others will. Finally, when you are ready, present your case.

## Assess Context

Context is the whole situation, background, or environment relative to a particular event, personality, and so forth (Neufeldt, 1991). How we interpret the information we receive from our senses is related to the context in which they occur. For example, we interpret the significance of shortness of breath differently if we know a client has known heart disease than if we know that client just hiked up a mountain. Language also occurs in a context (Chaffee, 1994). In speaking, context is the setting in which the words are spoken and to which they refer. In writing, context is the group of words surrounding the specific word under study.

Understanding context will help you determine the meaning of what is going on if you attend to the available clues. Look at how context changes the meaning of the word *discharge*.

1. The client has a foul *discharge* from his wound.

2. It is okay to *discharge* the client from the hospital.

3. When the S-A node *discharges,* its impulse is conducted both into the A-V node and into the Purkinje fibers.

With each sentence, the meaning of the word changed, which illustrates the importance of context.

Nonverbal communication is also part of context. Eye contact, gestures, and posture may affect what is heard. The significance of nonverbal communication may vary in different cultures. For example, Hispanic clients may nod their heads up and down when asked if they understand medical instructions. A health care provider may interpret the nodding as an indication of understanding; however, the nodding may be only a gesture of courtesy (Babcock and Miller, 1994).

## Detect and Exploit Labels

Labeling is the way in which a concept, event, or group is framed. One intent may be to represent a complex concept, event, or group in a brief, easy-to-communicate way. For example, the myriad of changes in the health care system supported by nurses can be captured under the label, "Nursing's Agenda for Health Care Reform." It is a catchy phrase, and it aligns nursing with the reform movement. None of the components of Nursing's Agenda for Health Care Reform are identified in the title, thus minimizing the possibility of others immediately rejecting nursing's direction for reform. Another intent of labeling may be to alter a stereotype, exemplified by changing labels from "handicapped" to "physically challenged" or "differently abled."

Labels can also be used to misrepresent a concept, event, or group and arouse negative emotions. Negative labels, also know as loaded terms (Hughes, 1992), may take the form of name calling, mud slinging, and controversial phrases (epithets). Consider the contrasting mental images that occur with these phrases: angels of mercy, hard-hearted nurse, lawless youth, patriot, traitor, emotionally disturbed person, and mature adult. These labels express approval and disapproval without giving supporting evidence to sustain that judgment.

How a concept, event, or group is labeled helps shape our attitude toward it. Consider a speech made by former Colorado Governor Lamb who commented on the disproportionately high amount of money the United States spends on caring for the elderly in the last year of life—disproportionate when compared with the amount of money spent on the young through such programs as well baby care. The comments generated much discussion across the nation and were subsequently captured by the label that the elderly had a "duty to die." Labeling Mr. Lamb's remarks with these words set a tone for discounting and rejecting his intended meaning. A different label would have resulted in a different understanding of his meaning. How would the discussion have been different had his comments been labeled "humane treatment for the elderly," "pro-choice for eldercare," or "fair share for children"?

When a client is characterized as fussy, complaining, good, or cooperative, she or he is being labeled. When a client is labeled, nurses tend to alter their interactions with the client, based on the labels they have heard. The client may then respond in a way that confirms and reinforces the label, thus perpetuating the behavior.

Consider how administrators frame and label situations. The administrator of one home health care agency reported that the balance sheet showed a loss for the past year. She declared that nursing personnel costs were too high and staff would have to be downsized (reduced). Instead of accepting the administrator's frame, several nurses examined the financial records. They separated administrative personnel costs from nursing personnel costs and discovered a disproportionately high ratio of administrators to nurses when compared with the ratio of administrators to nurses at other comparable home health care agencies. The nurses also discovered that revenue could be increased if billing practices were changed to reflect more accurately the actual time nurses spent with clients. By thinking creatively and investigating carefully, the nurses were able to challenge how the administrator framed the situation. The nurses reframed the situation based on their findings. They relabeled the situation a "revenue enhancement opportunity."

This example also illustrates how labels can be exploited for a positive use. To exploit is to take advantage of a situation. It can be done in a positive, productive way or an unethical way. When you get into a nursing management or leadership position, you must learn to exploit labels. Nurse leaders are responsible for creating a vision of how things can be on a specific nursing unit, in a home health care agency, or in the profession itself. When nurse leaders describe their visions to others, they should choose labels that will inspire others to form positive attitudes and energize them to make the visions reality.

## SUMMARY

Refining your thinking is yet another aspect of thinking critically. When you learn to make important distinctions in the process of interacting with clients, families, colleagues, and administrators, you refine your thinking. Through reflection you develop new insights and understandings and find meaning in experiences. You enhance reflection by giving yourself time to think. You may do this in solitude and with others. Journal keeping is another excellent method for enhancing reflection.

Reflect on your language. Language is the tool through which you express your thoughts. Frame your thoughts into a message that expresses your intent. Reflection and language are reciprocal processes. Writing your thoughts helps you think clearly. Reflecting on the material in your journal helps refine your thinking. When you make the effort to choose language that conveys your thoughts clearly and precisely, you think clearly and precisely. Labeling can be used positively. By thinking creatively and clearly, you can use labels to frame situations to your advantage.

# EXERCISES

## Exercise 1

**Purposes:** *Distinguish between important concepts*
*Promote reflection*

### DIRECTIONS

Distinguish between the following concepts:

1. Person and idea
2. Taste and judgment
3. Fact and interpretation
4. An idea's validity and the quality of its expression
5. Truth and belief
6. Stereotype and individuality
7. One's own frame of reference and other frames of reference
8. Thinking by choice and thinking by habit

Recall an interaction or experience in which you made or failed to make the distinction for each one. If you failed to make a critical distinction, replay the interaction or experience in your mind. How would you do it differently?

## Exercise 2

**Purposes:** *Promote reflection*
*Experience the value of writing in a journal to promote reflection*
*Experience the insights gained in reading one's thoughts in retrospect*

### DIRECTIONS

Write in your journal about the following questions and statements:

1. Have you ever wanted to say something and could not find the right words to express your thoughts clearly? Describe the incident. Why did you have difficulty expressing yourself? What do you think was going on when this occurred?
2. If you have a mentor, why did you pick this particular person?
3. Complete the following sentences:
   a. "I find that it is easiest to read, write, and study when I . . ."
   b. "I do my best thinking when I . . ."

4. Reflect upon the following statement: "It wrecks concentration to go halfway through one book and then start another book without finishing the first."

5. What were you curious about today? How did you handle the curious moment?

# Exercise 3

**Purpose:** *Examine areas of ignorance*

## DIRECTIONS

Form small groups. Volunteer one person to present a case study of a client for whom she or he has cared. Follow your school's case study format. Discuss the following:

1. What is known and not known about the case.

2. What arouses your curiosity? What would you like to know more about? Write all the questions to which you would like answers.

# Exercise 4

**Purpose:** *Examine areas of ignorance*

## DIRECTIONS

Form small groups. Take turns presenting the aspect of nursing that each person finds most interesting. Discuss:

1. What you think you know about it,

2. What you think you know about it but do not actually know, and

3. What you do not know about it and are aware of your ignorance.

Which questions would make good nursing research studies? Why?

# Exercise 5

**Purpose:** *Create clear and precise language from vague statements*

## DIRECTIONS

Read the following statements. Identify the vague word or phrases by asking who, what, where, when, how, and why. Create a clear and precise statement in its place.

1. The client just picks at her food. She is so thin, but she thinks she is more attractive this way. She eats so little. She now wears dresses three sizes smaller than she did before.

2. Billy is getting in with the wrong crowd of kids and acquiring some genuinely bad habits. It will not be long before he is picked up by the police for being a trouble-maker. He is so immature. When will he grow up?

3. The client is confused. He is more confused now than he used to be. The staff found him wandering around and directed him to return to his room. He just kept on doing what he was doing and ignored them. Maybe he should be sedated more.

## Exercise 6

*Purpose:*  *Develop skill in using clear and precise language*

### DIRECTIONS

1. Identify a concrete aspect of nursing and health care in which you are interested. Describe it verbally and in writing using clear and precise language.

2. Identify an abstract aspect of nursing and health care in which you are interested. Describe it verbally and in writing using clear and precise language.

## Exercise 7

*Purpose:*  *Reflect on language as a tool to foster critical thinking*

### DIRECTIONS

1. Describe an example from your experience in which using jargon, vague, or ambiguous language created a misunderstanding. What was the context? What words created the problem? What did you intend to communicate? What was heard? How was it heard? How did you determine that a communication problem existed? How did you correct it? Replay the incident. How would you do it differently?

2. Define the following words from a medical and a lay perspective:

Ambulate

NPO

BID

QD

Per Os

## Exercise 8

*Purpose:* *Develop skill in using clear and precise language*

### DIRECTIONS

Solicit two volunteers, one to role-play a nurse taking a health history from a client and another to play the role of the client. The remainder of the class should assume the role of unobtrusive observers.

**Nurse:**      You are taking a health history on a client and are ready to do a review of the body systems. Use the format you were taught and ask what you believe are appropriate questions. If you need help getting started, ask the following questions related to the gastrointestinal system as an example to stimulate your own questioning style.

1. Do you have any difficulty with your gastrointestinal tract?

2. Does your stomach hurt?

3. How often does your stomach hurt?

4. Do you have frequent stomachaches?

5. Do you have occasional stomachaches?

**Client:**      Decide on your gender, age, ability level, education, culture, and attitude toward health care providers. Answer the nurse's questions as you hear them, based on your beliefs.

**Observers:**   Note the language the nurse uses to ask each question and the language the client uses to answer. How do the client's answers differ depending on how the question is framed? Is the nurse's intended meaning accurately interpreted by the client? Are the questions sufficiently broad-based to accommodate the client's response? Are the questions leading? In what way? Do the questions limit the scope of the client's response? How? How would this exercise have been different had a real client been interviewed? A client from another culture?

## Exercise 9

*Purpose:* *Develop skill in using clear and precise language*

### DIRECTIONS

Read the following passages. Identify all vague words that need to be defined to promote effective communication. Then, rewrite the passages so the meaning is clear to you. When you have finished, share your rewritten passages with your colleagues and critique each others' responses.

1. Cindy, a 16-year-old client had come into the clinic with a chief complaint of not feeling well, with frequent and painful urination of short duration. After a careful workup, it was determined that she had cystitis, and a course of antibiotic therapy was prescribed. Cindy informed the nurse that she does not like to take drugs and will reluctantly take the medication only until she feels better. She further states that she uses only natural remedies, preferring to keep her body free of artificial chemicals and impurities.

2. A well qualified leader is an important asset in managing a nursing unit. The nurse manager is responsible for creating a positive atmosphere on the unit and on the other levels of the nursing hierarchy in the institution. A positive atmosphere enables staff to communicate freely, ask questions, make suggestions, and experiment with new ways of doing things. A positive atmosphere is essential to providing high quality nursing care. It keeps interpersonal conflicts to a minimum.

## Exercise 10

**Purposes:** *Develop awareness of the variety of meanings possible for words commonly used in health care*
*Illustrate the vagueness of terms thought to be commonly understood*

### DIRECTIONS

Divide into small groups. Without conferring with each other, write down five words you think of when you hear each of the following terms: health, illness, nurse, and caring.

Compare your list with those of others in your group. Tally the number of times the same word appeared for each term. How many different words were identified for each term? How did the meaning of each word vary among members of the group?

Have each individual describe his or her meaning of each word. What is your reaction to the different words you heard? What did you learn from this exercise?

## Exercise 11

**Purpose:** *Recognize ambiguity*

### DIRECTIONS

Below is a list of words commonly used in health care that are ambiguous. Identify two distinct meanings for each. Use the dictionary or discuss it with colleagues if you are unsure.

| | | |
|---|---|---|
| drug | pain | headache |
| stress | breech | risk |
| depressed | labor | eliminate |
| critical | material | tension |
| degree | exercise | discharge |
| motor | mass | feel |
| reform | | |

## Exercise 12

**Purpose:** *Recognize labels*

### DIRECTIONS

Read the following statement, identify the labels, and discuss those circumstances in which you would agree and disagree with the statement. Reframe the word *drug* in ways that are both positive and negative. Rewrite the sentences that reflect your intent to inform, persuade, and inspire.

Drug use in the United States is on the rise. Because so many people use them, all drugs should be legalized and made freely available to those who want them.

## REFERENCES

Adams, K. (1990). *Journal to the self.* New York: Warner.

Ailinger, R.L. (1982). Hypertension knowledge in a Hispanic community. *Nursing Research, 31*(4), 207-210.

Babcock, D.E., and Miller, M.A. (1994). *Client education: Theory and practice.* St Louis: Mosby.

Blum, D.E. (1993, January 27). Arizona professor offers curriculum on ignorance to give medical education a wake-up call. *The Chronicle of Higher Education,* p. A21.

Bradley-Springer, L. (1993). Discovery of meaning through imagined experience, writing and evaluation. *Nurse Educator, 18*(5), 5-10.

Browne, M.N., and Keeley, S.M. (1994). *Asking the right questions* (4th ed.). Englewood Cliffs, N.J.: Prentice Hall.

Chaffee, J. (1994). *Thinking critically* (4th ed.). Boston: Houghton Mifflin.

Dewey, J. (1933). *How we think.* Chicago: Henry Regnery.
————. (1916). *Essays in experimental logic.* Chicago: University of Chicago.

Engel, S.M. (1994). *With good reason: An introduction to informal fallacies* (5th ed.). New York: St. Martin's Press.

Halpern, D.F. (1984). *Thought and knowledge: An introduction to critical thinking.* Hillsdale, N.J.: Lawrence Erlbaum Associates.

Hughes, W. (1992). *Critical thinking.* Lewiston, N.Y.: Broadview.

Johannsen, J.M. (1993). Update: Guidelines for treating hypertension. *American Journal of Nursing, 93*(3), 42-49.

Kim, J.C.S. (1994). *Introduction to logic.* New York: McGraw-Hill.

Laing, M.K. (1994). Letting the healing begin. *American Journal of Nursing, 94*(8), 48-50.

Malone, R. (1994). 'Disturbing trend' cites health care as a commodity and patients as consumers. *The American Nurse, 26*(8), 20.

Mirin, S.K. (1981). *The nurse's guide to writing for publication.* Wakefield, Mass.: Nursing Resources.

Moore, B.N., and Parker, R. (1992). *Critical thinking* (3rd ed.). Mountain View, Calif.: Mayfield.

Neufeldt, V. (1991). *Webster's new world dictionary* (3rd ed.). New York: Webster's New World.

Ruggiero, V.R. (1991). *The art of thinking* (3rd ed.). New York: Harper Collins.

Samuelson, R.J. (1993, October 4). Health care. *Newsweek,* pp. 31-35.

Schon, D.A. (1983). *The reflective practitioner: How professionals think in action.* New York: Basic Books.

Snow, L.F. (1991). Folk medical beliefs and their implications for the care of patients: A review based on studies among Black Americans. In G. Henderson and M. Primeaux (Eds.), *Transcultural health care* (pp. 78-101). Menlo Park, Calif.: Addison-Wesley.

————. (1983). Traditional health beliefs and practice among lower class Black Americans. *Western Journal of Medicine, 139*(6), 820-828.

Wassman, R., and Rinsky, L.A. (1993). *Effective reading in a changing world.* Englewood Cliffs, N.J.: Prentice Hall.

Weber, B. (1994, August 4). United takes charge of baggage. *Rocky Mountain News,* p. 4a.

# Thinking Creatively

Chapter 5

## OVERVIEW

Chapter 5 considers creative thinking and examines several questions: What is creative thinking? How is it different from critical thinking? Is it good thinking? When should we use it? Is it a gift, or can we develop it in ourselves? Can we promote it among our colleagues, team members, and children? Throughout the chapter we apply examples of the use of creative thinking to general life situations and to nursing.

## CREATIVE AND CRITICAL THINKING

What is creative thinking? It is the combination of knowledge and imagination (Ruggiero, 1991). Creative thinking occurs when the conscious thinking of the left brain and the spontaneous patterning and imaging of the right brain merge. The right side of the brain offers unusual connections and alternatives to the left brain, which orders and sequences the connections and images into a comprehensible perspective (Springer and Deutsch, 1981). More comprehensive physiological explanations of this intellectual process have emerged since technologically sophisticated equipment allow us to monitor and better understand the normal human brain in action (Raichle, 1994).

Creative thinkers are willing to be "different." Artists are considered creative thinkers. They have the most liberty to be unconventional in appearance and actions. Creative thinkers are more open than many people to ideas that may contradict their own. They are more willing to accept risky ideas. They are resourceful and hardworking. The notion of the creative genius lying around waiting for an inspiration is a myth. Thomas Edison said, "Genius is one percent inspiration and ninety-nine percent perspiration" (Adler, 1990).

Widely recognized creative people such as Albert Einstein, Marie Curie, and Margaret Mead described themselves as doing their most creative work when they experienced a deep, single-minded, trancelike intensity of being totally immersed in their work—a phenomenon known as the "flow experience" (Csikszentmihalyi, 1990). Nurses have described similar experiences when they have had a "good COR," or a "good day" when "everything went right," or they were able to pick up and respond to many slight cues and "catch things" before they got out of control.

Amabile (1990) found that most people are more prolific when they are exploring for internal satisfaction. Like the person who climbs a mountain "because it's there," the creative person commences and persists in an activity, idea, or production because the creator cannot wait to see the results.

In retrospect the idea that earns the label "creative" is one that can stand the scrutiny of critical thinking and appears logical and valuable once it has come into existence.

## Comparison of Creative and Critical Thinking

How is creative thinking different from critical thinking? One way of differentiating the two is to use the sponge and filter analogy (Browne and Keeley, 1994). Critical thinking uses the filter approach: we evaluate the clarity of argument, tease out hypotheses, check for consistencies, and note the congruence of the logic from one step to the next. We look for flaws; we take a cautious view of the statements offered in defense of the position. In creative thinking we take the sponge approach: we absorb every idea, every bit of information on anything, any thought, and every angle, no matter how seemingly unrelated.

Another way to differentiate between these two processes is to view creative thinking as the kind of thinking to use when you construct a hypothesis, and critical thinking as the kind to use when you test that hypothesis. The creative thinker is characterized by the ability to tolerate and even welcome alternative, parallel, and even paradoxical hypotheses.

Critical thinking is sometimes characterized by the attitudes of doubt, tentativeness, and caution. When you think critically, you question all assumptions usually made by people when they think. You assume that all of the data are not in and the case is not closed. You adopt a wait-and-see attitude. You base your conclusions on the evidence at your disposal. When you think creatively, you may take some sort of intellectual leap; you invest time, money, energy and maybe face difficulties to carry out an experiment before the idea is well tested or guaranteed to pay off. In Table 5-1, words frequently associated with critical thinking are compared with words frequently associated with creative thinking.

One of the characteristics of the creative phase is setting aside the law of noncontradiction. According to binary logic, things cannot be and not be at the same time. Thinking critically requires you to focus on one thing at a time. Creative thinking requires you to entertain apparent contradictions simultaneously. You may merge items, events, and ideas that seem contradictory.

The story of the blind men who each perceived the animal they were touching differently illustrates the importance of creative thinking. In this story one man thought the animal was short and fat like a tree trunk, and another man perceived the animal to be long and thin like a snake. They argued about their perceptions. If a creative thinker had been among them, perhaps that person would have asked how they might both be right, or hypothesize that each of them had discovered a piece in a large puzzle: the animal they were feeling was an elephant.

Table 5-1   **Contrasts Between Critical Thinking and Creative Thinking**

| CRITICAL THINKING | CREATIVE THINKING |
| --- | --- |
| Selective | Generative |
| Orderly | Messy |
| Predictable | Unpredictable |
| Follows a path | Creates a path |
| Direction is clear | Direction is murky |
| Analytical | Provocative |
| Step by step | Leaps forward, backward, and sideways |
| Enforces rules | Breaks rules |
| Reasons stated | No good reason |
| Well thought out | Spontaneous |
| Most likely next step | Least likely next step |
| Probabilities | Possibilities |
| Judgmental | Playful |
| Evaluative | Tinkering |
| Why | How |
| Method oriented | Process oriented |
| Congruency | Contradiction |

The critical thinker compares what is proposed with what he or she believes to be true or is known. The creative thinker compares what he or she thinks with what he or she conjectures might be another truth.

In addition to projecting an attitude of open-mindedness and willingness to tolerate or even welcome divergent points of view, the creative thinker challenges any solution as only a possible answer. The creative thinker has a penchant for trying to generate alternatives and to restructure current patterns. Discovering the unknown appeals to creative thinkers.

## Appraisal

Is creative thinking good thinking? Marzano and colleagues (1988) believe that creative thinking is an essential component of good thinking. They, along with others (Ennis, 1985; Paul, 1990), integrate critical and creative thinking into a unified model. "All good thinking involves both quality assessment and the production of novelty. Critical thinkers generate ways to test assertions; creative thinkers examine newly generated thoughts to assess their validity and utility. The difference is not of kind but of degree and emphasis" (Marzano, et al., 1988, p. 17).

Critical reasoning is particularly important for weighing long-term decisions such as practicing a particular lifestyle. When the consequences of the decision may be costly and lengthy, the individual should engage in careful and deliberate critical thinking.

Creative thinking is complementary to critical thinking; it is needed when known solutions fail and when change occurs quickly. Like critical thinking, creative thinking has limited usefulness, but when it is needed, there is no substitute. Many nurses report that they are not encouraged to think creatively during their basic education. Following rules is the emphasis. Fortunately this idea is changing (Demetrulias and Shaw, 1985).

## APPLICATIONS OF CREATIVE THINKING

When should we use creative thinking? Creativity plays an important role in helping us view the ways in which nursing care evolves. Our definitions of health, nursing, and health care delivery will shape our behavior and our responses to what we encounter.

Creative thinking can serve critical thinking when we imagine the future and how we want that future to be. Creativity is coming to be valued as an essential component of change and constructive progress. It is as valuable as knowledge and techniques, both of which are becoming more accessible as our communication systems improve.

A situation in which creative thinking might help involves Mrs. Kaye, a 92-year-old female with extensive Mohs surgery. The flesh of the woman's nose was gutted almost to the mucus cells of her nostrils. Some cartilage was also shaved to remove cancer cells. There was enough skin on the top and sides to pull together with stitches. The cartilage is still exposed and after five weeks there is still no sign of granulation over the cartilage. A home nurse is visiting everyday to inspect the wound, cleanse the skin, and apply antibacterial ointment and a bandage. The nurse is frustrated because the woman is not learning to dress her own nose and because her healing time is slow. Some creative options to consider—look in an old "five and ten" for a magnifying mirror, write the directions in print, 3/4 of an inch high, send a colleague to do therapeutic touch on the woman (or learn yourself), assign the client to show you pictures of noses. If she forgets—ask colleagues to bring in pictures of noses and every day ask her which ones she prefers. Both spiritual nursing (therapeutic touch) and psychological nursing (age appropriate focused concentration) might boost the woman's healing powers. Look at the woman's pills—she refuses to take any more. Can the nurse find a multivitamin to take instead of the magnesium or potassium with a similar dosage?

Critical thinking works better when facts are known or can be learned. Theoretically, facts about the past and present are available, and hypotheses about these events can be tested. Future events, however, are uncertain. We can extrapolate and predict on the basis of analysis of the past, but we cannot be sure. Critical thinking is conducted with an attitude of caution and desire for information to support or refute the hypothesis.

Creative thinking is less cautionary than critical thinking. Creative thinking does not rely on certainty as a way of preparing for the future. Many kinds of thinking take courage. While the critical thinker must show courage to take in evidence and stick to a particular conclusion in spite of its lack of popularity or disruption of personal beliefs, the creative thinker must make predictions about the future, act on hunches, and experience the results.

The creative thinker applies what she or he learns in another discipline to her or his own discipline. Further, the creative thinker often sees lessons in everyday life that can be applied to her or his area of creative focus. In the above example about Mrs. Kaye, the nurses would be experimenting with several variables at once with no guarantee that they would work.

## Characteristics of Creative Thinking

Creativity is a great motivator, because it makes work more interesting. While thinking creatively we generate options and alternative approaches and envision the future. Creative thinking is characterized by an attitude of interest in everything and a generalized playfulness toward ideas. The creative thinker searches for new ideas and manipulates knowledge and experience as if they were toys.

Sometimes a playful attitude can help solve a problem. For example, consider the young nurse who was unable to manage the computer at work. When she watched the ease with which the computer was manipulated by little children, she felt like she was a failure. A colleague suggested that she turn the computer into a toy and play with it like the children did. Altering her frame of reference allowed the young nurse to release her fears of making mistakes and looking foolish; rather, she shifted her focus and was able to be comfortable with the computer and to have fun while learning. In general, children are less afraid than adults to make mistakes or to look foolish.

By changing your perspective, branching out on a particular path, meandering off a particular path of focus, and playing with knowledge, you may come up with a new idea, solution, or tactic to handle an argument or problem. For example, consider the community health office that was growing rapidly. The supervisor met with the staff to present a problem that was a mixed blessing. The company had expanded so rapidly that the staff needed to expand. At this point, however, they could not afford to move again. A new nurse, Elisa, would augment the evening staff. Because all of the offices were full, someone would have to share an office. Until that time everyone had a separate office. After considering drawing lots and the rule "last hired, first to share," the group decided that Mario, the day nurse with the earliest shift, would share his office. Because Elisa would be working the evening shift, the group reasoned that the pair were less likely to be in each other's way. Mario countered with a proposal to convert a storage area into an office. He even offered to organize the stored items and to paint the new office. Mario used creative thinking to handle the problem.

The creative thinker, like the artist, looks at the same thing that everyone else looks at; however, the creative thinker perceives these same objects differently. The painter sees more detail and color in the leaves, more shapes in the clouds, than others less artistic. The vocalist hears shades of tonal differences that are lost on the ordinary ear. The creative person perceives the same stimuli as others, but responds to them differently. While a person may think about an idea and the logical consequences of following that line of thought, the person in a creative phase thinks about that one idea, turns it around backward and argues the other way, and then turns it sideways and argues a whole different direction from a whole new set of premises.

In the musical play *Fiddler on the Roof,* Tevya, a Jewish father, tries to reconcile his obligations to fulfill tradition, while granting his daughters their personal choices in life mates. In very amusing and touching scenes, he argues with himself using the phrase "on the other hand" to indicate his shifts in reasoning. Finally in a dream he finds a way out of the most complicated predicament—reneging on his pledge to give one of his daughters to a man who could make his life easier.

Tevya illustrates what happens to us when we enter conflict. He solved his dilemma by entertaining paradoxical ideas until a solution emerged. When we need to generate new ways to accomplish our objectives, we may need to reexamine our own traditional way of thinking. For example, many registered nurses find satisfaction in primary nursing. They believe it to be the only safe way to provide good care at the bedside. Yet we are being confronted with the reality that nurse extenders will take over many of those tasks. Most of us find it very difficult to relinquish our beliefs whether or not they are based on objective evidence. By entertaining all of the variables without judgement (we must make more use of nurse extenders, we must lower costs, we must protect client safety) we may be able to offer creative experiments.

## Uses for Creative Thinking

Creative thinking is very useful when what we know and what we know how to do are not working, including the rules of reason, common sense, gravity, and routine. The creative thinker is willing to think wildly, without having any idea where her or his path of thinking may lead. Deliberative cognition is temporarily held in abeyance. Focused thinking (Paul, 1990) is set aside in favor of association that is considered undisciplined. DeBono (1992) believes that creative thinking does not have to be undisciplined. He believes that structures should be present to help thinkers focus on the problem; however, many constructive ideas appear when the thinker is not focused on a problem. For example, people often come up with ideas and solutions when just taking a walk. In all fairness, creative thinking can appear undisciplined, particularly during certain phases. Creative thinking can indeed be characterized by undisciplined association that bypasses previous paths and rules, to allow new associations and new pathways to originate (Baer, 1993).

Creative thinking may be used for crisis intervention, such as when an important piece of equipment fails to function properly while it is being used with a very sick individual, or when administrative personnel announce that they intend to cut the nursing staff. The crisis might occur as you enter a new developmental phase within your family: you discover that your child has a pronounced rash just as you leave for work or that your elderly parent who lives in another state is confused when you make your regularly scheduled phone call. Crises occur in many forms and they vary in severity. All crises prevent us from using our usual problem-solving techniques; however, we cannot ignore or delay dealing with the crises. We must act immediately. We must use creative thinking to find a solution to the problem.

For example, consider the instructor who began a weekly seminar with an exercise designed to promote relaxation and centering. The students appreciated the exercise because it allowed them to unwind from traffic and other cares to focus on their clinical concerns. One student, however, volunteered that at this particular time, she was unable to relax. She was frustrated. She had difficulty identifying her source of frustration, and the other students' suggestions on how they soothed themselves were not helpful. She was obviously irritated, sitting with her arms folded. She confessed to trying to pick a fight with her husband and noted her son's puzzled looks at her "weird" behavior. The instructor recognized the need to address the student's frustration right on the spot. She distributed a box of salt water taffy to the group, inviting them to throw the candy at each other. Amid a good bit of throwing and hilarity, the energy in the room changed, and the frustrated student was able to get in touch with what frustrated her.

In this situation, the instructor, after seeing that one line of intervention (soothing) was not being helpful, used creative thinking to lead the group in the opposite direction (a fight). The instructor helped the frustrated student focus on her anger. This harmless and silly way to express anger freed up the student from being stuck. She and her peers then had a meaningful discussion about caring for a client whose values conflict with the care giver. One advantage of creative thinking is that it offers the freedom to look beyond the one right answer. The answers we find are integrally related to the question we ask. To find another answer, we ask different questions.

## PROMOTING CREATIVE THINKING

Is creative thinking a gift, or can we develop it in ourselves, our children, our clients, and our staff? All people are creative in different ways. Some people are more creative in certain areas than others, and some people seem to be creative in everything they do. Creative thinking may be more conspicuous or significant in some individuals. For example, the leaders who constructed the Magna Carta and the constitution of the United States were creative in a long-lasting and historically significant way. These accomplishments are of greater historical significance than the manufacture of the bobby pin. Like many other human traits, creative thinking seems to come easier to certain individuals. Indeed, some of us may be born with much natural creative talent. If we were aware of creative thinking, its value, and if we knew how to promote it in ourselves, our students, our assistant personnel, and our clients, we could use it to benefit ourselves and others. How creativity is defined and valued is greatly influenced by the context in which it emerges. If our environment demands or asks for creativity and rewards it, more creative actions emerge (Albert, 1990; Albert and Runco, 1990; Csikszentmihalyi, 1990). An environment that exposes you to different ways of thinking will raise your chances of being creative (Rosella, Regan-Kubinski, and Albrecht, 1994).

### Notice Your Own Creativity

Natural creative thinkers may believe that how to be creative is obvious. They may believe that everyone thinks like they do or that everyone can see what they see.

Others who admire creative individuals may assume they themselves are not creative. Both assumptions could be wrong. Only by allowing yourself to be creative can you establish how much capability you really have.

The amorphous command or even permission to be creative, however, may not be helpful to some people, even if they wished to learn. Boden (1991) noted that creativity is unpredictable. You increase your chances of being creative if you develop positive attitudes and practice thinking creatively (Russ, 1993). The more ideas you come up with, the more chance you have of being creative. Your first thoughts are more likely to follow the paths you think you know or the probabilities you have learned to expect. What you think you know is defined by the rules and by the frame of reference you learned to use when thinking in general and about specific topics. You confine yourself when you limit your thinking according to these rules and the accompanying assumptions.

To become creative in your thinking, you need to move beyond the usual, let go of the most logical path, be willing to experiment with various paths, throw out the central concepts and ideas involved, and start with a new set of assumptions and possibilities (Leff and Nevin, 1990). Emphasize possibility thinking. The possibility thinker is willing to start with premises that appear absurd to others and thus lie fallow. The possibility thinker often makes assumptions that appear unlikely and follows through, using logical processes to discover where the assumptions might lead. The exercises at the end of this chapter encourage this process.

Creative thinking may be promoted through a number of channels that are connected to the mind, namely the senses. You can promote your creativity by talking about creativity itself, or you can have fun being creative about a problem you encounter. To increase your creative thinking abilities, let go of your inhibitions, fear of being wrong, seeming ridiculous, judgments, and the idea of seeking *the* one right answer. Paul (1990) claims that a tolerance for backtracking, self-contradiction, and zigging and zagging are necessary to creative thinking.

## Be Open to New Ideas

Thinking creatively necessitates a particular set of attitudes and methods to treat information. The creative thinker can approach information with an attitude of experimentation and openness to novelty. The solution to a problem may be found by turning the problem upside down or sideways. For example, in Australia a private phone company made its reputation by charging one price for a phone call rather than by a price per minute. The company's charging scheme caused a dilemma: people were staying on the phone too long, eating into the company's profits. Because company officials did not want to change their method of charging per call, they devised a solution: to make the hand pieces very heavy by putting lead in them so callers would tire and terminate their calls.

The creative thinker focuses on results—not the method used to achieve the results. The creative thinker may tinker around with some information when she or he notices a particular effect. If the effect is useful, the thinker is delighted. In retrospect she or he will examine the activities that led to the effect in an effort to repeat it. When you encounter a mistake or an unexpected event, try redefining the situation as a new possibility. In sewing, a mistake is a new design. In cooking, it is the base for a new recipe.

Consider the implications of creative thinking for Dolores, a home health nurse who became involved with Virginia, a client who suffered incapacitating pain from sciatic nerve involvement. Virginia was in such pain that she could not shop for groceries or drive herself to the medical clinic. During her assessment of Virginia's health, Dolores learned that Virginia was constantly asked by the physician and the physical therapist what caused her hip injury. She insisted that she had not done anything. Dolores also noted that Virginia looked frail. In addition, she learned that Virginia's husband, who had required years of intense physical care, had died within the past year. Virginia was lonely and welcomed company. As she listed all of the guests who had come from out of town, she confided that she was ready to collapse. Dolores hypothesized that developing an inflamed sciatic nerve allowed Virginia to do just that—collapse.

Dolores suggested to Virginia that perhaps her body had gone on strike from being overworked with too much company. Virginia admitted that she had never thought of that. They spent the rest of their session considering options: writing a pro and con list of effects of having company, listing the traits of "relaxing company" and "exhausting company," and findings ways to graciously refuse visitors.

Before leaving Dolores developed a form and asked Virginia to fill it in (see the Differentiating Types of Guests box below). The purpose of the form was to enlist Virginia to think on her own behalf and to continue taking some responsibility for some social

---

**Differentiating Types of Guests**

1. Why have company?

| Pros | Cons |
| --- | --- |
| _____ | _____ |
| _____ | _____ |
| _____ | _____ |

2. Guest that are comforting and refreshing do:

_____

_____

3. Guest that are thoughtless and exhausting do:

_____

_____

4. Gracious ways to head off or refuse company:

_____

_____

_____

variables that might be affecting her health. Follow-up could be conducted over the phone or at the next visit. If Virginia showed an interest in further exploring such options, Dolores could engage Virginia in some role plays, particularly on practicing refusals to certain company. In this example the nurse used creative thinking to detect a possible pressing issue and to get the client to use critical thinking in addressing the issue. During subsequent visits, the nurse could help the client use creative thinking in role playing to develop refusal skills.

## Try Activities that Promote Creative Thinking

Creative thinking is a basic part of good thinking. You can develop some skill at it with training just as you can develop further skill in critical thinking. An example of promoting creativity is the annual contest for paper airplanes, first sponsored by the magazine *Scientific American*. Experts in the field of aerodynamics and interested amateurs compete in this contest. The contest allows its participants to tap into the "creative child within" and produce new ideas.

***Brainstorming.*** Brainstorming is a group problem-solving technique that involves the spontaneous contribution of ideas from all members of the group (*Webster's Collegiate Dictionary*, 1993). Participants set aside consequences and practicalities during the hatching phase. The rules for the initial brainstorming phase include *not* filtering the practicality of any idea that occurs. The group builds on unusual and absurd ideas, spiraling off in many directions instead of critiquing them. The group leader encourages fantasy, visionary thinking, and impracticality. After exploiting all of the possibilities, the group looks for ramifications of these ways. When the group has exhausted its time limit or its ability to elaborate on the ideas it has created, it then focuses on finding ways to make these possibilities into probabilities, using criteria that the group has established: cost-effectiveness (time, money, and energy) and investments that show the most promise of producing the greatest gain. The group then starts prioritizing and setting up time lines for doing pilot projects. Brainstorming has been used particularly by groups that must anticipate the future and set up plans for a time and circumstances that are not yet present.

***Divergent Thinking.*** Divergent thinking skills can be taught, encouraged, and nurtured. They appear to have a positive influence on the increase of creative thinking (Guilford, 1967). Instructions such as "Think of as many ways as you can to use intravenous tubing" is an example of encouraging divergent thinking. Another example is "Draw all the things that you have studied in your anatomy book or that you have seen in your clinical experiences that include a circle." After all of the ideas have been exhausted, ask yourself such questions as "How can I change or reverse it? What else could it be or do if I added to, subtracted from, or combined it with something else? What would occur if I made it bigger, smaller, thinner, or weaker?" For instance, list all of the safe self-injections spots that an athlete can reach. This question might produce a variety of responses. You could elaborate on it by then answering the questions: "What if the person were stiff? Obese?"

***Analogies.***   Creating and completing analogies promote divergent thinking. Try completing the sentence "I am like an ocean because . . ." or "I am like a mountain because . . ." Tasks that require the generation of a variety of possible paths promote creative thinking.

***Mind Mapping.***   A mind map, which promotes associative thinking, is a tangible representation of stream of consciousness thinking. Mind mapping can be done with balloons or with branches and involves five steps. Step 1 is to find a large surface on which to write, such as cardboard or a large piece of newsprint. Step 2 is to write down a central idea or problem and draw a balloon around it. Step 3 is to record all of the impressions that come to mind that the word or central idea evokes; circle them, and draw lines from them to the central theme. Step 4 is to go back to each initial impression and elaborate on it; record specific thoughts, observations, and questions that occur to you; draw balloons around them; and draw lines attaching these new thoughts to the stimulus. Step 5 is to go back to each new thought and add to it. Continue the process until you run out of time, space, energy, or ideas.

Mind mapping promotes divergent thinking and system thinking, which specifies that everything is connected to everything else. Using branches such as you might find on a tree or bush instead of balloons is an alternate way of promoting this kind of thinking. Figs. 5-1 and 5-2 are examples of mind maps.

The Torrance tests for creative thinking attempt to measure the capacity for creative thinking by evaluating the amount of fluency, flexibility, elaboration, and originality that an individual is able to produce in response to the test questions (Gowan, Khatena, and Torrance, 1981). Fluency refers to the number of responses the individual can produce. Flexibility refers to the number of different categories into which the responses fit. Elaboration refers to the amount of embellishment that the individual does to each item, such as adding corners to it, inserting items into it, or designing it to serve several uses. Originality refers to the amount of responses that are novel or unique, unlike the responses of everyone else.

Although divergent thinking has played a very important role in the development of theories of creativity, it should be kept in proper perspective. Some people believe integrative thinking is the essential characteristic of creative thinking (Songxing and Guozheng, 1989). No singular type of thinking can be the essence of creative thought. How could it, when by its very definition creative thinking means new and novel ways of thinking?

## Promote Creative Thinking

Self-regulation is an individual's ability to modify physiological activity, behavior, or cognitive processes (Pesut, 1990). Self-monitoring is careful and deliberate attending to your own thinking, feeling, and doing. Self-evaluation means comparing your own performance with a set of criteria, standards, or expectations of a desired outcome. Self-reinforcement is the administration of a set of contingencies you have chosen to shape your own behavior in a desired direction.

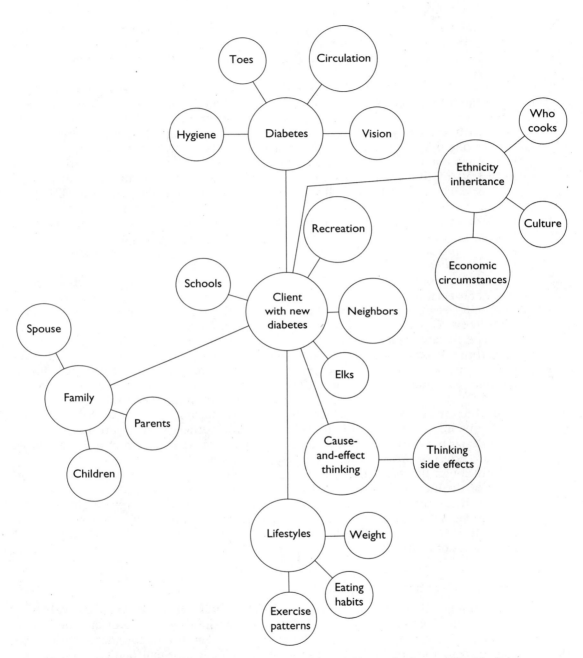

**Fig. 5-1** This mind map illustrates issues of concern for a client newly diagnosed with diabetes mellitus. The concerns are grouped in beginning clusters.

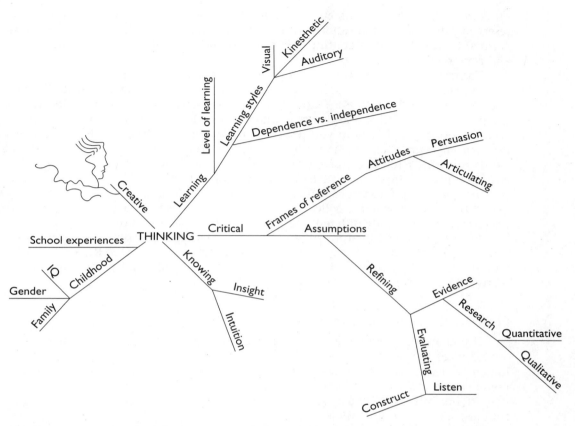

**Fig. 5-2** Branching associations allow you to relate certain concepts to each other. This is an example of the associations you might make with the work *thinking*. Thinking is the original stimulus. The other words are associated with it.

You may promote creative thinking by using free association, visualizing, and synthesizing unrelated ideas. One way of viewing all thinking is that it is a dynamic balance between divergent and convergent thinking (Songxing and Guozheng, 1989). Another way you may promote creative thinking is to pay attention to yourself and reward yourself when you recognize that you are thinking creatively. Congratulate yourself whenever you act creatively to meet a particular goal. Celebrate with your peers when you have achieved a goal or done something creative in the service of your goal. Call your own thoughts creative aloud. Treat yourself when you complete a specified task creatively. For an example illustrating the significance of recognizing and reinforcing creative thinking, consider the nurse who was raised in a conservative home where modesty was prized. The nurse tended to be on the reserved side, which affected her relationship with clients and coworkers. She made friends with a very outgoing colleague, who sometimes talked about her own "brilliant thoughts." The reserved nurse found that after a while, she also started calling her own thoughts "brilliant," which led to a continued confidence that enabled her to deal with clients and coworkers effectively.

To promote creative thinking in yourself, try to capture your thoughts in your journal, even if they do not seem immediately useful to you. You may write or draw your thoughts (Adams, 1994). Think about a pattern of thinking and behavior that in the past had merit but no longer fits you currently. Reflect about it in your journal. Seek out other people whom you respect but who have a viewpoint that is very different from yours. Quiz them and listen carefully. Try to grasp the meaning of their words from their frame of reference. Listen carefully at work to several people discussing the same situation. Notice how widely disparate their perceptions can be. Collect newspapers, photographs, problems, stories, anecdotes, themes, and ideas suggested by children, clients, colleagues, and others. Collect articles from papers and magazines that illustrate different ways of looking at the same situation.

Read some more literature on what has been learned about how the mind works. Learn to think from a culturally diverse frame of reference (Rosella, Regan-Kubinski, and Albrecht, 1994). Any particular way of looking at things is only one from among many other possible ways.

## Promote Creative Thinking in Others

If you are the leader at a brainstorming meeting, go last or first and offer really absurd ideas to keep the more timid or politically attuned members from trying to match your ideas instead of offering their own original creations. If you are a group member and anticipate attending such a meeting, dream up your own ideas before you attend; otherwise, you may become set on the suggested path and fail to contribute your own original thoughts.

To promote creativity in others such as assistive personnel, clients, teammates, and children, expect creativity. Ask for it. Create scenarios such as "Here is a problem. Let us think of 20 things we could do about it." Ask questions designed to generate a variety of possible solutions, rather than presenting the problem as if there is only one correct response (Carroll and Howieson, 1991). Conduct brainstorming sessions. Reinforce creative thinking and problem solving when you see or hear it. Try to let go of defensiveness and negative programming. Do not compare yourself or others unfavorably with someone who is creative. Try to celebrate the creative person's unique talents. Do not respond with answers such as "It will not work because . . ." or "We tried that, and it did not work." Try to respond with a positive and welcoming enthusiastic attitude. An atmosphere of positive expectations and warmth improve creative thinking and problem solving (Greene and Noice, 1988). Capture the ideas on the chalkboard or large sheets of newsprint for everyone to see. Draw lines between thoughts that are spun off other thoughts (such as in a mind map). Develop the idea and related ideas as far as possible. Only after the creative energy of everyone has subsided, ask how these parts or ideas can be put to use. Ask the group what problems they can anticipate and how they might vault those hurdles. Take note of the talents in your group and make use of them. You may have skeptical colleagues who could think of problems with any notion they hear. Tell them it is their job to anticipate problems and possible obstacles. In any size group there are usually very practical members who are good at solving problems or finding ways to actualize possibilities. Call on these people to help surmount obstacles, or think of ways around anticipated difficulties. If you find the whole idea strange, read deBono's (1970) recommendations for lateral thinking. His "different hats" is a useful structure for getting started.

Another way to promote creativity is to shift the point of focus. Pay close attention to some aspect of a construct that is ordinarily ignored. For example, when one nursing unit was being redesigned, the medical personnel went to the unit where the clients were housed, instead of clients being transported to where the care givers were stationed (Porter-O'Grady, 1994).

***Encourage Creativity in Children.***   When a care giver responds joyfully to a baby, the care giver is promoting creativity by encouraging the baby to listen, create, performs and enjoy his or her own sounds (Moore, 1990). Babies perceive and create musical sounds at the earliest stages of life. Parents can encourage experimentation and provide an environment rich with new possibilities by singing with and to the child, tapping on toys with a spoon, and allowing the child to play with the pots and pans.

According to Moore (1990), the principle motivators during early childhood are play and self-satisfaction. If you wish to promote creativity in older children, give them tasks that require a variety of possible solutions, such as "See how many size squares you can divide these squares into." "How many ways can you calculate to get the answer 30?" Avoid giving problems for which there is only one correct answer, such as "What is the answer to 15 + 15?"

***Check with Reality.***   When promoting creativity in children, you need to balance it with reality checks. If a child is creatively adding numbers and comes up with the wrong answer, the child needs to be told that he or she is wrong and to be shown how to do it correctly. Some people conclude that spontaneous, free association is an easier substitute for careful, laborious, and intensive mental work; however, it is not. Free association is a valuable step in the process of good thinking and problem solving, but it will not provide a complete solution.

A creative thought or action is not always useful. How do you distinguish between nonproductive creative thinking and productive creativity? Going with a creative idea for fun just because it is fun is different from corralling ideas to produce something that is effective and constructive. The former is a distraction, a source of amusement. It may not actually be productive in itself. That sort of personal expression is fine and a worthwhile recreational activity, because you are more likely to think better when you are refreshed. It can also get a group or individual who is stuck to get off dead center. Eventually, you need to filter your idea through critical thinking. In other words, eventually you have to apply holistic thinking. Creative thinking is incomplete without critical thinking and vice versa.

To be creative is wonderful, but when a person's health is in jeopardy, you need to process your ideas quickly. To think long and critically about anticipating emergencies and developing plans of action that take into consideration most of the likely problems is wise. A recurring emergency should have a protocol worked out by experts who have experience in dealing successfully with such crises. Your job in such a situation is to get training ahead of time and accede to the commands of the designated leader—not to think creatively. A crisis is a time of unified and smooth, efficient action in response to a well thought out plan. Perhaps during the rehash of such a situation, questions and options can be considered.

When you function as the leader of a nursing care team, you must observe carefully what kind of thinking and behavior your assistive personnel exhibit. You will want to accurately assess their level of maturity, values, and communication levels, and the reinforcement they have had for thinking creatively in the past (Harrington, 1990). You may need to be very creative in detecting the personnel's strengths and areas for improvement and in deciding what methods of communication work best with each person (Porter-O'Grady, 1994).

As the workplace and our world become more diverse, we will find creative thinking an ever-increasing necessity. As the pace of change accelerates and familiar structures crumble, we must take chances by creating new structures before we have enough evidence to reasonably support a particular path of thinking. In fact, if we had perfect information in a particular situation, our need for sophisticated thinking would be lessened. Unfortunately, we cannot obtain data about the future.

In a highly competitive environment, doing things better or more efficiently may not be enough. Cutting costs by slashing employment numbers may be hazardous to client safety. We may need to rethink and restructure the work rather than just reduce numbers. Whatever the solution, health care costs are too high. Our nation cannot pay the medical bill. Nurses can either help invent solutions or continue to expect others to solve the problems. We are more likely to be part of the solution if we can think creatively and then evaluate our ideas with the other thinking skills of checking assumptions, using logic, and anticipating consequences. If nurses are to help articulate the dangers of slashing employment numbers, we must present ideas in a positive manner that appeals to the values of the decision makers, and we must present concrete suggestions for addressing those values.

## SUMMARY

Creative thinking is neither inferior to nor superior to critical thinking; they are vital companions. Both aspects of thinking are characterized by curiosity and open-mindedness. Creative thinking is a useful, enjoyable, exciting way to think. It is a very useful tool for solving problems when all of the facts are unknown, the problems are ongoing, the conflicts cannot be permanently resolved, and the environment in which the problems occur keep changing. To think critically, apply the rules. To think creatively, break the rules!

# EXERCISES

The following exercises may be done alone or with others. You may write them in your journal, or you may be assigned to discuss them in class or with a group of peers.

## Exercise 1

**Purpose:** *Practice freeing yourself from self- or system-imposed limits on your thinking*

### DIRECTIONS

Identify an inefficient situation at work. Imagine that those in charge tell you the situation must be the way it has always been handled to meet their requirements.

1. Ask yourself the following questions and try to answer them in an unusual way.

   ▼ Why is it done this way today?

   ▼ Must it be done this way?

   ▼ What are your barriers to change?

   ▼ Have you considered a different way? Describe.

   ▼ What do you think of this other explanation for what is going on?

   ▼ What if we added _____ to it?

   ▼ What if we simplified it by _____?

2. Find a colleague whom you respect and who is knowledgeable in the situation. Ask your colleague the above questions and listen carefully to his or her answers.

3. What new knowledge or perspective did you gain from this interaction?

## Exercise 2

**Purpose:** *Expand your awareness of situations amenable to tinkering*

### DIRECTIONS

Produce some ideas to reduce costs, shorten the number of days in the hospital or return appointments to a clinic or return home visits, produce a safer cleaning product, shorten telephone calls, speed up the checkout procedure, reduce the frequency of staff turnover, reduce losses to theft, prevent condensation, or address some other problem you have noticed.

## Exercise 3

**Purpose:** *Become aware of and challenge an assumption*

### DIRECTIONS

Argue *against* the following statement: "If it ain't broke, don't fix it."

## Exercise 4

**Purpose:** *Deepen your awareness of the circumstances that promote your own creativity*

### DIRECTIONS

Describe a recent creative idea pertinent to your play. Answer the following questions:

1. How long ago did it happen?
2. How did the idea emerge? Were you just fooling around? At play while observing something? In the middle of the night? While you were at work? While you were researching a problem?
3. How often do such processes occur?

## Exercise 5

**Purpose:** *Deepen your awareness of your own creative processes*

### DIRECTIONS

Describe a recent creative idea pertinent to your work. Answer the following question:

1. How long ago did it happen?
2. How did the idea emerge? Was it at work while you were observing the problem? In the middle of the night? While you were at play? While you were researching the problem? Other?
3. How often do such processes occur?

## Exercise 6

**Purpose:** *Expand your awareness of how you break free of an intellectual block, barrier, or rut*

### DIRECTIONS

Describe a recent creative idea that solved a conflict you had with someone. Answer the following questions:

1. How long ago did it occur?

2. How did the idea emerge? During the argument itself while listening to your opponent? While you were at play? In the middle of the night? While you were at work? While you were researching the problem? Other?

3. How often are you able to do that?

## Exercise 7

**Purpose:** *Expand your awareness of the influence of previous experience on creative problem solving*

### DIRECTIONS

Break into groups based on your length of time in nursing. Problem solve together on the following dilemma: You are working in the emergency department when three people come into the unit at once from a fire disaster, all needing moisturized oxygen. All of the wall units are in use for seriously ill individuals except two. What do you do?

1. Each of you come up with a brainstorming list. At this point they do not have to be practical ideas.

2. After each group has generated three ideas, get together and share your thoughts.

3. Ask the instructor to record any new possibilities that the interchange produces.

4. If time permits, prioritize the ideas. Discuss the influence of previous experiences on the ideas generated.

## Exercise 8

**Purpose:** *Experiment with the process of generating group synergy*

### DIRECTIONS

Form into groups and take 5 minutes to identify your group with a symbol or name that signifies a trait or interest you share in common.

1. Study a splotch and generate as many meanings as possible to explain the splotch.

2. Decide on prize winners (e.g., most creative, most numerous, most expensive, most colorful).

3. Decide on prizes (e.g., being sung to, receiving a 2-minute massage, a piece of candy, a funny nose).

4. Decide on acceptance activities (e.g., song of thanksgiving, return massage, bowing and curtseying [European style], bowing and pointing hands [Oriental style]).

## Exercise 9

**Purpose:** *Compare and contrast creative and critical thinking*

### DIRECTIONS

Differentiate creative thinking and critical thinking by listing characteristics that are diametrically opposed to one another.

1. Discuss which kind of thinking is better and justify your response.
2. Discuss ways in which such diametrically opposed traits could be synthesized.

## Exercise 10

**Purpose:** *Distinguish between playful trivia and goal-directed creativity*

### DIRECTIONS

Describe three creative experiences you have had or you have witnessed that you consider worth noting. Answer the following questions:

1. Why do you call them creative?
2. Why were they significant (as opposed to trivial, not worth noting)?
3. What conditions, in your opinion, added to the possibility that the creative moment could emerge?

## Exercise 11

**Purpose:** *Become aware of ways to capture your creative ideas and to reinforce yourself for creativity*

### DIRECTIONS

Think of a creative activity you have done and write about it in your journal. Select a creative activity that you can recall completely, such as one of the most creative things you have done or one that is recent. The point is to recall it in the fullest possible detail.

1. Name it.
2. Why do you perceive it to be creative and not routine?
3. Why did you pick this project rather than another?
4. Did you know what you wanted to accomplish as you attempted to complete the tasks?
5. What did you think were your chances for success as you began?

6. Did those ideas change during the project?

7. How long did it take from conception of the idea to its completion?

8. How did your environment influence your getting the idea, working on it, completing it, etc. Did someone else give you the idea inadvertently or suggest it to you?

9. How did your environment respond to your exploratory efforts? With encouragement? With discouragement such as: "That's crazy? Why are you wasting my time, energy, or money? Why bother? I want an answer now! Just give them what they want. That's not important. Stop that and do this. I want your attention, your time, and energy for me, or my interests."

10. Did you do it all by yourself or did you receive help?

11. Did you work together or each take a piece of the task? Did you plan it together or did you "run into" each other during the task and decide you could get farther together?

12. What emotions did you encounter during your process? Excitement, tedium, fear, frustration, discouragement, uncertainty, or fear of reception in your ecosystem?

13. If you ran into discouragement or boredom, how did you keep yourself going at that time?

14. In retrospect what were the events that spurred you on the most? Interfered with your progress the most?

15. What did you learn from all this?

# Exercise 12

***Purpose:*** *Use humor to expand your own or another's frame of reference*

## DIRECTIONS

Make up a joke or alter a saying that shows a switch in perceptions. Consider the following example.

A little child who was praying wanted to ask God for a million years. The child asked God how long a million years are. "To you my son, it is a million years, but to me it is only a second," said God. The child asked, "How much is a million dollars to you?" God responded, "It is only a penny to me." The child asked, "Could I have a penny?" And God said, "Yes son, but you'll have to wait a second."

## Exercise 13

**Purpose:** *Gain awareness of the game strategy as a mind-expanding activity*

DIRECTIONS

Get into groups and complete the following steps:

1. Select a letter of the alphabet.
2. Add one letter to it to make a word.
3. Add one more letter to it to make another word using the previous letters.
4. Repeat this procedure as many times as you can. Each time you enlarge the word, you must use all of the letters in the previous word in any order you choose.
5. The group that creates the most words in the allotted time wins.

| | |
|---|---|
| t | h |
| it | ha |
| bit | hat |
| abit | hath |
| habit | that's |

## Exercise 14

**Purpose:** *Experiment with an activity to warm up a lethargic or stuck group*

DIRECTIONS

Repeat Exercise 13 but use building materials instead of letters. The group that builds the highest tower before it crashes wins. You may not support the tower with your hand or other structures.

## Exercise 15

**Purpose:** *Experience symbolically the phenomena of varied perceptions of the same stimulus*

DIRECTIONS

Break into small groups and complete the following steps:

1. Choose a simple figure and draw it.
2. Draw clones of that figure.
3. Combine that figure as many ways as you can think of with its clones.

4. See how many other figures you can create by the way you combine all of the clones.

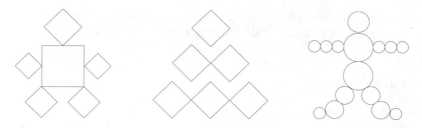

5. See the example.

6. The group with the most (numerous, complex, beautiful, colorful, imaginative) figure(s) wins.

# Exercise 16

**Purpose:** *Experiment with expanding the visual perceptions of a common figure*

## DIRECTIONS

Draw (or receive from the instructor) a page full of circles. Using each circle create as many scenes as possible, relevant to your profession. What have you seen in nursing, anatomy books, and nurseries that you could associate with a circle or draw with a circle? Draw these items or phenomena using the circles.

# Exercise 17

**Purpose:** *Become aware of self-limiting assumptions*

## DIRECTIONS

1. Look at the figure made of dots.

.     .     .

.     .     .

.     .     .

2. Go through all of the dots with four straight lines without repeating yourself or retracing your steps and without lifting your writing implement.

3. Draw a small mark in the middle of a page and a circle around it without lifting your writing implement off the paper. The surrounding circle may *not* be connected to the dot on this drawing.

## Exercise 18

**Purpose:** *Become aware of the many processes involved in developing and testing assumptions and communicating these using the game strategy*

<u>DIRECTIONS</u>

Invent a new dot game.

1. Make up the rules.
2. Solve it to suit yourselves.
3. Give the game to the next group.
4. See how long it takes them to solve it.
5. Note how they solved it. Did they solve it in the same way you did? Did they break any rules you stated? Did they break any rules you assumed but did not state? Did they stymie themselves by obeying (assuming) any rules you did not impose?
6. Discuss what you have learned.

## Exercise 19

**Purpose:** *Experiment with a game as a strategy for learning one aspect of reasoning*

<u>DIRECTIONS</u>

Read the following vignette and solve the problem. If you are a visual learner, you may wish to use visual aids to help you keep track of the players (such as three pennies and three dimes).

Three missionaries and three cannibals are on this side of the river. It is filled with piranhas. You have only one boat that only holds two people. They all know how to row.

Get them across the river without leaving more cannibals than missionaries on either side.

## Exercise 20

**Purpose:** *Experiment with an alternative method of communication*

<u>DIRECTIONS</u>

Make up an analogy. Relate it to something in nursing. If you experience difficulty getting started try the following examples:

▼ A nurse moving from novice to expert is like a ripening apple. (See Chapter 2, Thinking and Learning.)
▼ A rumor is like a snowball rolling down hill.

▼ A nurse who uses only one way of thinking is like a monkey whose hand is trapped in a jar as long as he tries to remove a fistful of nuts from the jar.

▼ Changing your eating habits is like clearing a garden of weeds.

# Exercise 21

***Purpose:*** *Experience at the symbolic visual level a shift in your frame of reference*

## DIRECTIONS

1. Draw a picture or word that changes depending on which way you look at it or frame it. Think of a way you might use this to make a point in nursing (with a colleague, peer, or client).

2. If you think of a great word or picture but cannot think of a use for it, teach it to a classmate and ask for help finding an application.

3. If you cannot think of a word or picture, use the vase/profiles model. Depending on how you view it, the picture is a vase or two profiles.

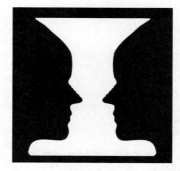

# Exercise 22

***Purpose:*** *Become aware of your own values about the process of creative thinking*

## DIRECTIONS

Read the following and then respond.

Some authors believe that the undisciplined mind, wandering around in a morass (dry or drugged) is not creative and productive; creativity is a product of the disciplined and focused mind. Other authors urge you to pay attention to your "fringe thoughts" that may seem quite random or unconnected at first. How can you tell ahead of time if you are just randomly wandering around or if you are thinking in a creative and productive manner?

## Exercise 23

**Purpose:** *Apply the creative thinking process to a possible improvement at work*

Bring in a piece of equipment you use at your work every day. Describe what is good and bad about it. Describe how you would change it.

## REFERENCES

Adams, K. (1994). *Mightier than the sword.* New York: Warner.

Adler, D.A. (1990). *Thomas Alva Edison: Great inventor.* New York: Holiday House.

Albert, R.S. (1990). Identity, experiences, and career choice among the exceptionally gifted and eminent. In M.A. Runco and R.S. Albert (Eds.), *Theories of creativity* (pp. 13-34). Newbury Park, Calif.: Sage.

Albert, R.S., and Runco, M.A. (1990). Observations, conclusions and gaps. In M.A. Runco and R.S. Albert (Eds.), *Theories of creativity* (pp. 255-269). Newbury Park, Calif.: Sage.

Amabile, T.M. (1990). Within you, without you: The social psychology of creativity and beyond. In M.A. Runco and R.S. Albert (Eds.), *Theories of creativity* (pp. 61-91). Newbury Park, Calif.: Sage.

Baer, J. (1993). *Creativity and divergent thinking.* Hillsdale, N.J.: Lawrence Erlbaum Associates.

Boden, M.A. (1991). *The creative mind.* New York: Basic Books.

Browne N., and Keeley, S. (1994). *Asking the right questions: A guide to critical thinking* (4th ed.). Englewood Cliffs, N.J.: Prentice Hall.

Carroll, J., and Howieson, N. (1991). Recognizing creative thinking talent in the classroom. *Roeper Review, 14*(2), 68-71.

Csikszentmihalyi, M. (1990). The domain of creativity. In M. A. Runco and R. S. Albert (Eds.), *Theories of creativity* (pp. 190-212). Newbury Park, Calif.: Sage.

deBono, E. (1992). *Serious creativity.* New York: Harper Collins.

————. (1970). *Lateral thinking.* New York: Harper and Row.

Demetrulias, D.M., and Shaw, R.J. (1985). Encouraging divergent thinking. *Nurse Educator, 10*(6), 12-17.

Ennis, R.H. (1985). A logical basis for measuring critical thinking skills. *Educational Leadership, 43*(2), 44-48.

Gowan, J., Khatena, J., and Torrance, E.P. (1981). *Creative ability.* Dubuque, Iowa: Kendall/Hunt Publishing Co.

Greene, T.R., and Noice, H. (1988). Influence of positive effect upon creative thinking and problem solving in children. *Psychological Reports, 63,* 895-898.

Guilford, J.P. (1967). *The nature of human intelligence.* New York: McGraw-Hill.

Harrington, D.M. (1990). The ecology of human creativity: A psychological perspective. In M.A. Runco and R.S. Albert (Eds.), *Theories of creativity* (pp. 143-169). Newbury Park, Calif.: Sage.

Leff, H.L., and Nevin, A. (1990). Dissolving barriers to teaching creative and meta thinking. *Teacher Education and Special Education, 13* (1), 36-39.

Marzano, R.J., Brandt, R.S., Hughes, C.S., Jones, B.F., Presseisen, B.Z., Rankin, S.C., and Suhor, C. (1988). *Dimensions of thinking.* Alexandria, Va.: Association for Supervision and Curriculum Development.

Moore, J.L.S. (1990). Strategies for fostering creative thinking. *Music Educators Journal, 76*(9), 38-42.

Paul, R. (1990). *Critical thinking.* Rohnert Park, Calif.: Sonoma State University.

Pesut, D.J. (1990). Creative thinking as a self regulatory megacognitive process—a model for education, training and further research. *The Journal of Creative Behavior, 24*(2), 105-109.

Porter-O'Grady, T. (1994). Working with consultants on a redesign. *American Journal of Nursing, 94*(10), 33-37.

Raichle, M.E. (1994). Visualizing the mind. *Scientific American, 270*(4), 58-64.

Rosella, J.D., Regan-Kubinski, M.J., and Albrecht, S.A. (1994). The need for multicultural diversity among health professionals. *Nursing and Health Care, 15*(5), 242-246.

Ruggiero, V.R. (1991). *The art of thinking: A guide to critical and creative thought* (3rd ed.). New York: Harper Collins.

Russ, S.W. (1993). *Affect and creativity.* Hillsdale, N.J.: Lawrence Erlbaum Associates.

Songxing, S., and Guozheng, L. (1989). Integrative thinking is the essential characteristic of creative thinking. In *Chinese Studies in Philosophy* (vol. 21, no. 2). White Plains, N.J.: M.E. Sharpel.

Springer, S.P., and Deutsch, G. (1981). *Left brain, right brain.* New York: W.H. Freeman.

*Webster's collegiate dictionary.* (1993). Springfield, Mass.: Merriam-Webster, Inc.

# *Evaluating Quantitative Evidence*

Chapter **6**

## OVERVIEW

Chapter 6 focuses on what you, the nurse consumer of research, need to know to apply critical thinking to the evaluation of evidence derived from nursing quantitative research. The chapter provides a basis for you to determine if quantitative research reports are sufficiently strong to warrant application to your practice setting by presenting an organized format to guide your thinking and discussing the reasoning process required to critically evaluate evidence.

Chapter 6 begins with a discussion of scientific reasoning and how this particular way of reasoning is applied to nursing research. Scientific reasoning is an attempt to discover the relationship between that which is observed and the explanation for it. The conclusions from scientific reasoning guide your beliefs and actions as they relate to your professional nursing practice.

## SCIENTIFIC REASONING

Science and technology have had a profound impact on the way we live. They affect how and what we eat, how we transport ourselves, how we communicate, and our present state of personal and community health. Science and technology have also affected the practice of modern nursing. Today hospitals are replete with different types of electronic equipment that allow health care providers to monitor the progress of clients in ways that were unheard of only a few years ago. New diagnostic tools are continually being developed to allow physicians to evaluate different organ systems of the body while the organ systems are functioning, observing what was once not observable. New advances in efficacious medications and therapeutic treatments, designed to help us maintain health and prevent illness, are now widely available.

What makes these advances possible? How have they come about? How have we benefited so dramatically by them? What kind of reasoning do scientists use to bring about these remarkable achievements? What is the scientific basis of nursing practice? This chapter looks at the application of reasoning to the scientific method and to nursing research, and how this kind of reasoning has made many of the advances in science and technology possible.

The scientific method is a search for explanations, or "reasoning that moves from observable facts of experience to reasonable explanations for those facts" (Bandman and Bandman, 1995, p. 60). "The world is constructed in a complex web of causal relationships that can be discovered through systematic investigation" is an assumption that underlies the scientific method (Chaffee, 1994, p. 594).

Anyone can use the scientific method, not just scientists. Bandman and Bandman (1995) believe that nurses engage in scientific reasoning when they use the nursing process to deliver client care and when they use the problem-solving process to solve other kinds of problems that occur in managing a nursing unit. This suggests that an overlap in how we apply reasoning to the complex array of experiences found in the practice of nursing occurs.

The scientific method is an organized, systematic approach for discovering causal relationships (i.e., discovering the relationship between what is observed and its explanation). The scientific method also allows users to test the accuracy of the conclusions drawn (Chaffee, 1994). According to Chaffee, the scientific method consists of

1. Identifying an event or relationship between events to be investigated,

2. Gathering information about the event (or events),

3. Developing a theory or hypothesis to explain what is happening,

4. Testing the theory or hypothesis through experimentation, and

5. Evaluating the theory or hypothesis (p. 594).

In this chapter we apply these steps to nursing research.

## EVIDENCE AS RESEARCH FINDINGS

Evidence is something that tends to prove another thing. It provides the grounds for a belief (Neufeldt, 1991). Research-based evidence supports beliefs and actions. Research evidence that is carefully evaluated, pertinent to the issue at hand, and similar to findings in other studies adds a level of credibility not found in other types of evidence. For example, credible research evidence suggests that sponge baths are ineffective to reduce fevers and may even be harmful to clients (Herder, 1994), yet nursing textbooks still recommend sponge baths as a nursing intervention to treat fever and nurses still use them in practice. This example presents two sides to the issue about the use of sponge baths to treat fever. One side has the weight of research-based evidence on it; the other has the weight of textbook authority and personal opinion as evidence. How will you choose which evidence to believe and what action to take in your practice? You must determine if the research is credible, if textbooks are completely accurate, and evaluate the importance of personal opinion and experience on any given nursing intervention.

The nurse consumer is surrounded by reports in newspapers and on television that purport to give the latest scientific information about a topic. We live in an age in which research findings are widely disseminated. Consider the following headlines: "Tylenol overdoses can harm liver" (Tylenol Overdoses, 1994), "The truth about self-esteem" (Kohn, 1994), and "Madness tied to creativity, study reveals" (Madness, 1987). If you interpreted the headlines at face value without reading the reports, you

**Critical Thinking Skills Associated with Evaluating Evidence**

▼ Evaluate evidence derived from quantitative and qualitative research
▼ Evaluate evidence derived from the assessment of clients
▼ Make appropriate inferences based on evidence derived from research and clients
▼ Assess research for its relevance to clinical practice
▼ Participate in systematic and accurate data collection

would be misled about the real meaning of the headlines. The consumer of research should critically examine such reports and discard the spurious ones. The box above lists the critical thinking skills associated with evaluating evidence.

### Definition of Research

Research is the careful, systematic investigation in some field of knowledge. Research is undertaken to discover or establish facts or principles (Neufeldt, 1991). Research in the scientific sense is a process in which a problem is identified; a structure is created for the study, which includes the research design and sample; data are collected and analyzed; and the findings described and conclusions made. Nursing research is the application of scientific reasoning to phenomena of interest to nurses (i.e., clients, families, health, illness, nursing, and the environment).

### Purpose of Nursing Research

The purpose of research in nursing is twofold: research (1) improves the nurse's clinical judgment and decision making, thereby improving the quality of nursing care provided to clients, and (2) helps to develop a unique body of nursing knowledge for the advancement of the profession. To achieve these purposes, the nurse must learn how to use critical thinking skills to evaluate nursing research and, where appropriate, to incorporate the findings into clinical practice (Brockopp and Hastings-Tolsma, 1995). When research improves practice, nursing strengthens its scientific and humanistic foundation and advances its status as a profession. The nurse must keep pace with the rapid advancements in health care technology and the changing political and economic health care environment, and be aware of the strong reliance on quantitative and qualitative research as the basis for professional practice.

## THE NURSE AS A CONSUMER OF RESEARCH

All nurses should be intelligent consumers of research (Creasia, 1991). Brockopp and Hastings-Tolsma (1995) define the research consumer as one who "determines the quality and merit of a given research report through systematic review and critique" (p. 44). As a consumer of research, you will evaluate the significance of the research problem to determine its applicability to your clinical practice. With further study you will learn to assess the merits of the research design for its suitability to the research problem and assess whether or not the findings apply to your clinical setting. With practice and careful analysis, you will learn to distinguish between good and poor research. The most critical step in being a good consumer of research is to determine whether or not the findings are sufficiently credible and compelling to warrant changing your clinical practice.

Specific guidelines for the participation of nurses in research vary according to educational level. Although role expectations for nurses differ depending on educational preparation, the researcher role is integral to the practice of all nursing. All nurse graduates, including those from associate degree programs, are expected to embrace the importance of nursing research, identify problem areas in clinical practice that need further study, participate in data collection activities, and use the findings in nursing practice.

As their educational preparation advances, baccalaureate students are expected to understand the steps of the research process, evaluate research, assess the results for relevance to practice, and refine practice accordingly. Master's and doctoral degree students have even greater responsibilities for nursing research. They participate in research proposal development; that is, they develop the theoretical framework, select the research design, implement the design, and evaluate the findings. In addition, doctoral students develop new methods of scientific and humanistic inquiry and theoretical explanations for nursing phenomena (American Nurses' Association, 1981; LoBiondo-Wood and Haber, 1994b).

The quality of research reports differs. Research reports need to be scrutinized before their findings are implemented into clinical practice. All research studies have strengths and weaknesses, and the nurse consumer of research should carefully analyze and evaluate these. Research reports should be supported with additional studies that find similar results before they should be considered for implementation into clinical practice. The nurse consumer of research should determine the relevance, significance, feasibility, and applicability of research reports to clinical practice.

## FORMAT FOR RESEARCH REPORTS

To become an informed consumer of research, you need to know how critical thinking skills help you read and evaluate a research report. At this point in your experience, you may be overwhelmed by the initial appearance of a research report and find it difficult to read. You may need to read a report several times to fully grasp the content and the significance of the conclusions. Learning to read critically and efficiently will facilitate your ability to think critically about research.

You may find it easier to comprehend a research report if you break it down into its component parts. Once you understand each of the parts and how they relate to one another, you will be able to assimilate the entire report. You can learn to review research reports quickly to determine their relevance to your personal interests and to your practice area. Research reports follow a characteristic format and usually include the following section headings (adapted from Wilson, 1993, p. 34):

1. Abstract
2. Introduction
   a. Problem
   b. Purpose
   c. Review of the literature
   d. Theoretical or conceptual framework
3. Method
   a. Subjects
   b. Design
   c. Materials (data collection)
   d. Procedure (data analysis)
4. Results (findings)
5. Discussion
6. References

## Abstract

The abstract is a summary of the pertinent aspects of the research study. An abstract includes a purpose, questions or hypothesis, a description of the study population, an overview of the data collection and analysis procedures, and a summary of the significant findings.

A good, well-written abstract sometimes includes all you need to know about the research. The following is an example of an abstract.

The purpose of this study was to determine the safety and efficacy of 2% nitroglycerin ointment to facilitate venous cannulation. In a double-blind experimental design, 80 adult subjects were randomly assigned to receive a 2% nitroglycerin ointment or a placebo ointment prior to cannulation. Variables measured before and after ointment application included heart rate, electrocardiogram, vein size, and presence of headache. No statistically significant differences were found in vein size or adverse effects following nitroglycerin ointment application (Griffith, James, and Cropp, 1994, p. 203).

This abstract contains the essential information you need to know to determine whether you wish to read the entire report. This research report, which is reproduced in Appendix B, will be used as an example throughout the remainder of this discussion.

## Introduction

The introduction usually includes a brief description of the problem, a statement of the purpose for the study, a brief review of the pertinent literature, and a theoretical or conceptual framework. The example research study above began with the identification of the problem. The researchers noted that medication administration and many diagnostic procedures require venipuncture and that many techniques have been advocated to facilitate venipuncture. The researchers then focused on a recommendation that topical nitroglycerin ointment should be applied to dilate veins and facilitate venous access. The researchers noted that minimal data exists to support this recommendation.

The researchers briefly reviewed the literature and summarized other research reports related to this topic. They concluded the introduction with the purpose of their research: "to determine the safety and efficacy of topical nitroglycerin ointment application to facilitate venous cannulation" (p. 203).

## Method

The method section of a research report includes a detailed discussion of the sample, the type of research design used, the materials (instruments) used to record the findings, and the procedures followed to carry out the study. This amount of detail must be included so that others can replicate the study.

An example of a detailed discussion of the sample is the following:

> Eligibility criteria included absence of cardiovascular disease, no current cardiac medications, a systolic blood pressure greater than 100 mm Hg, and no previous allergies to medications. Subjects included 50 females and 30 males. Forty subjects received topical nitroglycerin ointment, and 40 received placebo ointment. Subjects ranged in age from 21 to 69 years, with a mean age of 41.3 (SEM ±1.3) years. Forty subjects were normal volunteers, and 40 subjects, who had interstitial lung disease, were admitted for diagnostic bronchoscopy (Griffith, James, and Cropp, 1994, p. 203).

The researchers used a double-blind experimental design. They formed two groups: an experimental group that received the nitroglycerin ointment treatment and a control group that received the placebo ointment. A double-blind design is one in which neither the subjects nor the researchers know who receive the experimental treatment. The researchers identified and described the instruments they used to record each of the findings (blood pressure, heart rate and rhythm, headache pain, vein diameter, and plasma nitroglycerin). They also described the accuracy of each measurement instrument. For example, they measured the plasma nitroglycerin as follows:

> Plasma nitroglycerin samples were analyzed by trained personnel using a mass spectrometer (Model 5988A, Hewlett-Packard, Atlanta, GA) following manufacturer's specifications. Mass range is 10 to 1000 atomic mass unit (amu), with an accuracy of ± 0.13 amu (Griffith, James, and Cropp, 1994, p. 204).

Typically, this section of a research report includes a discussion of the reliability and validity of the measurement instrument(s).

The report also described the procedures that the researchers followed to carry out the study. They randomly assigned the research subjects to one of two groups. One group received the 2% nitroglycerin ointment treatment, and the other received a placebo ointment treatment. The research report provided a detailed description of how each group was treated in terms of ointment application and data collection.

## Results

Results should include the findings from the study. In the previous example, the researchers presented a factual summary of the differences between the two groups on each of the variables they measured (blood pressure, headaches, plasma nitroglycerin levels, heart rate and rhythm, and mean vein size) after applying the ointments. They also reported one unanticipated occurrence, erythema at the site of ointment

Table 6-1   **Example of a Descriptive Statistics Summary***

**Description of the Physiological Variables Across Phases of the Heel Stick Procedure**

| VARIABLE | MEAN | STANDARD DEVIATION | MAXIMUM RANGE | MINIMUM RANGE |
|---|---|---|---|---|
| **BASELINE DATA** | | | | |
| Maximum heart rate | 149.04 | 14.20 | 194.00 | 117.00 |
| Mean heart rate | | | | |
| standard deviation | 4.19 | 2.30 | 9.40 | 0.50 |
| Minimum oxygen saturation | 94.54 | 3.78 | 100.00 | 80.40 |
| Mean oxygen saturation | | | | |
| standard deviation | 1.00 | 0.80 | 3.60 | 0.10 |
| Intracranial pressure difference | 5.73 | 4.89 | 19.20 | 0.00 |

I *Modified from Stevens BJ and Johnston C: Nurs Res 43(4):228,1994.

application. The researchers reported no statistically significant difference between the two groups, which means the treatment (2% nitroglycerin ointment) was not efficacious in aiding venous access.

Many nurse researchers will summarize their findings in tables, graphs, or figures (see Table 6-1 for an example). This format provides an easily understandable summary of data, and it allows you to examine the data for yourself.

## Discussion

The discussion section includes an interpretation of the results and what they mean in relation to the purpose of the study and the literature review. In the nitroglycerin ointment example, the researchers discussed the results in depth and put them in the larger context of the results obtained by other nurse researchers (as reported in the literature review). The discussion section concludes with recommendations for further research. In the nitroglycerin ointment example, the nurse researchers recommended that further study should "focus on patients with extremely poor venous access" (p. 206).

## References

The last section of a research report contains a complete list of all references cited in the report such as books, articles, monographs, and personal communications. The references provide the theoretical context for the study from which the interested reader may pursue further information. References should always include complete bibliographic information. References should follow a specified style. The American Psychological Association editorial style is commonly used in nursing publications.

# FORMAT TO EVALUATE QUANTITATIVE RESEARCH

To evaluate a research report requires more systematic, rational, in-depth thought than does a review of a report. The latter can be done quickly, whereas the former requires full concentration and sufficient time. Evaluation, which challenges the higher levels of the cognitive processes, requires a knowledge of the research process and the subject matter.

You may apply critical thinking to the evaluation of a research report by using a questioning format. The questions focus your thinking on each component of the research process and illuminate the reasoning of the nurse researcher. Learning to ask the right questions and evaluate the answers are important critical thinking skills.

## Format to Evaluate Quantitative Research

The box below provides an organized format to evaluate evidence derived from quantitative research, focusing on the major components of quantitative research. It identifies critical questions with each component to think about and to ask about the research report. Each component is discussed in depth.

## Problem

To think critically about the problem of a quantitative research report, you need to determine what the problem is.

***Is it Identified?***    The problem is usually identified in the introductory paragraph of the research report with a brief statement that establishes the context for the study and the significance of the study. For example, Munro, Creamer, Haggerty, and Cooper (1988) identified stress as an important factor in determining susceptibility to coronary heart disease. This statement set the context for their study about the effect of relaxation therapy on post-myocardial infarction clients' rehabilitation. Lierman, Young, Powell-Cope, Georgiadou, and Benoliel (1994) noted that advancing age was the greatest risk factor in the development of breast cancer. They studied the effects of education and support on breast self-examination in older women.

---

 **Format to Evaluate Quantitative Research***

**PROBLEM**
- ▼ Is it identified?

**PURPOSE**
- ▼ Is it relevant to nursing?
- ▼ Is it relevant to your interests?

**RESEARCH QUESTION OR HYPOTHESIS**
- ▼ Is it stated precisely and unambiguously?

**Format to Evaluate Quantitative Research—cont'd**

**LITERATURE REVIEW**

▼  Is it relevant to the question or hypothesis?
▼  Is it comprehensive with sufficient depth and breadth?
▼  Is it placed within the context of other related studies?
▼  Is the theoretical framework described?

**RESEARCH DESIGN**

▼  Is it identified and described?
▼  Is it appropriate for the problem?

**RESEARCH SAMPLE**

▼  Is the sample representative of the population under study?
▼  How are the subjects selected?
▼  How are the subjects assigned to groups (experimental design)?
▼  Is informed consent obtained?

**DATA COLLECTION**

▼  Are the data collection methods and instruments described?
▼  Does the data collection procedure adequately answer the research question or hypothesis?
▼  Are the reliability and validity of the research instruments described, and are they acceptable?

**DATA ANALYSIS**

▼  Are the results presented?
▼  Are the statistical procedures appropriate to the research question or hypothesis and to the type of data collected?
▼  Is the meaning of the statistical procedures discussed?

**DISCUSSION OF FINDINGS**

▼  Do the data answer the research question or hypothesis?
▼  Do the data support the researcher's interpretation and conclusion?
▼  Are other conclusions possible?
▼  Are the limitations noted?
▼  Are the implications for education, practice, and theory appropriate to the research design and results?
▼  Are recommendations for further research made?

*Modified from Brockopp DY and Hastings-Tolsma MT: Fundamentals of nursing research (ed. 2), Boston, 1995, Jones and Bartlett; LoBiondo-Wood G and Haber J: Nursing research methods, critical appraisal, and utilization, St Louis, 1994, Mosby; and Jacox A and Prescott P: Am J Nurs (11/78), 1882-1889.

## Purpose

To think critically about the purpose of a quantitative research report, ask the following:

▼  Is it relevant to nursing?

▼  Is it relevant to your interests?

***Is it Relevant to Nursing?***   First look at the statement of purpose to determine its relevance to nursing and to your own interests. The purpose statement is in the abstract and also in the introduction section of the written report. The purpose statement is a concise explanation of the intent of the research. The following are examples of purpose statements.

> The purpose of this study was to determine if low-intensity aerobic exercises, specific to muscles of the knees and ankles, would improve muscle strength, flexibility, and balance among sedentary elderly persons, as compared with elderly persons who did not participate in this intervention (Mills, 1994, p. 207).

> The purpose of this study was to describe the premature infant's physiological responses to an acute painful stimulus and to determine how these responses are influenced by the infant's behavioral state and severity of illness (Stevens and Johnston, 1994, p. 226).

Both purpose statements clearly identify the nature of the study and the study population. From these purpose statements, you can quickly determine if the study is relevant to your practice interests. If your interests are in geriatric nursing, you might not be interested in the second study.

The phrase "relevance to nursing" may include studies that are pertinent to nursing practice, nursing education, nursing research, and nursing theory. This chapter focuses on research that is relevant to clinical practice; however, education, research, and theory development are important to the advancement of nursing as a profession.

Although the research examples in this chapter come exclusively from nursing research journals, research published in nonnursing journals may also have relevance to nursing practice. For example, Knowles' (1990) research on the adult learner has contributed to our understanding of how adults learn. Knowles, an educator, is frequently cited in nursing texts that discuss health education and teaching adults in clinical practice areas. When you review research in nonnursing journals, review reports thoroughly to determine their relevance to nursing and your interests.

***Is it Relevant to your Interests?***   Only you know if research is relevant to your interests. To keep up with the research in all areas of nursing is impossible. You will find it more reasonable and less exhausting to narrow your interests to a few specific areas and then continually update your knowledge in these areas. If you adopt the philosophy that life is a continuous learning process and that life offers an unending array of learning opportunities, you will pursue your interests, wherever they may lead.

## Research Question or Hypothesis

The research question may be stated either as a question or as an hypothesis. It identifies the variables under study and the nature of the population. A single study may have more than one research question or hypothesis. To think critically about the research question in a quantitative research report, you need determine if it is stated well.

**Is it Stated Precisely and Unambiguously?**   Regardless of whether a research question or hypothesis is used, precise and unambiguous language should be used. To be stated precisely means that key words are strictly defined and accurately used throughout the report. To be stated unambiguously means that key words have only one meaning. Recall from Chapter 4 that a word or statement is ambiguous when it has more than one meaning. There should be no doubt in your mind about the meaning of the question or the hypothesis.

**Research Questions.**   Consider the following examples of research questions. Stuifbergen and Becker (1994) examined the usefulness of Pender's Health Promotion Model to explain the occurrence of health promoting behaviors among adults with disabilities. Their specific research questions were:

1. What combination of cognitive-perceptual factors and modifying factors best predicts reported health-promoting behaviors among adults with disabilities?

2. How do adults with disabilities perceive their abilities to perform health-promoting behaviors? (p. 4)

McKeever and Galloway (1984) sought to determine the nature and frequency of menstrual cycle alterations following nongynecological surgery in adolescent and adult females. Their research questions were:

1. How is menstrual cycle length affected by surgery performed under general anesthesia in adolescent and adult females?

2. What is the relationship between menstrual cycle phase at the time of surgery and the onset of the first postoperative menses?

3. What is the relationship between the extent to which hospitalization is stressful and postoperative menstrual cycle length alterations?

4. How do women perceive menstrual cycle length alterations following nongynecological surgery? (p. 42)

**Research Hypothesis.**   The hypothesis is a statement that something is true (Weiss, 1993). It expresses what the researcher expects to find (Jacox and Prescott, 1978). A hypothesis is a statement such as "Subjects who participate in natural childbirth classes will experience less pain and anxiety during labor and delivery than subjects who do not participate." Data gathered will either support or not support the statement.

Kolanowski (1990) posed the following hypotheses:

1. Elderly persons exposed to broad-spectrum fluorescent lighting will exhibit less motor activity than those exposed to warm white fluorescent lighting.

2. Elderly persons exposed to broad-spectrum fluorescent lighting will report a lower level of activation than those exposed to warm white fluorescent lighting (p. 181).

Krouse and Roberts (1989) studied the impact of enhanced client participation in the nurse-patient interaction in the process of decision making. Their hypothesis was:

Individuals who participate in an actively negotiated process of decision making with the practitioner, when compared with those who participate in either a traditional or a partially negotiated approach, will:

1. perceive more control over their care and have fewer feelings of powerlessness,

2. express greater agreement with the recommended treatment plan, and

3. demonstrate greater satisfaction with care (pp. 719-720).

In each of these examples, the research questions and the research hypotheses are stated precisely and unambiguously. Every research report will provide a precise definition for each of the key terms used in the study. This eliminates any confusion or ambiguity about the meaning the nurse researcher intended.

## Literature Review

The literature review uncovers important information that influences the direction of a research study. The literature review identifies what is known and unknown about a particular topic or problem. It pinpoints the gaps that exist in the literature and the consistencies and inconsistencies that are present. The literature review exposes unanswered questions about the topic or problem. It describes the strengths and weaknesses of the theoretical and conceptual approaches, the research designs, and data collection methods of earlier research studies. It helps the nurse researcher generate useful research questions, select an appropriate research design, and identify appropriate data collection methods. It also reveals if there is a need to replicate a well-designed study or to refine an existing one (Miller, 1994).

To think critically about the literature review of a quantitative research report, ask the following:

▼  Is it relevant to the question or hypothesis?
▼  Is it comprehensive with sufficient depth and breadth?
▼  Is it placed within the context of other related studies?
▼  Is the theoretical framework described?

***Is it Relevant to the Question or Hypothesis?***   The literature review should be current and relevant to the research question or hypothesis. Examine the reference list to see what it tells you about the literature sources used to support the study. Are the literature sources published or unpublished (conference presentations, master's theses, doctoral dissertations)? Are the sources data-based literature (reports of completed research studies) or conceptual literature (nonresearch material such as reports about theories, concepts, and models) in both print and nonprint (audiovisual materials) forms? Are the literature sources from refereed or nonrefereed journals? Are the literature sources primary or secondary sources? Answers to these questions will give you a sense of the quality of the research (Miller, 1994).

Journal articles are most frequently cited in research reference lists. Journals are more up-to-date than books and, therefore, are the best place to look for the results of current research. Become familiar with nursing journals and the types of articles that they publish. The journal references should be from refereed ones. Articles published in refereed journals have been through an internal and external peer review process before they are accepted for publication (Miller, 1994). Publication in a refereed journal adds a measure of credibility to the article, although it does not mean the research itself has met all the criteria for good research. Some popular refereed nursing research journals are *Nursing Research, Research in Nursing and Health, Advances in Nursing Science, IMAGE: Journal of Nursing Scholarship,* and *Western Journal of Nursing Research.*

The nurse researcher should use primary sources rather than secondary sources in the literature review. The term *primary source* means that the author is the person who conducted the research or who developed the theory. The term *secondary source* means that the author is not a direct observer or participant in the research or theory development; rather, the secondary source author writes about the work of the primary source author. It is always preferable to use primary sources of information. Using a secondary source may be necessary when the primary source is unavailable and when different perspectives for critical analysis are desired. Then secondary sources can provide useful thoughts and perspectives about the topic that you would not otherwise have considered. Secondary sources are also useful because they combine knowledge from a variety of primary sources into a single publication such as a textbook (Borg and Gall, 1989; Miller, 1994).

***Is it Comprehensive with Sufficient Depth and Breadth?***   The literature review should have sufficient depth and breadth so that a reader can thoroughly understand the research problem. It should include all of the important published scholarly (database and conceptual) literature about the research problem. The nurse researcher should go back in time a sufficient number of years to trace and develop the context for the research problem. A literature search may extend back 10 years or more as would be appropriate to the topic (Miller, 1994).

***Is it Placed within the Context of Other Related Studies?***   One purpose of the literature review is to identify what is known about the current research problem. The critical evaluation and clear reporting of this information establishes the context for the research report. The literature review should show how the study fits with what is already known about the problem and what contribution the study makes to this body of knowledge.

***Is the Theoretical Framework Described?***    Research is conducted within the context of a theoretical framework, and this framework should be clearly identified and described in the review of the literature. The theoretical framework gives meaning to the research problem by providing the theoretical rationale for it. The theoretical framework summarizes what is known in the field of inquiry. Thus, the theoretical framework becomes the foundation for the research study. It is upon this foundation that concepts are defined, the relationship among the variables is identified, the research questions or hypotheses are posed, the research design is selected, the data collection methods are developed, the findings are interpreted, and the generalizations are made. The theoretical framework is like the frame of a house, which forms the foundation upon which a house is built. Like a road map, the theoretical framework leads the way to the final destination. The framework provides guidance and direction to all aspects of conducting the research study (Feldman, 1994).

For example, recall earlier in this chapter the hypothesis posed by Krouse and Roberts (1989), who studied the impact of enhanced client participation in the nurse-patient interaction in the process of decision making. The purpose of their study was:

> To assess the difference between traditional patient-provider interaction and varying degrees of negotiated styles within a simulated clinical environment. Three types of interaction were compared according to time involved and patient satisfaction, feelings of powerlessness, feelings of control, and willingness to comply with prescribed treatment (p. 719).

The accompanying theoretical framework for this study examined the related theories and concepts about the traditional patient-provider interaction and negotiated styles of patient-provider interaction. The authors discussed the nature of patient-provider interactions, the concept of negotiated interactions, and the desirability of greater patient participation. The authors also defined the types of interactions (traditional approach, partial negotiation, and active negotiation), agreement with the plan (compliance), patient satisfaction, powerlessness, and control within the context of the theoretical framework.

When you evaluate the theoretical framework, you should assess whether the concepts and their definitions, and the research questions or hypotheses, are consistent with the framework. You should also note whether the literature review provides sufficient breadth and depth to support the theoretical framework. Perhaps the best way for you to grasp and understand theoretical frameworks is to read reports of nursing research.

## Research Design

Three common types of research design are experimental, quasiexperimental, and nonexperimental. As a consumer of research, you can assess the research design by having a basic understanding of the three types of designs. To think critically about the research design of a quantitative research report, ask the following:

▼  Is it identified and described?
▼  Is it appropriate for the problem?

***Experimental Research Design.***   The purpose of the experimental research design is to test theories about cause and effect relationships. It uses a deductive approach and is the most powerful research design available for this purpose (Borg and Gall, 1989). It is an appropriate design to use in nursing because nursing is concerned primarily with developing nursing interventions that help restore health and promote wellness. It is useful to evaluate the outcomes of nursing interventions and to demonstrate their efficacy and cost-effectiveness (Grey, 1994b; Tanner, Imle, and Stewart, 1989).

The true or classic experimental design is structured to test cause and effect relationships. Fig. 6-1 illustrates its basic structure, showing a nursing intervention as the experimental treatment. The experimental design requires at least two groups, an experimental group and a control group. Both groups must be alike so that the nurse researchers can study the impact of the treatment or nursing intervention. The purpose of the design is to compare the two groups on the dependent variable after they have experienced the manipulation of the independent variable (Brockopp and Hastings-Tolsma, 1995).

The dependent variable is the effect, or outcome, under investigation. Review the experimental research design used in the research report entitled "Evaluation of the Safety and Efficacy of Topical Nitroglycerin Ointment to Facilitate Venous Cannulation" in Appendix B. In this report, the dependent variable is the facilitation of venous cannulation as measured by vein size. The independent variable is the cause or the condition that the nurse researcher manipulates (Wilson, 1993). In our example report, the independent variable is the 2% nitroglycerin ointment treatment given to the experimental group. The control group received a placebo ointment.

Grey (1994b) describes three essential characteristics of experimental designs: (1) random assignment to a group, (2) control, and (3) manipulation. First, subjects are randomly assigned to either the experimental group or the control group. Random

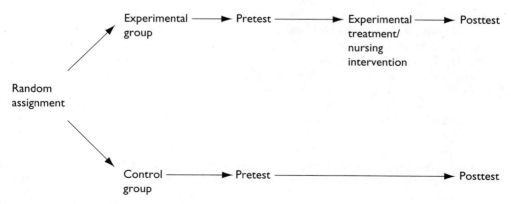

**Fig. 6-1** True or classic experimental design.

Modified from Grey M: Experimental and quasiexperimental designs. In LoBiondo-Wood G and Haber J (Eds.), Nursing research: Methods, critical appraisal, and utilization (ed. 3), St Louis, 1994, Mosby.

assignment is a method to distribute the research subjects between the experimental group and the control group. It minimizes the differences between the groups before the experiment begins; that is, of those research subjects selected to participate in the study, each subject has an equal chance of being in each group. In the experiment to test the safety and efficacy of topical nitroglycerin ointment, subjects were randomly assigned to the experimental group and control group (see Appendix B).

Second, control over the variables is an essential characteristic of experimental designs. Control is achieved by holding all variables constant and by manipulating only the independent variable. It is also achieved by the random assignment of subjects to groups, the use of the control group as the comparison group, and the careful preparation of and meticulous compliance with the established experimental protocols.

The third characteristic of experimental designs is manipulation. Manipulation refers to the action of the independent variable, or the experimental treatment or nursing intervention. In our example report, the manipulation was the 2% nitroglycerin ointment that the experimental group received that the control group did not. All other variables were held constant.

Internal and external validity may affect the credibility of the results of experimental studies. Internal validity refers to whether or not the independent variable accounted for the difference in the dependent variable. Threats to internal validity include history, maturation, testing, instrumentation, mortality, and selection bias. Threats to internal validity occur while the experiment is in progress (LoBiondo-Wood, 1994b).

History could be a factor if something else happens during the experiment that could account for the results. For example, suppose the nursing intervention was a skin care protocol that was studied using a group of nursing home residents. In spite of the nurse researcher's efforts to follow the protocol, family members of some clients would massage their loved one's skin with lotion when they came to visit. If the skin care protocol were found to be a statistically significant nursing intervention, you would have to ask if the actions of the family members had any effect on the results of the study.

Maturation should be considered if developmental, biological, or psychological maturation could influence the results. For example, consider adolescent research subjects who were exposed to an educational intervention about human sexuality that spanned a period of 6 months. At the conclusion of the intervention, the researcher found that a statistically significant improvement in the knowledge level of the adolescents occurred. The researcher had to question if the result was due to the educational intervention or due to the maturation of the subjects that occurred during the 6 months.

Testing could be a factor if the pretest and posttest occur too close in time; that is, the pretest could sensitize the subjects to the research topic and thus create an effect on the posttest. Instrumentation could be a factor if there are changes in how the variables are measured or how data collection observations are made. Mortality could be a factor if subjects drop out of the study and those who remain are not similar to those who drop out. Selection bias is a factor when random assignment of subjects to experimental and control groups is not used.

*External validity* refers to whether or not the results can be generalized to other populations and other environmental conditions. Threats to external validity are the *effect of selection,* the *reactive effects,* and the *effect of testing.* The *effect of selection,* or how the sample of subjects is selected, impacts the generalizability of the research findings. For example, if hospitalized clients are used, the findings may not be generalizable to nonhospitalized clients. The *reactive effect* refers to how the very act of participation in a research study can impact the results. Subjects may feel special about being in the study and may respond differently than they otherwise would, which may impact the findings. The *effect of testing* refers to the impact of the pretest on the subjects. Just as pretesting can affect internal validity, it can also affect external validity. The pretest itself primes subjects about the nature of the study (Jacox and Prescott, 1978; LoBiondo-Wood, 1994b).

Although the experimental design is the best design to establish cause and effect relationships, it is not the most commonly used design in nursing. The design is difficult to implement because of the number of variables that must be controlled. Sick clients in busy health care settings require individualized care and rapid adjustments to accommodate their conditions. These critical adjustments complicate achieving the requisite level of uniform control needed for this design and contribute to the impracticality of its use. For this reason, variations on the experimental design have been developed. We will now look at only one variation, the quasiexperimental design. Information about other experimental designs may be found in nursing research textbooks.

**Quasiexperimental Research Design.** The quasiexperimental design and the experimental design are alike in that they both involve manipulation of the independent variable; that is, they both require the introduction of a treatment or nursing intervention. The quasiexperimental design is different from the experimental design in that it lacks one of the other two characteristics of the experimental design. It may lack either randomization or a control group; usually, randomization is lacking (Brockopp and Hastings-Tolsma, 1995; Grey, 1994b). Because of this, quasiexperimental design has greater flexibility for use in nursing research but less control over intervening variables.

Different quasiexperimental designs are available. The one commonly used in nursing is the nonequivalent control group design. It is identical in structure to the experimental design (see Fig. 6-1), except that in the nonequivalent control group design, the subjects are not randomly assigned to an experimental group and a control group.

To illustrate the quasiexperimental design, consider the study conducted by Munro, Creamer, Haggerty, and Cooper (1988). They studied the physical and psychosocial effects of a specific relaxation technique on clients in a cardiac rehabilitation program. They wanted to know if the client's behavioral style (Type A or Type B) influenced this relationship. The subjects were men with postmyocardial infarction who met the criteria for participation in the study, one of which was the ability to participate in the entire 12-week exercise program. The nurse researchers first recruited subjects for the control group. When the control group finished the

12-week exercise program, the nurse researchers then recruited subjects for the experimental group. Random assignment was not used to form the experimental group and control group. The nurse researchers formed the two groups as they did to avoid any interaction between the participants in the control group and the experimental group.

*Nonexperimental Research Design.* The purpose of the nonexperimental design is to describe what is, or what presently exists. Researchers seek to determine the characteristics of a sample of people or phenomenon of interest on one or more variables (Brockopp and Hastings-Tolsma, 1995). Nonexperimental research design is the most common type of design used in nursing research (Tanner, Imle, and Stewart, 1989).

LoBiondo-Wood and Haber (1994a) describe two types of nonexperimental designs: descriptive/exploratory survey studies and interrelationship studies. Descriptive/exploratory surveys are used to collect detailed descriptions about the existing variables such as age, sex, marital status, ethnicity, income, occupation, and religious affiliation. The descriptive/exploratory survey also answer questions such as:

▼ What are the attitudes of City Hospital nurses about caring for homeless clients?
▼ What are the favorite foods of residents at the Happy Hills Retirement Community?
▼ What are the most pressing health education needs of clients who have been newly diagnosed with hypertension?

Data are typically collected by questionnaire or interview.

An example of the descriptive/exploratory survey is Bresser, Sexton, and Foell's (1993) survey of clients awaiting coronary artery bypass graft surgery. The purpose of the study was to determine the clients' thoughts and feelings, particularly those clients whose surgical procedures had been postponed. Data were gathered through tape-recorded interviews. Clients whose surgery had been postponed expressed anger and disappointment.

Interrelationship studies come in several types, the most common being correlation. The correlation design allows the nurse researcher to describe the degree of the relationship between two or more variables. Correlation means that the variables "go together" to some degree (Glass and Hopkins, 1984). Correlation can be positive. For example, nurses who work overtime earn more money. Correlation can be negative (inverse). For example, experienced labor and delivery nurses know that usually the length of time in uncomplicated, low-risk labor decreases as the number of births a woman has had increases (Olds, London, and Ladewig, [1992]).

The magnitude of the relationship (correlation) is measured by a correlation coefficient that is discussed under analysis of data. What is critical to remember about correlational studies is that they cannot be used to either determine or infer causation. Because two variables are related to one another does not mean that one causes the other.

## Research Sample

How the research sample is drawn is of critical importance to understand the variable(s) under investigation and to infer generalizability of the findings beyond the sample population. Because it is impossible and impractical to test an entire population, the nurse researcher must select a sample that is representative of the population. How this sample is selected determines the generalizability of the research findings to the population from which it is drawn. To think critically about the research sample of a quantitative research report, ask the following:

▼ Is the sample representative of the population under study?
▼ How are the subjects selected?
▼ How are the subjects assigned to groups (experimental design)?
▼ Is informed consent obtained?

***Is the Sample Representative of the Population Under Study?*** Key words to understand are *population* and *sample.* The population, also called target population or universe, is the entire group under investigation. The sample is a smaller group drawn from the population. The population can be anything the nurse researcher wishes to study (e.g., people, medical records, events, institutions, and objects). For example, suppose that you want to determine if the stethoscope plays a significant role in the spread of infection in a hospital. You are curious about how effectively nurses and physicians clean their stethoscopes. To collect data you obtain cultures from the stethoscopes of both groups. Because it would take too much time and money to culture the stethoscope of every nurse and every physician in your hospital, you select a representative sample from both groups. If your sampling procedure is carefully designed and implemented, then you could generalize your findings to the entire population of nurses and physicians in your hospital.

***How Are the Subjects Selected?*** To define a population for study, the nurse researcher establishes eligibility criteria for participation. Sample selection may be related to age, gender, ethnicity, number of children, diagnosis, and so forth. In the research report found in Appendix B, Griffith, James, and Cropp (1994) established the following eligibility criteria: "absence of cardiovascular disease, no current cardiac medications, a systolic blood pressure greater than 100 mm Hg, and no previous allergies to medication" (p. 203). Establishing eligibility criteria helps to restrict the population to a homogeneous group of subjects (Haber, 1994).

Sampling strategies fall into two broad categories: probability and nonprobability sampling. Probability sampling is based on probability theory, meaning events occur by chance. Random selection in probability sampling means that each member of the population has an equal and independent chance of being included in the sample. Inferential statistics, or methods to draw conclusions about a population based on a sample, require random sampling from populations. Several probability sampling strategies exist; the most widely used is simple random sampling. The technique requires the use of a table of random numbers (Brockopp and Hastings-Tolsma, 1995; Haber, 1994; Weiss, 1993).

Nonprobability sampling is less rigorous but more feasible for the nurse researcher to achieve. Nonprobability sampling does not give each and every member of the population an equal and independent chance of being included in the sample. A sample may be selected because the subjects are accessible and convenient (convenience sampling), because the subjects can be selected who are proportionally representative of the population (quota sampling), and because the subjects represent a specific area of interest and random selection is not possible (purposive sampling). Nonprobability sampling tends to provide a less accurate picture of the population and limits the ability of the nurse researcher to infer generalizations about the population. Therefore, sampling bias exits when there is little confidence that the sample represents the population. Even with these drawbacks, most samples in nursing research are nonprobability samples. This sampling strategy is more feasible for the nurse researcher because random selection from the population is often impossible. As you think critically about a research report, note how the sample is selected and what generalizations the nurse researcher infers about the population (Brockopp and Hastings-Tolsma, 1995; Haber, 1994).

Although random sampling is the most desirable strategy, it is rarely possible to achieve in nursing research. For a variety of reasons related to the practice setting and the health status of clients, nurse researchers must rely on a convenience sample. As you think critically about the research report, expect the researcher to provide a description of the sample and how it is selected. Based on this information, you can assess the strengths and limitations of the sample (Tanner, Imle, and Stewart, 1989).

***How Are the Subjects Assigned to Groups (Experimental Design)?***    When more than one group is part of the research design, then how the subjects are assigned to the groups becomes important. Subject assignment is a critical issue to establish internal validity. With random assignment, each subject in the experiment has an equal and known probability (likelihood) of being assigned to the experimental group(s) and the control group (Grey, 1994b). Random assignment is the best technique to ensure initial equivalence between the groups. The procedure for random assignment, which is basically the same as obtaining a random sample from a defined population, can be accomplished using a table of random numbers (Borg and Gall, 1989).

***Is Informed Consent Obtained?***    Research subjects should fully understand the nature of the research study and their rights and responsibilities within it before participation. Research subjects must be free to decide to participate without fear of reprisal. The researcher should not include anyone in any research who has not given his or her informed consent (Brockopp and Hastings-Tolsma, 1995).

In the process of obtaining informed consent, the researcher must disclose certain information to the research subjects. For example, subjects should have a description of the purpose of the research, the procedures they will follow, the expected duration of their participation, the risks and discomforts they may encounter, the method for maintaining anonymity and confidentiality, and the persons whom they should contact for answers to their questions (Jackson, 1994).

Federal law requires that universities, hospitals, and other health care agencies that apply for grants or contract for projects or programs that use human subjects in biomedical or behavioral research must have institutional review boards. The review board is composed of qualified individuals who review research proposals and ensure that the research subjects are protected from undue risk and loss of personal rights and dignity. When you evaluate the research, you should note if the study was approved by the institutional review board and if informed consent was obtained from the research subjects. You should also be alert to any unethical research practices. For example, in the now famous Tuskegee syphilis research (1932-1973) many subjects (poor black males) were uninformed about the study's purpose and procedures. One group with syphilis was denied treatment to allow researchers to study the untreated disease (Jackson, 1994).

## Data Collection

How data are collected is the next major area to evaluate. Data collection must be objective and systematic. To be objective means that the data were not influenced by those who collected it. To be systematic means that the data were collected in the same way by all participants (Grey, 1994a). The goal of data collection is to obtain accurate information. To think critically about the data collection of a quantitative research report, ask the following:

▼ Are the data collection methods and instruments described?
▼ Does the data collection procedure adequately answer the research question or hypothesis?
▼ Are the reliability and validity of the research instruments described, and are they acceptable?

***Are the Data Collection Methods and Instruments Described?***   The selection of data collection methods and instruments should be appropriate to the problem, the research question or hypothesis, the definition of key concepts, the setting, and the population. The types of data collection methods are physiologic or biologic measurement, observation, interviews, questionnaires, and records or available data (Grey, 1994a). Each has its advantages and disadvantages.

Physiological or biologic measurement is the most precise method for data collection. Examples of biologic measures include heart rate, blood pressure, blood cholesterol levels, and specific microorganisms' identification. Instruments to measure these include a heart monitor, sphygmomanometer, stethoscope, syringe, and other laboratory equipment. Consider the physiological data collected by Stevens and Johnston (1994). To assess the premature infant's physiological response to an acute painful stimulus (heel lance procedure), the nurse researchers recorded heart rate and oxygen saturation using a pulse oximeter placed on the infant's foot. They assessed intracranial pressure using a Ladd Intracranial Pressure Monitor via a fiber-optic sensor secured on the anterior fontanelle.

Observation, as a data collection method, requires skill and training on the part of the observer. Observation may yield more accurate quantitative data than that obtained on standardized tests, questionnaires, and interviews because these rely on self-report, and subjects often bias the information they provide. Audiotape or video-tape recorders make observation data more accurate (Borg and Gall, 1989). For example, suppose a nurse researcher were interested in comparing the classroom learning styles of Asian and Hispanic clients who participate in health education classes. The classes could be videotaped, and the nurse researcher could observe and record the frequency of selected behaviors such as asking questions, seeking further information, and verbalizing personal experiences with health problems. If observation were used, a systematic plan for the observations and recording of data would have to be in place. If more than one person participated in data collection, the nurse researcher would have to describe how consistency among the observers was ensured.

Interviews and questionnaires are the dominant data collection methods used in survey research. Both methods rely on information that is obtained directly from the subjects. Data may be collected between the nurse researcher and the subjects by face-to-face interview, the telephone, or written questionnaire. The questions may be open or closed ended. As with observation data, if more than one person participates in the interview, the nurse researcher should describe how he or she maintained consistency between interviewers.

The written questionnaire gathers information about the client's knowledge, attitudes, beliefs, and feelings. The usefulness of the questionnaire depends upon the client's ability to read and comprehend the survey questions, his or her willingness to put a response in writing, her or his concern (or lack thereof) about the destination and purpose of the questionnaire, and the client's willingness to be honest. People tend to answer what they know they *should* do instead of what they actually do.

Written questionnaires and written measurement instruments such as standardized tests are frequently constructed to yield subscores and an overall score. For example, to investigate the health-promoting behaviors of African-American women, Ahijevych and Bernhard (1994) administered the Health-Promoting Lifestyle Profile. The profile assessed the likelihood of subjects to engage in health-promoting behaviors by measuring the frequency of health-promoting behaviors on a four-point scale that ranged from "never" to "routinely." The subscales were self-actualization, health responsibility, exercise, nutrition, interpersonal support, and stress management. The instrument yielded an overall score and subscale scores.

The last type of data collection method discussed here is the examination of records or other available data. Here the nurse researcher is using information that is already available to answer the research question. Sources of such data might be hospital records, client records, nursing care plans, and census data.

***Does the Data Collection Procedure Adequately Answer the Research Question or Hypothesis?***    If the purpose of the study is to investigate a biological problem, then appropriate biological data should be collected. For example, when Griffith, James, and Cropp (1994) investigated the efficacy of the nitroglycerin ointment to facilitate venous cannulation, they measured the vein diameter using electrocardiogram calipers. To ensure objectivity, a second investigator placed the caliper against a millimeter ruler to obtain the numerical reading of the caliper measurement.

If the purpose of the study is to investigate a psychosocial problem, such as adolescent loneliness, then pertinent psychosocial data should be collected using an appropriate psychometric instrument. Sometimes instruments and tools are not available to measure the specific variable in which the researchers are interested. In this case, the researchers may create their own instruments. If they develop their own instruments and tools, expect a sufficient description about them to allow you to make a judgment about their reliability and validity.

### Are the Reliability and Validity of the Research Instruments Described, and Are They Acceptable?   To provide credible results, the nurse researcher needs reliable and valid data collection instruments. To evaluate the reliability and validity of the research instruments requires in-depth knowledge about instrument development and statistical methods. An overview of reliability and validity is provided here, but you will need further in-depth information to assess these adequately. Reliability and validity are issues for all data collection instruments, be they paper-and-pencil instruments, direct observations, or structured interviews.

Reliability of an instrument refers to its level of stability and internal consistency over time (Borg and Gall, 1989). For example, suppose subjects with high blood pressure participate in a study to test the effects of a new antihypertensive drug. The nurse researcher assesses the blood pressure daily for 2 months to determine the drug's effectiveness. Each day as the nurse obtains the blood pressures, she notices wide fluctuations in the readings of individual subjects, fluctuations that she does not believe represents each client's true vasomotor state. Assuming the blood pressure in the subjects is actually stable (though elevated), she should suspect that faulty calibration of the measurement instrument (sphygmomanometer) is the cause of the fluctuations. If the sphygmomanometer is not reliable, how can accurate blood pressure readings be obtained? How does the researcher know if the drug is effective? The data obtained from faulty measurement instruments is unreliable. This error is called measurement error. The reliability of paper-and-pencil instruments must be evaluated in a similar manner.

Reliability has three characteristics that are commonly evaluated: stability, internal consistency, and equivalence. Stability, or the degree to which subjects' responses change over time, is measured by test-retest reliability using a correlation coefficient. Internal consistency reliability, or the extent to which all subparts measure the same characteristic, is commonly measured by either Cronbach's alpha or the Kuder-Richardson formula, which are statistical tests that yield a coefficient. Equivalence is an issue when different observers use the same instrument to collect data at the same time. To ensure equivalence among their observations, researchers calculate interrater reliability (Brockopp and Hastings-Tolsma, 1995). As you think critically about research, you need to look for and evaluate these characteristics in the research report.

Tests for both stability and internal consistency are reported as a reliability coefficient that has a range of 0 to 1.00 (the expectation is that the direction is positive), in which 1.00 represents a perfect correlation between variables. Reliability coefficients usually fall between 0.40 and 0.90. A reliability coefficient above 0.70 is considered adequate according to Nunnally, 1978 (cited in Tanner, Imle, and Stewart, 1989). The nurse researcher should report the reliability coefficient on all standardized tests and on all instruments developed by the researcher. For example, recall the Health-Promoting Lifestyle Profile used by Ahijevych and Bernhard (1994) to investigate the health-promoting behaviors of African-American women. The researchers reported that the alpha coefficients on the individual subscales ranged from 0.70 to 0.90 and that the alpha coefficient for the total instrument was 0.92. Thus the support for the reliability of this instrument is very strong.

Validity of an instrument refers to the degree an instrument measures what it purports to measure (Borg and Gall, 1989). The five types of validity by which to judge instruments are (1) content validity, (2) face validity, (3) predictive validity, (4) concurrent validity, and (5) construct validity (Brockopp and Hastings-Tolsma, 1995). All are different ways to ensure that the instrument measures that which it is supposed to measure. A full discussion of validity is beyond the scope of this text. Validity, although an important feature to establish the credibility of instruments, is difficult to achieve and is less frequently discussed in research reports than is reliability. Often there is some mention of at least content validity. The nurse researcher should report the attempts to achieve validity or the lack thereof.

As a critical thinker, you will need to continue developing your ability to evaluate the relative merits of data collection methods and instruments and become more comfortable with the concepts of reliability and validity.

## Data Analysis

Analysis of the data involves the presentation of the results of the research and an examination of the statistical procedures used. To think critically about the data analysis of a quantitative research report, ask the following:

▼ Are the results presented?
▼ Are the statistical procedures appropriate to the research question or hypothesis and to the type of data collected?
▼ Is the meaning of the statistical procedures discussed?

***Are the Results Presented?***   The data analysis is the portion of the research report that presents the results (findings) of the investigation. The next section of the research report, the discussion of findings, presents the interpretation of the results. The results should be presented objectively and in a straightforward manner, and data should be provided for each research question or hypothesis. A table or figure may be used to illustrate the results of the investigation.

If tables and figures are used, they should be titled so that the reader knows exactly what the data represent. If figures are used, the horizontal and vertical axes should be clearly labeled. A legend (key) should accompany a figure if symbols are used to indicate stages, or if lines are used to indicate the progress of different groups.

The meaning and format of the table or figure should be clearly understandable. Only pertinent summaries should be presented in the research report.

Data may be quantitative or qualitative; that is, data may be expressed in numbers or words. Quantitative data are numerical information such as that obtained from the measurement of quantities (e.g., height, weight, hemoglobin, blood pH, uric acid level, and liver enzyme levels such as SGOT and LDH). The data fall out on a continuum (i.e., on a continuous scale). Qualitative data are nonnumerical information (e.g., gender, ethnicity, leadership style, blood type, eye color, and diagnosis). Qualitative data sort people or items into separate, or discrete, classes (Weiss, 1993).

***Are the Statistical Procedures Appropriate to the Research Question or Hypothesis and to the Type of Data Collected?*** The two major categories of statistical techniques are descriptive and inferential. Descriptive statistics are used to depict the data. The most commonly used descriptive statistics are the mean, median, range, and standard deviation, which are measures of central tendency (mean, median) and the variability of scores (range, standard deviation) for the sample. Descriptive statistics take large amounts of data and convert them into information that is manageable and have meaning for the research consumer. Descriptive statistics summarize how a group scored on the variable of interest (Borg and Gall, 1989; Brockopp and Hastings-Tolsma, 1995). See Table 6-1 on p. 147 for a partial summary of the data presented by Stevens and Johnston (1994), who studied the physiological responses of premature infants to a painful stimulus. For illustration purposes, only the baseline data for the infants are shown.

Table 6-1 shows the mean, standard deviation, and range of scores (highest and lowest) of the baseline data collected by the nurse researchers. Baseline data collected are the maximum heart rate, mean heart rate standard deviation, minimum oxygen saturation, mean oxygen saturation standard deviation, and intracranial pressure difference. The study included a total of 138 premature infants, which gives the findings more credibility than if the sample size were only 20. Descriptive statistics summarize the large amount of data collected on each infant.

Inferential statistics are used to make inferences about a population based on the results obtained from studying a sample selected from the population. This inference is possible based on techniques that determine, within specified levels of confidence, if the results of the study occurred because of the manipulation of the independent variable or if they occurred by chance. Inferential statistics answer questions about the differences between groups (i.e., the difference between the experimental group and the control group in an experimental research design). Inferential statistics allow the nurse researcher to make an inference from the sample population to a larger population from which the sample is drawn.

For example, Cupples (1991) studied the effectiveness of preadmission preoperative education for clients having coronary artery bypass graft surgery. She hypothesized that both preadmission and postadmission preoperative education would result in "(1) higher preoperative knowledge levels, (2) lower levels of postoperative anxiety, (3) more positive postoperative mood states, and (4) more favorable physiologic recoveries" among the clients (p. 655). The experimental group received both preadmission and postadmission preoperative education. The control group received only routine postadmission preoperative education. She found that the experimental group had a statistically significant higher level of preoperative knowledge, more positive mood states, and more favorable physiological recoveries than the control group. She found no statistically significant difference in the level of postoperative anxiety between the two groups.

Table 6-2 presents the purpose of some commonly used statistics. These are descriptive and inferential statistics with which the nurse consumer of research should be familiar. They are the numerical basis upon which the nurse researcher reasons about the relationship between variables. The critical thinker must understand statistical reasoning to evaluate evidence derived from research.

The mean or median shows what the average subject in the study is like. The range of scores shows the largest and smallest scores of the subjects on the variable of interest. The range ignores the spread of scores between these two extremes. The standard deviation is a measure of the dispersion (variability) of scores about the mean. Standard deviation, along with the mean, gives a good description of the subjects in the study. Scores that are +3 and –3 standard deviations from the mean are furthest from the mean (in the tails of the normal curve) whereas scores that are +1 or –1 are closest to the mean (Borg and Gall, 1989).

Correlation coefficient is a descriptive measure in mathematical terms of the strength and the direction of the relationship between two variables. The correlation coefficient can be used for either descriptive or inferential studies. The most commonly used statistic is the Pearson product-moment correlation coefficient (Pearson's *r*), also known as the linear correlation coefficient. The value always lies somewhere between the range from –1.0 through 0 to +1.0. Zero means no relationship between

Table 6-2   **Purpose of Commonly Used Statistics***

| STATISTIC | PURPOSE |
| --- | --- |
| Mean or median | To represent what the typical or average subject is like. |
| Range of scores | To indicate how spread out the scores are. |
| Standard deviation | To show the variability around the mean of the scores in a distribution. |
| Pearson correlation | To reflect the degree of relationship between two variables. |
| Chi square | To reflect a relationship between two variables for categorical data. |
| t-test | To determine if a difference between the mean scores of two groups exists. |
| Analysis of variance | An extension of the t-test to test if significant differences among mean scores of three or more groups or with two or more independant variables occur. |

*Modified from Tanner CA, Imle M, and Stewart B: Guidelines for evaluation of research for use in practice. In Tanner CA and Lindeman CA (Eds.), Using nursing research, New York, 1989, National League for Nursing.

the two variables exists; –1 means a perfect negative relationship exists; and +1 means a perfect positive relationship exists. The + and – signs indicate the direction of the relationship. A negative score means the relationship is inverse (i.e., a high score on one variable is associated with a low score on the second variable). For example, the amount of pain the premature infants experienced with the heel lance procedure decreased as the time following the procedure increased. A positive score means that a high score on one variable is accompanied by a high score on the second variable. For example, an increase in pain is accompanied by an increase in heart rate (Glass and Hopkins, 1984; Weiss, 1993).

Chi square is a measure of the relationship between two variables for categorical data (Borg and Gall, 1989). For example, a nurse researcher wanted to study febrile children less than 2 years old. The nurse researcher placed the children in two categories, those with a temperature below 103°F and those with a temperature at 103°F and above. After forming these categories, the nurse researcher counted the number of children in each category who had convulsive seizures. The nurse researcher used chi square to determine if a statistically significant difference in the number of seizures between the two categories of children occurred.

The t-test is used to determine if a difference between the means of two groups exists. For example, a nurse researcher wanted to know if preoperative education had a positive effect on the recovery time of clients undergoing surgery. The nurse researcher randomly assigned subjects to an experimental group and a control group. The experimental group received the preoperative education, and the control group did not. The nurse researcher determined the mean recovery time for the two groups and used a t-test to determine if the magnitude of difference between the two means was significant.

The t value, which reflects the probability of that great a difference occurring by chance alone, is reported as a level of significance, or probability ($p$). A statistically significant finding means that the finding is unlikely to have happened by chance. The p 0.05 level of significance means the nurse researcher would obtain this result by chance alone only 5 or fewer times in 100; that is, the nurse researcher would reach the wrong conclusion only 5 or fewer times in 100. The p 0.01 level of significance means the nurse researcher would obtain this result by chance alone only 1 time in 100; that is, the nurse researcher would reach the wrong conclusion only 1 time in 100 (Grey, 1994c; Weiss, 1993).

Analysis of variance (ANOVA) is essentially the same as the t-test except it is more sophisticated. It can determine if three or more sample means are significantly different from one another. Analysis of variance considers the variation among all groups, rather than testing each pair of means separately. Analysis of variance yields an $F$ value, which is analogous to the t value (Borg and Gall, 1989; Grey, 1994c). Ultimately, the results of the analysis of variance and the t-test mean the same thing. For example, Peterson (1991) used analysis of variance to study client anxiety before cardiac catheterization. Peterson randomly assigned the clients to one of three groups. Clients in group one constituted the control group; clients in group two received an educational intervention to reduce anxiety; and clients in group three received a social intervention to reduce anxiety. The educational ($p = 0.001$) and social ($p = 0.0005$) groups had a significant drop in anxiety levels when compared with the

Table 6-3   **Commonly Reported Statistical Findings**\*

| STATISTICAL TEST | EXAMPLE OF REPORTED FINDINGS |
| --- | --- |
| Mean | $M = 118.28$ |
| Standard deviation | $SD = 62.5$ |
| Pearson correlation | $r = -0.39, p < .01$ |
| Chi-square | $\chi 2 = 2.52, df = 1, p < .05$ |
| t-test | $t = 2.65, p < .01$ |
| Analysis of variance | $F = 3.59, df = 2, 48, p < .05$ |

\*From LoBiondo-Wood G: Analysis of the findings. In LoBiondo-Wood G and Haber J (Eds.), Nursing research: Methods, critical appraisal, and utilization (ed. 3), St Louis, 1994a, Mosby.

control group. No significant difference between the drop in anxiety levels of the social and educational groups occurred ($p = 0.623$).

Table 6-3 presents some examples of how these statistics are reported in a research report. Note that the level of significance, in addition to the t-test, is also reported for the Pearson correlation, the analysis of variance, and the chi square. The interpretation of the $p$ level is the same as that described in the discussion of the t-test. *df* stands for degrees of freedom. It is a statistical term that factors in an estimate of variance between the true population mean (when it is unknown) and the sample mean.

***Is the Meaning of the Statistical Procedures Discussed?***   You need a basic knowledge about statistics to understand the statistical reasoning found in research reports; however, you do not have to be a master of statistical procedures. The researcher should identify which findings are statistically significant and discuss the meaning of the significance in the discussion of findings section of the report. The consumer of research should be able to distinguish between statistically significant and statistically insignificant results quickly.

## Discussion of Findings

The last section of the research report, the discussion of findings, is perhaps the most interesting part. In this section the nurse researcher interprets and assigns meaning to the data. You should read the discussion of findings, critically and analytically, always entertaining the possibility that other interpretations may be possible. To think critically about the discussion of findings of a quantitative research report, ask the following:

▼ Do the data answer the research question or hypothesis?
▼ Do the data support the researcher's interpretation and conclusion?
▼ Are other conclusions possible?
▼ Are the limitations noted?

▼ Are the implications for education, practice, and theory appropriate to the research design and results?

▼ Are recommendations for further research made?

**Do the Data Answer the Research Question or Hypothesis?**    The discussion of the findings section should begin by directing the attention of the reader back to the purpose of the research and the research question or the hypothesis. The discussion and interpretation of the findings should relate directly to them. Consider how the discussion of findings section begins in the example research report (Griffith, James, and Cropp, 1994).

This study evaluated the safety and efficacy of topical nitroglycerin ointment application to facilitate venous cannulation. This is the first study to report plasma drug levels in evaluating the technique. Despite the finding that topical application of 2% nitroglycerin ointment was safe to use, vein size did not increase significantly (p. 205).

The authors return to the purpose of the research, the unique contribution of this particular study, and the significance of the findings.

**Do the Data Support the Researcher's Interpretation and Conclusion?**    The nurse researcher interprets the results and draws conclusions based on her or his interpretations. Neither the nurse researcher nor research consumer should conclude that a significant result is a "fact" or that the research study proved something. The results provide descriptive information about a phenomenon of interest and may identify possible relationships among the variables. Significant results are meaningful only within the context of a specific study (Brockopp and Hastings-Tolsma, 1995).

The discussion of findings section is similar to the concept of a capstone. The discussion of findings ties together all of the component parts of the research study. The research report should relate the results to the theoretical framework and discuss whether the results supported the framework. Any additional findings or relationships not previously anticipated should also be included in the discussion (LoBiondo-Wood, 1994a).

Insignificant results do not indicate that the study was a failure or should not have been done. Insignificant findings can be important. All good research, regardless of the significance of the findings, contributes to the unique body of nursing knowledge. If the findings are not significant, the nurse researcher should reflect on the theoretical framework and reevaluate her or his earlier thinking processes (LoBiondo-Wood, 1994a). Expect the nurse researcher to provide an explanation of the insignificant finding. Factors such as the sample size being too small or too heterogeneous, the data collection methods or instruments being invalid or insensitive, or the intervention not being strong enough could affect the outcomes (Tanner, Imle, and Stewart, 1989).

**Are Other Conclusions Possible?**    When you reflect on the logic of the nurse researcher's conclusions, ask if other conclusions could be supported by the data. Are the data misleading in any way that cause the nurse researcher to draw a faulty conclusion? Avoid taking statements at face value; expect the nurse researcher to offer persuasive support for them (Brockopp and Hastings-Tolsma, 1995). If the researcher used an experimental or quasiexperimental research design, ask if something other than the treatment or nursing intervention could have affected the results. Consider the possibility that other intervening variables may be a factor in producing the results.

***Are the Limitations Noted?*** All research has weaknesses and limitations. They should be reported and discussed within the context of the research design, the sample, the data collection methods or instrument, and the analysis. The discussion should be factual in nature, not fault-finding (LoBiondo-Wood, 1994a).

***Are the Implications for Education, Practice, and Theory Appropriate to the Research Design and Results?*** The nurse researcher must be careful to make only appropriate generalizations. Inferences should not be made beyond the confines of the research design. The results of nonexperimental research designs are not generalizable; the findings are applicable to the research sample for that particular study. The findings of experimental research designs must be generalized appropriately, and only within the context of that particular research study (i.e., generalizations must be confined to the population from which the sample was drawn). For example, the statistically significant findings about the impact of aerobic exercises on muscle strength and flexibility on elderly subjects should not be generalized to middle-aged adults. Research reports that overgeneralize should alert the critical thinker to question the conclusions. LoBiondo-Wood (1994a) noted that generalizations are appropriate if they make inferences within the confines of the research design and are limited to a particular situation and a particular time.

The research report should identify the implications for education, practice, and theory as appropriate. The critical thinker should analyze and evaluate research reports that recommend a change in clinical practice. Tanner, Imle, and Stewart (1989) offer three guidelines to evaluate the applicability of research to practice. First, consider the similarity between the research sample and the practice setting and your own. If these are similar, evaluate how the sample is selected and whether it is representative of the target population. If random selection is used, you might assume the findings are applicable; however, recall that random selection in clinical research is rarely possible. If random selection is not used, you must rely on the researcher's description of the sample to determine the similarity of the sample and setting to your own.

Second, compare the staff who implemented the procedures in the study and your own staff. How similar are they? Will any special training be required for your staff? Titler et al. (1994) found that staff nurses who are included early in the process of implementing a change in nursing practice help facilitate the change. They become advocates for it.

Third, consider whether the study has been replicated and, if so, in what kinds of settings? If it has been replicated, and the findings are consistent across studies, then you can have more confidence in the results. Since few nursing research studies have been replicated, consider replicating the study in your practice setting and draw your own conclusions about the costs, risks, and benefits. Once you have concluded that it is appropriate to implement the findings of the research-based nursing practice, Titler, Kleiber, Steelman, Goode, Rakel, Barry-Walker, Small, and Buckwalter (1994) recommend you first implement the new practice on a pilot unit. This allows you to evaluate the feasibility of the practice further, monitor the impact of it on clients to minimize possible adverse effects, and revise it if necessary.

***Are Recommendations for Further Research Made?***   A research report usually points out areas for further investigation. A good research study generates more questions than it answers. When you reflect on the research study, determine what questions you have, what questions were not answered by the study, and what you would do differently if you had to conduct the study again. Answers to these questions point out directions for further research.

The research report should be written clearly, and the language should be readily understandable. The report should flow logically from one section to the other without unnecessary repetition. It should be thorough and include all information essential to understand the research purpose, problem, theoretical framework, design, sample, data collection, analysis, and discussion. Each part of the research process should be consistent with all other parts and contribute to the whole of the study.

## SUMMARY

Reasoning, as it is applied to scientific inquiry, follows a systematic process to investigate the relationship between that which is observed and the explanation for it. Nursing research is the application of scientific reasoning to the systematic investigation of nursing problems. The conclusions, or findings, then become the evidence you need to support a change to improve clinical practice or to justify further study. Nursing research also contributes to the expansion of the unique body of nursing knowledge.

The evaluation of evidence from quantitative nursing research requires critical thought and a systematic process to ensure thoroughness. The questioning format we propose in this chapter encourages thoroughness. Evaluating nursing research is an expectation of graduates from all nursing programs at the associate degree level and beyond. Nurses are expected to be informed consumers of research and be capable of evaluating reports to determine their relevance to clinical practice, a process that requires a sophisticated level of critical thinking.

# EXERCISES

## Exercise 1

**Purpose:** *Become familiar with nursing research journals*

### DIRECTIONS

1. Go to the library and browse through some nursing research journals (e.g., *Nursing Research, Research in Nursing and Health, IMAGE: Journal of Nursing Scholarship,* and *Western Journal of Nursing Research*). You may look up a research report referred to in this chapter, or you may find one that interests you. Evaluate it using the format presented in this chapter.

2. Complete a topic search using the library's computerized databases. Select a topic in which you are interested and find a research report about it that is published in a nursing research journal.

   Do not be intimidated by an unduly, sophisticated-looking article or discouraged by any initial difficulty you may have in reading and understanding it. Education is a process of becoming familiar with the unfamiliar. Consider this as just another fun challenge for you in a long list of challenges that you have already successfully mastered.

3. Report back to the class about the article you selected and why it was interesting to you. Briefly summarize your evaluation for your colleagues.

## Exercise 2

**Purpose:** *Practice thinking like a researcher*

### DIRECTIONS

1. Repeat Exercise 1, except select an article from a nonnursing research journal. How does that research article compare with the nursing research article?

2. Report back to the class about the article you selected and why it was interesting to you. Briefly summarize the differences you found between the nursing and nonnursing research reports for your colleagues.

# Exercise 3

**Purpose:** *Evaluate a report of a research study found in a newspaper*

## DIRECTIONS

1. Find a report of a health-related survey in a daily newspaper widely circulated in your community. What questions would you want answered before you support the conclusions of the researchers?

2. Bring the report to class and share your evaluation with your colleagues. What questions, other than the ones you identified, do your colleagues want answered?

# Exercise 4

**Purpose:** *Evaluate a quantitative research report*

## DIRECTIONS

Complete a full evaluation of the quantitative research report in Appendix B. Use the format presented in this chapter. Discuss your analysis in class with your colleagues who have also evaluated it. On which items is there full agreement? Disagreement? Why? Defend your views in those instances where significant disagreement occurs.

# Exercise 5

**Purposes:** *Conceptualize a nursing research study using the quantitative approach*
*Create a theoretical framework to conduct the research*

## DIRECTIONS

Divide into small groups. Identify an area for study that is of interest to the group. Engage in the following activities:

1. Brainstorm researchable questions or hypotheses and create a brief paragraph to serve as the theoretical framework.

2. Discuss which type of research design would be most appropriate to use and which type of data would best answer the research question or hypotheses.

3. Define the population of interest and determine how the research sample will be drawn.

4. Select appropriate statistical tests and create a sample table to show the results.

5. Interpret the results, draw conclusions, and identify implications.

When you have completed this assignment, reflect on the following:

- ▼ What areas were the most and the least difficult for the group?
- ▼ Do all members of the group agree on the most and the least difficult areas?
- ▼ How did the group get beyond the difficult areas?
- ▼ What reasoning skills were essential in conceptualizing and conducting nursing quantitative research?
- ▼ What role would each member of the group like to play if it were possible to carry out the research?

## Exercise 6

**Purpose:** *Articulate an explanation and defense for your research*

### DIRECTIONS

Role-play your appearance before the research committee in a health care agency. The purpose of the committee hearing is twofold: first, to explain what you will study and how you will study it, and second, to request permission to conduct the study in this agency.

The class should assume the role of committee members who seek further information and clarification about your study. They should conclude the role play by making a judgment about whether or not you should be given permission to conduct the study in their agency.

## Exercise 7

**Purpose:** *Apply your knowledge of statistics*

### DIRECTIONS

Analyze the meaning of the following numerical tables. Explain what the data mean.

1. Table 6-4 (adapted from Aaronson and MacNee, 1989) shows the birth weight of infants and the amount of weight gain by the mothers during pregnancy.

2. Table 6-5 shows the demographic and functional characteristics of older Hispanic immigrants (adapted from Ailinger, Dear, and Holley-Wilcox, 1993).

3. Recall the study conducted by Cupples (1991). She hypothesized that subjects having coronary artery bypass graft surgery who received both preadmission and postadmission preoperative education would have (1) higher preoperative knowledge levels, (2) lower levels of postoperative anxiety, and (3) more positive postoperative mood states. What does Table 6-6 tell you about the findings relative to the hypotheses?

### Table 6-4   **Descriptive Statistics of Study Variables***

| VARIABLE | MEAN | STANDARD DEVIATION | RANGE |
| --- | --- | --- | --- |
| Birth weight (g) | 3,556.0 | 556.0 | 1,040.0 to 7,216.0 |
| Weight gain (lb) | 33.5 | 10.0 | −2.5 to 63.5 |

*Modified from Aaronson LS and MacNee CL: Nurs Res 38(4):223-227, 1989.

### Table 6-5   **Demographic and Functional Characteristics***

| DEMOGRAPHIC | ORIGINAL (N=156) | REINTERVIEWED (N=76) | DECEASED (N=30) | UNABLE (N=38) | REFUSED (N=12) |
| --- | --- | --- | --- | --- | --- |
| **GENDER** | | | | | |
| Female | 106 | 44 | 22 | 28 | 12 |
| Male | 50 | 32 | 8 | 10 | 0 |
| **AGE** | | | | | |
| Mean | 66 | 66 | 69 | 63 | 65 |
| Standard deviation | 8.94 | 8.94 | 9.52 | 9.49 | 7.34 |
| **YEARS IN THE UNITED STATES** | | | | | |
| (Mean) | 13 | 14 | 12 | 9 | 17 |
| **COUNTRY OF ORIGIN** | | | | | |
| South America | 62 | 28 | 12 | 18 | 4 |
| Cuba | 40 | 22 | 7 | 6 | 5 |
| Central America | 38 | 16 | 10 | 11 | 2 |
| Other | 16 | 10 | 1 | 3 | 1 |
| **FUNCTIONAL AREA** (Good to excellent rating) | | | | | |
| Social | 71 | 38 | 8 | 10 | 4 |
| Economic | 42 | 22 | 4 | 8 | 4 |
| Mental | 79 | 44 | 4 | 13 | 4 |
| Physical | 53 | 27 | 5 | 7 | 5 |
| ADL | 89 | 45 | 7 | 15 | 7 |

N = 156
ADL = Activities of daily living.
*Modified from Ailinger RL, Dear MR, and Holley-Wilcox P: Nurs Res 42(4):240-244, 1993.

Table 6-6    **Independent t-tests for Outcome Measures: KQ, STAI, and POMS TMD Scores***

| VARIABLE | MEAN | STANDARD DEVIATION (SD) | DEGREES OF FREEDOM (DF) | t | PROBABILITY (P) |
|---|---|---|---|---|---|
| **KQ SCORES** | | | | | |
| Experimental group | 18.74 | 1.34 | 38 | 3.87 | <0.001 |
| Control group | 16.85 | 1.66 | | | |
| **STAI SCORES** | | | | | |
| Experimental group | 32.80 | 7.91 | 38 | 1.20 | 0.24 |
| Control group | 36.96 | 13.2 | | | |
| **POMS TMD SCORES** | | | | | |
| Experimental group | 10.40 | 20.69 | 38 | 2.31 | 0.03 |
| Control group | 36.00 | 45.09 | | | |

*KQ: Coronary Artery Bypass Graft Surgery Knowledge Questionaire (given preoperatively)

STAI Scores: State anxiety scale of the State-Trait Anxiety Inventory (assesses the transitory condition of perceived anxiety; given postoperatively)

POMS TMD Scores: Profile of Mood States (to measure postoperative mood states) as expressed by the TMD score (a total mood disturbance, a single, global estimate of affective state)

From Cupples SA: Heart Lung 20(6):657, 1991.

# Exercise 8

**Purpose:** *Debate an issue*

## DIRECTIONS

Debate the following issues:

1. Statistical thinking leads to stereotyping people.

2. Scientific reasoning is the best way to discover new knowledge.

# Exercise 9

**Purpose:** *Reflect and write in your journal*

## DIRECTIONS

Reflect and write in your journal about the following:

1. What are you curious about? Make a list of questions for which you would like answers and about which the answers are now unknown.

2. Think about the clients for whom you have cared and your nursing interventions. Generate researchable questions about the situations. Which would be the most important to investigate? Least important?

3. Based on your present level of knowledge, what gaps in the unique body of nursing knowledge can you identify? Compare your list with your colleagues.

## REFERENCES

Aaronson, L.S., and MacNee, C.L. (1989). The relationship between weight gain and nutrition in pregnancy. *Nursing Research, 38*(4), 223-227.

Ahijevych, K., and Bernhard, L. (1994). Health-promoting behaviors of African-American women. *Nursing Research, 43*(2), 86-89.

Ailinger, R.L., Dear, M.R., and Holley-Wilcox, P. (1993). Predictors of function among older Hispanic immigrants: A five-year follow-up. *Nursing Research, 42*(4), 240-244.

American Nurses' Association. (1981). *Guidelines for the investigative function of nurses.* Kansas City, Mo.: Author.

Bandman, E.L., and Bandman, B. (1995). *Critical thinking in nursing* (2nd ed.). Norwalk, Conn.: Appleton and Lange.

Borg, W.R., and Gall, M.D. (1989). *Educational research: An introduction* (5th ed.). New York: Longman.

Bresser, P.J., Sexton, D.L., and Foell, D.W. (1993). Patients' responses to postponement of coronary artery bypass graft surgery. *IMAGE: Journal of Nursing Scholarship, 25*(1), 5-10.

Brockopp, D.Y., and Hastings-Tolsma, M.T. (1995). *Fundamentals of nursing research* (2nd ed.). Boston: Jones and Bartlett.

Chaffee, J. (1994). *Thinking critically* (4th ed.). Boston: Houghton Mifflin.

Creasia, J.L. (1991). Professional nursing roles. In J.L. Creasia and B. Parker (Eds.), *Conceptual foundations of professional nursing practice* (pp. 73-86). St Louis: Mosby.

Cupples, S.A. (1991). Effects of timing and reinforcement of preoperative education on knowledge and recovery of patients having coronary artery bypass graft surgery. *Heart & Lung, 20*(6), 654-660.

Feldman, H.R. (1994). The theoretical framework. In G. LoBiondo-Wood, and J. Haber (Eds.), *Nursing research: Methods, critical appraisal, and utilization* (3rd ed., pp. 142-159). St Louis: Mosby.

Glass, G.V., and Hopkins, K.D. (1984). *Statistical methods in education and psychology* (2nd ed.). Englewood Cliffs, N.J.: Prentice Hall.

Grey, M. (1994a). Data collection methods. In G. LoBiondo-Wood and J. Haber (Eds.), *Nursing research: Methods, critical appraisal, and utilization* (3rd ed., pp. 344-364). St Louis: Mosby.

————. (1994b). Experimental and quasiexperimental designs. In G. LoBiondo-Wood and J. Haber (Eds.), *Nursing research: Methods, critical appraisal, and utilization* (3rd ed., pp. 213-230). St Louis: Mosby.

————. (1994c). Inferential data analysis. In G. LoBiondo-Wood and J. Haber (Eds.), *Nursing research: Methods, critical appraisal, and utilization* (3rd ed., pp. 404-423). St Louis: Mosby.

Griffith, P., James, B., and Cropp, A. (1994). Evaluation of the safety and efficacy of topical nitroglycerin ointment to facilitate venous cannulation. *Nursing Research, 43*(4), 203-206.

Haber, J. (1994). Sampling. In G. LoBiondo-Wood and J. Haber (Eds.), *Nursing research: Methods, critical appraisal, and utilization* (3rd ed., pp. 286-312). St Louis: Mosby.

Herder, S. (1994). Sponge baths for fever: A waste of nursing time. *American Journal of Nursing, 94*(10), 55.

Jackson, B.S. (1994). Legal and ethical issues. In G. LoBiondo-Wood and J. Haber (Eds.), *Nursing research: Methods, critical appraisal, and utilization* (3rd ed., pp. 313-343). St Louis: Mosby.

Jacox, A., and Prescott, P. (1978, November). Determining a study's relevance for clinical practice. *American Journal of Nursing,* 1882-1889.

Knowles, M. (1990). *The adult learner: A neglected species* (4th ed.). Houston: Gulf.

Kohn, A. (1994). The truth about self-esteem. *Phi Delta Kappan, 76*(4), 272-283.

Kolanowski, A.M. (1990). Restlessness in the elderly: The effect of artificial lighting. *Nursing Research, 39*(3), 181-183.

Krouse, H.J., and Roberts, S.J. (1989). Nurse-patient interactive styles: Power, control, and satisfaction. *Western Journal of Nursing Research, 11*(6), 717-725.

Lierman, L.M., Young, H.M., Powell-Cope, G., Georgiadou, F., and Benoliel, J.Q. (1994). Effects of education and support on breast self-examination in older women. *Nursing Research, 43*(3), 158-163.

LoBiondo-Wood, G. (1994a). Analysis of the Findings. In G. LoBiondo-Wood and J. Haber (Eds.), *Nursing research: Methods, critical appraisal, and utilization* (3rd ed., pp. 424-437). St Louis: Mosby.

———. (1994b). Introduction to design. In G. LoBiondo-Wood and J. Haber (Eds.), *Nursing research: Methods, critical appraisal, and utilization* (3rd ed., pp. 192-211). St Louis: Mosby.

LoBiondo-Wood, G., and Haber, J. (1994a). Nonexperimental designs. In G. LoBiondo-Wood and J. Haber (Eds.), *Nursing research: Methods, critical appraisal, and utilization* (3rd ed., pp. 231-252). St Louis: Mosby.

———. (1994b). The role of research in nursing. In G. LoBiondo-Wood and J. Haber (Eds.), *Nursing research: Methods, critical appraisal, and utilization* (3rd ed., pp. 3-32). St Louis: Mosby.

Madness tied to creativity, study reveals. (1987, March 24). *Rocky Mountain News.*

McKeever, P., and Galloway, S.C. (1984). Effects of nongynecological surgery on the menstrual cycle. *Nursing Research, 33*(1), 42-46.

Miller, B.K. (1994). The literature review. In G. LoBiondo-Wood and J. Haber (Eds.), *Nursing research: Methods, critical appraisal, and utilization* (3rd ed., pp. 109-141). St Louis: Mosby.

Mills, E.M. (1994). The effect of low-intensity aerobic exercise on muscle strength, flexibility, and balance among sedentary elderly persons. *Nursing Research, 43*(4), 207-211.

Munro, B.H., Creamer, A.M., Haggerty, M.R., and Cooper, F.S. (1988). Effect of relaxation therapy on post–myocardial infarction patients' rehabilitation. *Nursing Research, 37*(4), 231-235.

Neufeldt, V. (1991). *Webster's new world dictionary* (3rd ed.). New York: Webster's New World.

Olds, S., London, M., and Ladewig, P. (1992). *Maternal Newborn Nursing* (4th ed.). Redwood City, Calif.: Addison-Wesley.

Peterson, M. (1991). Patient anxiety before cardiac catheterization: An intervention study. *Heart & Lung, 20*(6), 643-647.

Stevens, B.J., and Johnston, C.C. (1994). Physiological responses of premature infants to a painful stimulus. *Nursing Research, 43*(4), 226-231.

Stuifbergen, A.K., and Becker, H.A. (1994). Predictors of health-promoting lifestyles in persons with disabilities. *Research in Nursing & Health, 17*(1), 3-13.

Tanner, C.A., Imle, M., and Stewart, B. (1989). Guidelines for evaluation of research for use in practice. In C.A. Tanner and C.A. Lindeman (Eds.), *Using nursing research* (pp. 35-60). New York: National League for Nursing.

Titler, M.G., Kleiber, C., Steelman, V., Goode, C., Rakel, B., Barry-Walker, J., Small, S., and Buckwalter, K. (1994). Infusing research into practice to promote quality care. *Nursing Research, 43*(5), 307-313.

Tylenol overdoses can harm liver. (1994, December 21). *The Denver Post*, p. 4A.

Weiss, N.A. (1993). *Elementary statistics* (2nd ed.). Reading, Mass.: Addison-Wesley.

Wilson, H.S. (1993). *Introducing research in nursing* (2nd ed.). New York: Addison-Wesley.

# Evaluating Qualitative and Other Evidence

## Chapter 7

## OVERVIEW

Chapter 7 continues the discussion of the evaluation of evidence, which began in Chapter 6. This chapter describes how critical thinking applies to the evaluation of evidence derived from qualitative research conducted by nurse researchers. The discussion distinguishes between the philosophical and methodological differences of the quantitative and qualitative research approaches. Chapter 7 concludes with a discussion of evidence derived from sources other than research, such as the data derived from client assessment and evaluation.

This chapter's primary emphasis is on the reasoning process you need to critically evaluate qualitative research reports. Similar to the one discussed in Chapter 6, the format to apply critical thinking to the evaluation of qualitative research is organized, systematic, and uses a questioning strategy. The discussion focuses on what you, the nurse consumer of research, need to know to evaluate evidence derived from qualitative research. It provides a base for you to determine if the evidence is sufficiently strong to warrant application to your practice setting.

In Chapter 6, you learned about the critical thinking skills associated with evaluating evidence. They are to (1) evaluate evidence derived from quantitative and qualitative research, (2) evaluate evidence derived from the assessment of clients, (3) make appropriate inferences based on evidence derived from research and clients, (4) assess research for its relevance to clinical practice, and (5) participate in systematic and accurate data collection.

## QUALITATIVE RESEARCH

Qualitative research is gaining popularity in nursing. In the past, nurse researchers have primarily used quantitative methods of scientific inquiry to develop nursing's unique body of knowledge. The dominance of research reports with nonexperimental and experimental research designs using quantitative data that are published in nursing research journals attests this fact. Quantitative nursing research methods embrace the tenets of the scientific method and attempt to understand nursing science by studying its component parts (reductionistic thinking) as expressed by the language of mathematics (Carter, 1985). By studying the component parts, the researcher attempts to understand the whole. Objectivity is achieved by studying variables in isolation of their context and existing values as illustrated earlier in the discussion of quantitative research.

More recently, nurses have become interested in humanistic, qualitative research approaches that provide an entirely different theoretical and methodological orientation to research. The movement toward qualitative research is a significant paradigm shift in how nurse researchers think. The interest in qualitative approaches is based on the belief that they are more suitable to understand many nursing phenomena. Qualitative approaches focus on understanding the whole phenomenon rather than its component parts in isolation. Traditionally, nursing educators have taught a holistic view of clients, families, and society by emphasizing integratation of the biologic, psychologic, sociologic, cultural, and spiritual dimensions of humanness. Nursing focuses on the uniqueness of each individual and the importance of understanding the individual within his or her surrounding context (i.e., environment). The qualitative approach to inquiry encompasses the complex, holistic nature of nursing—an approach that examines the lived experiences of the individual within his or her environment. This conceptualization is consistent with general systems theory that describes the interrelatedness and interdependence of all phenomena. General systems theory teaches that a change in one part of the system creates changes in other parts. A growing number of nurse researchers believe that qualitative research provides an approach that more closely matches the "real world" of nursing practice.

Brockopp and Hastings-Tolsma (1995) define qualitative research as:

> . . . an inductive approach to discovering or expanding knowledge. It requires the involvement of the researcher in the identification of the meaning or relevance of a particular phenomenon to the individual. Analysis and interpretation of findings in this method are not generally dependent upon the quantification of observations (p. 235).

Qualitative research is an inductive reasoning process that generates new knowledge and understandings. In contrast, quantitative research is a deductive reasoning process that tests theories. The goal of qualitative research "is to document and interpret as fully as possible the totality of whatever is being studied in particular contexts from the people's viewpoint or frame of reference" (Leininger, 1985b, p. 5).

Qualitative research is an inclusive term and refers to more than 20 different kinds of research methods (Leininger, 1992). Table 7-1 illustrates the essence, foundation, and questions characteristic of the qualitative research of four commonly used methods.

## FORMAT TO EVALUATE QUALITATIVE RESEARCH

The Format to Evaluate Qualitative Research box on p. 182 contains one suggested format for the nurse consumer of research to apply critical thinking to the evaluation of qualitative research. Because of the differences among the many qualitative research methods, each method has its own way by which it is best evaluated. You should keep this in mind when using this format. The format asks specific questions to guide your thinking as you evaluate a qualitative research report. Knowing the right questions to ask and evaluating the answers are important critical thinking skills. A thorough, critical

Table 7-1   **Comparison of Qualitative Methods:
Essence, Foundation, and Questions***

| METHOD | ESSENCE OF METHOD | FOUNDATION | EXAMPLE QUESTIONS FROM PUBLISHED STUDIES |
|---|---|---|---|
| Phenomenological | Description of the "lived experience" | Philosophy | What is it like to be a provider of care in the NICU? (Swanson, 1990)<br><br>What are the essential features of self-transcendence in women with advanced breast cancer? (Coward, 1990) |
| Grounded theory | Systematic set of procedures used to arrive at theory about basic social processes | Symbolic interaction and the social sciences | How do care givers of family members with Alzheimer's disease experience bereavement? (Jones and Martinson, 1992)<br><br>How do patients with AIDS manage their illness? (Ragsdale, Kotorba, and Morrow, 1992) |
| Enthnographic | Descriptions of cultural groups or subgroups | Cultural anthropology | How do nurses from various health care settings perceive collaboration between indigenous and cosmopolitan health care systems? (Uphall, 1992)<br><br>What is the meaning of wellness to aging individuals? What factors contribute to wellness and aging? (Miller, 1991) |
| Historical | Systematic compilation of data to describe some past event | Philosophy, art, and science | How did philosophy, training methods, and settings establish the foundation of nursing education in America? (Davis, 1991)<br><br>How did nurses actively influence the development of ICUs through observation and triage, as well as seeking out necessary knowledge? (Fairman, 1992) |

*From Liehr PR and Marcus MT: Qualitative approaches to research. In LoBiondo-Wood G and Haber J (Eds.),
Nursing research: Methods, critical appraisal, and utilization (ed. 3), St Louis, 1994, Mosby.

# Format to Evaluate Qualitative Research*

**PHENOMENON OF INTEREST**

- ▼ Is the research focused on human experience within a natural setting?
- ▼ Is the research relevant to nursing?

**STUDY STRUCTURE**

### Research Question
- ▼ Does it specify a distinct process to be studied?
- ▼ Is it appropriate to the selected qualitative method?

### Researcher's Perspective
- ▼ Are the biases of the researcher reported?
- ▼ How was the literature review conducted and integrated into the study?

### Sample Selection
- ▼ Is the sample living the phenomenon of interest?
- ▼ Is the informant's context within the phenomenon of interest identified?
- ▼ Is the sample sufficient to tap all viewpoints on the phenomenon of interest and to saturate the concept(s)?

**DATA COLLECTION**

- ▼ Are data sources and methods described?
- ▼ Is the informant's consent an integral part of the data collection process?

**DATA ANALYSIS**

- ▼ What methods for data analysis were chosen? Why were they chosen?
- ▼ Does the researcher paint a clear picture of the reality and meaning experienced by the informant?
- ▼ Are concepts missing that you expected to find based on your clinical experience? Should the sample have yielded these concepts or would a different sample be needed?
- ▼ Are the relationships among the concepts supported by the data? Do the relationships make sense? Are other relationships possible?
- ▼ Have other professionals confirmed the researcher's interpretation?

**DESCRIPTION OF FINDINGS**

- ▼ Are examples provided that link the raw data to the researcher's synthesis?
- ▼ Are the findings linked to existing theory or literature?

---

*Modified from Liehr PR and Marcus MT: Qualitative approaches to research. In LoBiondo-Wood G and Haber J (Eds.), Nursing research: Methods, critical appraisal, and utilization (ed. 3), St Louis, 1994, Mosby; and Tanner CA, Imle M, and Stewart B: Guidelines for evaluation of research for use in practice. In Tanner CA and Lindeman CA (Eds.), Using nursing research, New York, 1989, National League for Nursing.

analysis of qualitative research requires extensive knowledge about the specific method-ological approach used by the nurse researcher. This format presents a beginning guide to evaluate qualitative research based on the five basic elements of qualitative research identified by Liehr and Marcus (1994).

## Phenomenon of Interest

To think critically about the phenomenon of interest of a qualitative research report, ask the following:

▼ Is it focused on human experience within a natural setting?
▼ Is it relevant to nursing?

Table 7-1 identifies the primary focus of each of the four commonly used quali-tative methods. Phenomenology focuses on the meaning of the lived experience for the individual. It examines the meaning and significance of the human experience (Ray, 1985). Grounded theory focuses on the basic social processes of the individual in interaction with others that are "grounded" in real life circumstances. The ethno-graphic method focuses on the lifeways or particular patterns of a cultural (or subcul-tural) group in its familiar environment in order to grasp what these mean to the members of the group (Leininger, 1985a). The historical method focuses on the sys-tematic examination of the past to include people, events, and occurrences. Ulti-mately the purpose of both qualitative and quantitative research in nursing is to improve the quality of nursing care delivered to clients and to continue to expand the body of nursing knowledge.

For example, Kondora's (1993) phenomenon of interest was the lived experi-ence of adult women survivors of childhood incest. Kondora used the phenomeno-logical approach. The purpose of her study was to reveal the personal journeys of childhood incest survivors by understanding their difficulties, their endurance, and their healing.

Kauffman (1994) used the ethnographic approach to examine the insider-outsider dilemma (i.e., the experience of "getting in" a poor black community). The purpose of her study was "to delineate the phases of getting in and suggest strategies for those researchers studying groups that differ from themselves" (p. 179). Both Kon-dora and Kauffman's research focused on the human experience, which is relevant to the practice of nursing.

## Study Structure

To evaluate the structure of the study, the consumer of research should evaluate the research question, the researcher's perspective, and the sample selection.

***Research Question.***    To think critically about the research question of a qualita-tive research report, ask the following:

▼ Does it specify a distinct process to be studied?

▼ Is it appropriate to the selected qualitative method?

The research question is based on the specific experience being investigated. Table 7-1 has examples of questions characteristic of each of the four approaches. The people Kondora (1993) studied were asked to respond to the following question: "What does it mean to you to be a survivor of childhood incest?" The interviews were unstructured and open-ended, and the women shared freely. After asking the research question, the nurse researcher encouraged the women to elaborate on their experiences by stating, "Tell me more about that," and "What did that mean to you?" Kauffman (1994) did not have a specific research question, which is a characteristic of quantitative research. Her purpose was to investigate the phases of getting into another cultural group.

With historical research, the investigator's topic may begin with a question or series of questions. Kruman (1985) posed the following questions to illustrate historical questions: "What role did Florence Nightingale play in the establishment of the modern nursing profession? What did she do that led historians to conclude that she was the first modern nurse? If, indeed, she was the first modern nurse, then how did she find a number of competent nurses to serve under her during the Crimean War?" Kruman noted that the perspective of the nurse researcher may change as she or he investigates a topic. The topic and questions may shift somewhat, which is acceptable. The initial set of questions, however, provides direction for the historical researcher.

To adequately judge whether the research question is appropriate to the selected qualitative method, you must complete further reading and study. Kondora's (1993) study about the lived experience of adult women survivors of childhood incest used the phenomenological approach, and Kauffman's (1994) study used the ethnographic approach to study a specific cultural community. Both were appropriate qualitative research approaches for the purposes of the investigators.

***Researcher's Perspective.***    To think critically about the researcher's perspective of a qualitative research report, ask the following:

▼ Are the biases of the researcher reported?

▼ How was the literature review conducted and integrated into the study?

Qualitative research methods attempt to make the researcher aware of his or her biases in the examination and interpretation of phenomena. Bias, a mental leaning or partiality (Neufeldt, 1991), is a problem in both qualitative and quantitative research. The slanting of data results in questionable research findings. The nurse researcher must be aware of her or his biases and make every attempt to identify and correct them to improve the reliability of the research findings. For example, to control bias in the historical approach, the researcher should seek to substantiate a document with another collaborating source (Brockopp and Hastings-Tolsma, 1995).

To control bias in phenomenological research, the researcher uses brackets [ ] to indicate a personal perspective or bias (Liehr and Marcus, 1994). Bracketing is a way to "hold in abeyance those elements that are irrelevant to nursing" (Ray, 1985, p. 89) and allow the client to fully express his or her reality. To understand brackets, recall how you learned to refine your therapeutic listening skills. You recorded what the client said and clearly separated it from your own thoughts and observations during the interview.

Control of bias is also a concern with the ethnographic method. With this method the nurse researcher becomes an interpreter who seeks to understand life from the perspective of the natives. The nurse researcher learns to be aware of his or her own biases and views and brackets them to set them aside in her or his attempt to understand others. Like the other qualitative methods, the researcher seeks to understand life from the individual's perspective, without imposing his or her own interpretation (Liehr and Marcus, 1994).

The review of literature takes a form and meaning in qualitative research that is different from quantitative research. The nurse researcher understands the phenomenon of interest but does not do an initial full review of the literature until the data are collected and analyzed. Delaying the literature review allows the nurse researcher to enter the research process with an open mind rather than with preconceived ideas about what to expect. Grounded theory is an exception to this way of conducting the literature review. Grounded theory uses an inductive-deductive reasoning process to generate theory; thus, the literature review is simultaneous with the collection and analysis of data. In this way, theory remains "grounded in" (connected to) the actual data (Brockopp and Hastings-Tolsma, 1995; Liehr and Marcus, 1994).

**Sample Selection.**   To think critically about the sample selection of a qualitative research report, ask the following:

▼  Is the sample living the phenomenon of interest?
▼  Is the informant's context within the phenomenon of interest identified?
▼  Is the sample sufficient to tap all viewpoints on the phenomenon of interest and to saturate the concept(s)?

In qualitative research, those in the research sample are referred to as people or informants (Leininger, 1985c). They are identified this way because they are directly involved in the phenomenon and thus enable the nurse researcher to study it. Because the purpose of qualitative research is to examine life from the perspective of those living it, you should evaluate the characteristics of the persons selected for study. All the informants must be representative of the phenomenon of interest; that is, they must be involved in the process being studied (Tanner, Imle, and Stewart, 1989). For example, if you are interested in studying women experiencing menopause, the sample should consist of women who are in the throes of menopause—not women who are beyond it. With historical research, data sources such as documents, informants, or observers of events, and artifacts such as photographs, may constitute the sample (Kruman, 1985).

A sensitivity to context is important to understand the meaning of the informant's communications. Recall that context refers to the informant's entire situation.

It includes biologic, psychologic, sociologic, cultural, and spiritual variables. Context is important because words have different meanings in different times and among people of different cultures. For example, consider what the word *health* might have meant to a nurse living in the late 1800s when infectious diseases were the primary cause of death. Today a nurse in the United States views health in terms of preventing lifestyle diseases such as cardiovascular disease and health problems associated with obesity. Health to a nurse practicing in the poverty stricken parts of Rwanda has a different meaning from that of the nurse practicing in the United States. Kruman (1985) reminds us that the historian must understand the meaning of words within the context of the times.

Sample size is not the issue in qualitative research as it is in quantitative research. In qualitative research, saturation is the issue. Saturation is achieved when the nurse researcher believes that all viewpoints have been examined and no new information is coming from additional informants. When additional informants simply confirm what has been previously stated, then saturation has been achieved for that concept or category of interest (Tanner, Imle, and Stewart, 1989). The sample size may have as few as five informants and still be considered accurate research.

As you evaluate the selection of informants and the findings of the study, ask whether they are consistent with your own experience or with people you know (e.g., close friends and colleagues). As a critical thinker, ask if you know clients who have experienced the phenomenon of interest but whose experiences and perceptions are different from those reported by the nurse researcher. If so, why did the researcher not discover these? Would a larger sample be needed? Would a different sample be required to include your client's experiences and perceptions?

Kondora (1993) selected her sample of adult survivors of incest by interviewing five women whom she recruited through notices posted in bookstores and in university classrooms. Kondora excluded women who had suicidal ideation, who had difficulty functioning within the previous year, and who had been hospitalized for acute emotional difficulties within the previous year. The researcher selected informants who were emotionally able to participate in the study. (See Appendix C for Kondora's study.)

## Data Collection

To think critically about the data collection of a qualitative research report, ask the following:

▼ Are data sources and methods described?
▼ Is the informant's consent an integral part of the data collection process?

The primary sources of qualitative data are researcher observation, informants' interviews, and document analysis (Wilson, 1993). Qualitative data are expressed in words rather than in numbers. Qualitative data may be field notes, audiotapes, and videotapes. If field notes are used, they should be prepared so that others may view and understand them. Audiotapes must be transcribed, and videotapes must be described for critical review by others. In qualitative research, those who gather the data are themselves the data collection instruments (Tanner, Imle, and Stewart, 1989).

Note that both qualitative and quantitative researchers use observation and interview. The qualitative researcher uses the information to gain insight into the phenomenon of interest, whereas the quantitative researcher converts the information into numbers that provide answers to the research questions.

For phenomenological research, qualitative data are collected by interview (structured or unstructured). The nurse researcher may also ask informants to respond to written questions. For grounded research, the researcher collects data by interviewing and observing the research informants interacting in a social setting. The researcher tapes and transcribes interviews and records observations as field notes (Liehr and Marcus, 1994). Field notes contain the who, what, where, and how of a situation with as little interpretation from the researcher as possible (Wilson, 1993).

For ethnographic research, the researcher collects data by observing or immersing himself or herself in the setting and by interviewing informants. Data collection occurs in the natural setting. Meaning is given to the data within the context of the culture. The researcher may also obtain life histories and collect artifacts representative of the culture (Leininger, 1985a; Liehr and Marcus, 1994). In Leininger's (1985a) ethnographic method, the nurse researcher observes, participates, and finally enters a phase of reflective observation whereby she or he looks back thoughtfully to recapture the total experience and to understand what transpired between the informants and the researcher. Informants are encouraged to clarify, verify, and confirm the data they provide so that the data are accurate and meaningful.

For historical research, data may be in the form of diaries, letters, manuscripts, newspapers, meeting minutes, legal documents, nursing notes, reports, maps, and books. Criticism of the data sources is part of the research process. For example, external criticism is an examination of the authenticity of the source (validity), and internal criticism is correctly interpreting the contents of the data sources (reliability). Historical researchers attempt to locate and use original, authentic sources (Brockopp and Hastings-Tolsma, 1995).

If the nurse researcher uses an interview guide, he or she should report how it was developed. If more than one person collects the data, the nurse researcher should report how the data were collected in a consistent way by each person. These procedures are true for both observations and interviews. Maintaining consistency in data collection is an issue of reliability, similar to the evaluation of the reliability of instruments in quantitative research. Maintaining consistency is especially important if no interview guides or observational tools are uses (Tanner, Imle, and Stewart, 1989).

The research report should present evidence that the informants agreed to participate in the research study. The women who participated in the study of adult survivors of incest (Kondora, 1993) were volunteers who were fully informed about the study and agreed to participate.

## Data Analysis

Analysis of the data is the next portion of the report to evaluate. To think critically about the data analysis of a qualitative research report, ask the following:

▼ What methods for data analysis were chosen? Why were they chosen?

▼ Does the researcher paint a clear picture of the reality and meaning experienced by the informant?

▼ Are concepts missing that you expected to find based on your clinical experience? Should the sample have yielded these concepts or would a different sample be needed?

▼ Are the relationships among the concepts supported by the data? Do the relationships make sense? Are other relationships possible?

▼ Have other professionals confirmed the researcher's interpretation?

Data analysis in qualitative research is primarily an inductive reasoning process as contrasted with the deductive reasoning process used to analyze data in quantitative research. In qualitative research, often the nurse researcher seeks to generate a theory, whereas in quantitative research, the nurse researcher seeks to test one. Brockopp and Hastings-Tolsma (1995) identify the following common processes to analyze data in qualitative research: identifying themes; verifying the selected themes through reflection on the data and discussion with other researchers or experts in the area; categorizing the themes (using existing or novel categories); recording of support data for categories; and identifying propositions (p. 255).

In qualitative research, the nurse researcher uses an interactive process between data collection and data analysis. The nurse researcher analyzes and reflects on the data. He or she may ask the informants to validate the data (i.e., confirm that it is accurate) and to provide further information (Ray, 1985). This process of validating the data with the informant is similar to the process of validating an instrument in quantitative research. It ensures the accuracy of the data.

In qualitative research the nurse researcher has a large amount of raw data from which she or he begins the methodical process of reflecting on the data and sorting, coding, and categorizing it according to the formal, systematic processes dictated by the specific research method. The process of coding and categorizing the data may be done manually or by computer. Raw data are examined line by line as the nurse researcher looks for themes and patterns. As themes and patterns emerge, they are given a concept or theme label (Brockopp and Hastings-Tolsma, 1995; Tanner, Imle, and Stewart, 1989). Table 7-2 illustrates the manual process of data analysis. During this process, the nurse researcher draws tentative conclusions. He or she will continue to modify and refine these conclusions as more data are collected and analyzed. This interactive process drives the direction of subsequent data collection.

For example, phenomenological data may be analyzed by any one of several slightly different techniques. The end result of all techniques is the production of an exhaustive description of the informants' lived experiences. Kondora's (1993) article, which gives excerpts about the lived experiences of the women in her study, is a good example of a descriptive report (see Appendix C).

In grounded theory, data collection and data analysis also occur simultaneously. As this interactive process continues, patterns begin to emerge, and the nurse researcher begins to develop hunches about them. These hunches are pursued in the

Table 7-2   **Data Analysis: Identifying Themes from Client Statement***

| THEMES | SELECT CLIENT STATEMENTS: EXPERIENCES OF JOB LOSS |
|---|---|
| Loss of control<br>Betrayal<br>Unpreparedness<br><br>Financial stress<br><br>Loss of self-esteem<br><br>Devastation | "I felt as though I was about to explode! I couldn't believe that <u>after 28 years of service to the company—of being loyal, honest, hardworking—that this could be the thanks I got. Nothing in my life prepared me for an event like this.</u> I always figured I would be the guy who got the gold watch and that I could retire with a <u>pretty good pension and a nice nest egg to fall back on.</u> Now, I have to <u>face the prospect of trying to get a job at my age and of </u>trying to tell my friends, neighbors, and colleagues. It's embarrassing and demeaning. I will <u>never get over this . . . it has ruined my life.</u> |

*From Brockopp DY and Hastings-Tolsma MT: Fundamentals of nursing research (ed. 2), Boston, 1995, Jones and Bartlett.

field. This interactive process is combined with an ongoing review of the literature. As the researcher progresses and discovers relationships, he or she uses them to develop an explanatory scheme or a model or theory (Liehr and Marcus, 1994).

As you evaluate a qualitative research report, compare the results and the researcher's conclusions with your own clinical experience with the phenomenon. Are they consistent? Are your insights and experiences with the phenomenon different from the researcher's? If they are not alike, in what ways do they differ? What would you have done differently had *you* been the researcher? How should the researcher structure the research study to include your insights and experiences? Is the problem with the sample? Is the problem with the researcher's perspective and biases? Is the problem with the data collection methods? Your insights, reflection, and analytical thinking processes are essential to evaluate both qualitative and quantitative research.

## Description of Findings

To think critically about the description of findings of a qualitative research report, ask the following:

▼  Are examples provided that link the raw data to the researcher's synthesis?
▼  Are the findings linked to existing theory or literature?

As you read the researcher's description, can you follow the logic (reasoning)? Qualitative research reports should include informant statements that provide support for the researcher's synthesis. For example, Dzurec (1994) studied 15 schizophrenic clients' experiences of power. She concluded that the essence of power is the client's connection with the environment or the people in it. She also concluded that the extent of power is determined by the client's personal awareness of this connection. Dzurec's reasoning process is evident in the following excerpt:

> When participants were asked to identify the kinds of choices they make on a day-to-day basis, the two themes of basic activities of daily living and interpersonal interactions were found. The interpersonal interactions theme further subdivided as those necessary to get along with others ("I follow rules. Everybody has to follow rules.") and those geared toward giving ("A lot of my choices are based on what would be good for children I work with."). Choices involving activities of daily living reflected a limited repertoire of mundane alternatives for participants. However, in light of their hospitalization or residence in a supervised facility, the choices they described generally represented an accurate assessment of the range of choices available to them. For choices regarding interpersonal interaction, some participants recognized a need to interact with others, and did so freely. Others expressed anxiety about interactions and described their inferior positions in social relations. Those participants who sensed a personal inferiority seemed to find themselves at the mercy of others. One said, "Well, I'm scared of people, that they'll hurt me and stuff. . . . Every time it seems like I try to do something it seems like I'm going backwards" (p. 156).

Dzurec concluded that people with schizophrenia might behave in ways that perpetuate their relative powerlessness because they perceive themselves as powerless. She linked her conclusion to the view of three other researchers.

The qualitative research report should also identify the implications for education, practice, and theory as appropriate. Tanner, Imle, and Stewart's (1989) guidelines to evaluate the applicability of research to practice apply as much to qualitative research as to quantitative research. To determine relevance, you should first compare the similarity between the research sample and the practice setting with your clients and practice setting. Next, you should compare the similarity between those who implemented the procedures in the study with your own staff to determine if special training would be required. Finally, you should determine if the study has been replicated in other settings. If it has not, consider replicating it in your institution to evaluate the costs, risks, and benefits.

Like the quantitative research report, the qualitative research report must be written clearly and be easily understood. The reasoning process of the nurse researcher must be evident as she or he relates the informants' responses with the literature. The qualitative research report should include all information essential to understand the phenomenon of interest, study structure, data collection, data analysis, and findings.

# THE NURSE'S ROLE IN DATA COLLECTION

## Participate in Systematic and Accurate Data Collection

The ability to systematically and accurately collect data is a critical thinking skill we associate with evidence. Given the importance of nursing research to the quality of nursing care delivered to clients and the advancement of the nursing profession, your participation in systematic and accurate data collection is essential.

Nursing traces its interest in research back to the time of Florence Nightingale, who was an advocate of disciplined inquiry. She knew the importance of asking specific questions to focus the thinking of the nurse and the client. For example, Nightingale instructed nurses to collect accurate data by asking specific questions rather than leading questions. To ask "How many hours of sleep has the patient had?" will yield more accurate information than to ask "Has the patient had a good night?" The answer to the first question will yield accurate information, and the answer to the second question will depend upon each client's perceptions and experience. She believed that making accurate observations was essential to being a good nurse (Nightingale, 1992). Nightingale advocated critical thinking by focusing on questions as a strategy to collect accurate data.

The nurse who participates in data collection activities for research purposes must be honest, reliable, and provide skilled, meticulous nursing care. According to Davis (1995), the nurse may participate in systematic and accurate data collection in a variety of ways such as: gain the client's cooperation and informed consent; educate the client; administer the treatment or nursing intervention; or schedule the client for appointments.

***Gain the Client's Cooperation and Informed Consent.*** The nurse may be responsible for working with the client to gain and maintain cooperation. As discussed previously, the researcher must obtain the client's informed consent to participate in the study. The client must understand that his or her participation in the study is voluntary. Informed consent protects the client from any unethical research practice. Once the client has agreed to participate in the study, he or she may need or want continuous interaction with the nurse. Frequently the nurse is the primary care giver or the contact person whom the client sees regularly. The client's full cooperation and continued participation are essential to the conduct of the research.

***Educate the Client.*** The nurse may need to educate the client about any number of things about which the client needs further knowledge. The nurse must draw upon his or her health education skills to teach the client. Accurate data collection may depend on the instructions the nurse gives to the client and the client's understanding of these instructions. The nurse's instructions must be clear and feedback about the client's level of understanding must be assessed as the teaching occurs. For example, a client may have a skin test performed on a Monday and be instructed to observe for the degree of redness, swelling, and pain at the test site. Forty-eight hours later the client must return to the clinic to have the nurse examine the site and interpret the results. To maintain the accuracy of data collection in this example, the client must understand what to observe and return to the clinic at the right time.

The nurse may do formal or informal health education with a client or a group of clients. She or he should know how to present the message clearly. She or he should have written materials and other audiovisual aids available as appropriate to explain complex procedures. It is absolutely essential to the outcome of the research that the client both understands the protocol and follows instructions.

### Administer the Treatment or Nursing Intervention.

The nurse may be the person who administers the treatment or nursing intervention. For example, an experimental group of clients receives a special treatment for decubitus ulcers. The nursing intervention is administered twice a day at 12-hour intervals. The nursing intervention has three steps that must be followed sequentially: (1) cleansing the skin with a special solution, (2) drying the skin, and (3) applying a therapeutic cream. Following the research protocol is essential to test the effectiveness of the intervention and the reliability of the results. The interventions must be done at the prescribed time and according to the prescribed procedure.

For the results to be meaningful, research protocols must be followed exactly. For example, if blood is to be drawn at 2-hour intervals, then it *must* be drawn every 2 hours and not every 2 1/2 hours. If precise intake and output must be monitored, the nurse must gain the client's cooperation and keep careful records. If a urine specimen is inadvertently discarded, the nurse must be reliable and report the incident to the researchers in whose study he or she is participating. To omit information or falsify research records in any way is unacceptable.

### Schedule the Client for Appointments.

The nurse may be the person responsible for scheduling the client for future appointments. The purpose of the appointments may be to see the health care provider, to obtain specimens for laboratory tests, to have special tests done such as computerized tomography (CT) scans and radiographs, and to have special procedures done such as venous infusion of medication. To be accurate, the collection of these data must be scheduled as prescribed by the research protocol. Some clients may live in outlying areas, which may complicate the client's participation. By thinking critically, the nurse can anticipate problems and create solutions. For example, consider the client who lives in a rural community, a long distance from the university health care center where the research is conducted. Certain laboratory tests, such as blood tests, could be done at the local hospital where the client resides if the proper arrangements were made. The nurse must anticipate and collaborate with personnel at the local hospital to be sure they understand what is to be done and when it is to be done. The nurse must make sure the client understands what he or she needs to do and how to cooperate. The nurse should follow through with the client and the personnel at the local hospital as appropriate.

Usually the client who participates in a research protocol must been seen or tested at regular intervals. The nurse should help the client to understand this and cooperate to fit the appointments into his or her routine of daily living. Holding to the prescribed appointment schedule is part of the nurse's role as a collector of data. For example, a client may need to have a CT scan every month to follow her progress to limit the growth of cancerous tumors. The nurse must see that these appointments are scheduled, that the client is aware of the date and time of the appointment, and that the client is aware of the importance of keeping the appointment.

## Record Data Accurately

The client's chart or medical or health record is a key communication link among the nurses, physicians, and other specialists who are involved in the client's care. The chart documents the nursing interventions and medical treatments the client receives and his or her physiological response to them. It should also document any significant health-related behavioral responses and verbal communication from the client that are in response to the nursing interventions and medical treatments. An example of a health-related behavioral response is a client's report of increased urination as a response to taking a diuretic. An example of a significant verbal communication is the client's report of symptoms such as headache or a bodily sensation such as feeling tense. Symptoms are a subjective response that a client reports, a response that cannot be measured objectively as with a thermometer. All responses should be documented in the client's chart as it indicates the client's progress relative to nursing interventions and medical treatments.

The client's chart is also the source of raw data that are used in nursing and medical research. This is true for both quantitative and qualitative research. If the raw data are incomplete or inaccurate, the accuracy of the findings of the research becomes questionable. The importance of the accurate recording of data, whether it is the simple recording of a blood pressure or the more sophisticated assessment of wound healing, cannot be overemphasized. Accurate raw data are the building blocks of research.

# OTHER SOURCES OF EVIDENCE

In Chapter 6, you learned the definition of evidence. Evidence is something that tends to prove another thing. It provides the grounds for a belief (Neufeldt, 1991). Evidence rarely provides conclusive proof to support beliefs and actions; instead, it provides degrees of support (i.e., it tends to prove or disprove). Evidence deals with probabilities that affect everyday living and client outcomes. For example, what are the chances that if you study hard for the next examination, you will get a better grade than you did on the previous exam? What is the chance that pneumonia in postsurgical clients can be reduced by having clients breathe deeply every 2 hours? To reflect an understanding of evidence as degrees of support, it is more accurate for you to ask, "Does the evidence provide strong support? Does it provide weak support?"

Research is not the only source of evidence; there are other sources upon which you may base your beliefs and actions. When you attempt to persuade another to consider your viewpoint and actions, you provide reasons supported by evidence to make your case. When others attempt to persuade you to consider their viewpoints and actions, they also will present reasons supported by evidence.

What other sources of evidence do we have in addition to research studies? Browne and Keeley (1994) identify intuition, authorities, personal experience, personal observation, case studies and examples, and analogies as additional sources of evidence. To Browne and Keeley's list we add the client as a source of evidence upon which nurses rely. Client-based evidence includes subjective and objective data from client assessment and evaluative data from a client's response to nursing and medical interventions. Data are the evidence from which conclusions can be inferred.

## Client-based Evidence

In clinical nursing practice, the client is the major source of evidence. For example, Ms. Weil, a 67-year-old woman, was admitted to the hospital for vascular surgery to remove the blockage in her left femoral artery. Subjective data included her report of pain in the left leg after ascending a flight of stairs, which first occurred 5 to 6 years ago following exercise. When the pain became progressively worse, Ms. Weil limited her activities. The nurse assessed the client and found that Ms. Weil's femoral pulse was weaker in the left groin than the right. The dorsalis pedis and posterior tibial pulses on the left were barely perceptible, whereas the same pulses on the right were normal. The left leg was cool to touch and pale when compared with the right leg. This objective evidence supported the medical diagnosis of blockage, which was subsequently treated by surgical removal. After surgery the nurse again assessed Ms. Weil and found that the pulses were strong and comparable on both sides. This example illustrates evidence as subjective and objective data derived both from client assessment and from the evaluation of the surgical intervention.

Client data can be both quantitative and qualitative in nature. Quantitative client data refers to numbers such as a pulse count of 80 beats per minute, an intake of 240 ml of fluid, and a blood glucose level of 84 mg/dl. The evidence is in the form of a quantity (i.e., something that can be measured). In contrast, qualitative client data are in word form. It may be the subjective experience with a health problem as reported by the client such as pain, nausea, and the impact of a health problem on the client's activities of daily living. While some health care providers attempt to measure this information on a quantitative scale (i.e., rate your pain on a scale of 1-10 with 1 being no pain and 10 being intense pain), the source of the numbers is based on the client's subjective response.

## Client-based Evidence and the Nursing Process

The nursing process is a systematic problem-solving approach the nurse uses to assess and evaluate clients. Based on the evidence the nurse obtains from assessing the client, the nurse establishes a nursing diagnosis, creates a plan for the delivery of nursing care, implements the nursing care plan, and evaluates the client's response to the nursing care. During the evaluation process, the nurse obtains evidence that shows the effectiveness of the plan. Using this evidence, the nurse modifies the plan to bring about the desired client response.

For example, Golda, a 50-year-old client undergoing cancer chemotherapy, was nauseated and anorectic (loss of appetite). She was losing weight unnecessarily; that is, her weight loss was not associated with her early cancer. Her weight loss was attributed to her reaction to the diagnosis (shock) rather than to the disease itself. To treat the nausea and anorexia, the nurse administered the antiemetic medication prescribed by the physician and ordered the client's favorite foods from the hospital dietary service. These interventions reduced the nausea but did not stimulate Golda's appetite. Based on this evidence, the nurse continued these interventions and added another intervention: the nurse invited Golda's family to bring in some of her favorite foods to supplement the hospital meals. They did this on a daily basis, rotating the responsibility among themselves. Golda was touched by her family's caring and delighted to have her favorite foods. She began to eat more and was able to regain her normal weight. Based on this additional evidence, the nurse evaluated the nursing care plan as effective.

The nursing process is dynamic and driven by the subjective and objective data derived from the client. The nurse assesses this client-based evidence continuously during all interactions with the client. The nurse uses this evidence to evaluate the effectiveness of the client's response to nursing and medical interventions. You may find a thorough discussion of the meaning of evidence related to specific health problems derived from client assessment and evaluation in basic medical, surgical, obstetric, pediatric, and psychiatric textbooks.

## SUMMARY

Critical thinking is required to evaluate evidence derived from qualitative nursing research and from other sources of evidence such as that obtained from clients. Research is the systematic investigation and reporting of evidence. The nurse, as a consumer of research, should critically evaluate a research report to determine its strengths and weaknesses and the relevance of the findings to clinical practice. The client is another valuable source of evidence that nurses use. Based on the evidence obtained from client assessment, the nurse establishes a nursing diagnosis, and plans, implements, and evaluates the nursing care.

Substantial philosophical and methodological differences exist between the research approaches taken by quantitative and qualitative researchers. The choice of which approach to use depends on a number of variables, including the purpose of the research and the nature of the research problem. One research approach is neither superior nor inferior to the other. Quantitative and qualitative research approaches simply represent different ways of looking at the world. Each approach has its place, and each has a substantial contribution to make to the improvement of client care and to the development of the unique body of nursing knowledge.

# EXERCISES

## Exercise 1

*Purpose:* *Evaluate a qualitative research report*

### DIRECTIONS

Complete a full evaluation of the qualitative research report in Appendix C. Use the format presented in this chapter. Discuss your analysis in class with your classmates who have also evaluated it. On which items is there full agreement? Disagreement? Why? Defend your views in those instances where significant disagreement occurred.

## Exercise 2

*Purposes:* *Conceptualize a nursing research study using the qualitative approach*
*Create a theoretical framework for conducting the research*

### DIRECTIONS

Divide into small groups. Identify an area for study that is of interest to the group. Engage in the following activities:

1. Brainstorm researchable questions and write a brief paragraph to serve as the theoretical framework.
2. Discuss which qualitative research method would be most appropriate to use and the type of data that would best answer the research question or hypotheses.
3. Define the population of interest and determine how the research sample would be drawn.
4. Speculate on what you expect to find.

When you have completed this assignment, reflect on the following:

▼ What areas were the most and the least difficult for the group?

▼ Do all members of the group agree on the most and the least difficult areas?

▼ How did the group get beyond the difficult areas?

▼ What reasoning skills are the most essential in conceptualizing and conducting qualitative nursing research?

▼ What role would each member of the group like to play if it were possible to conduct the research?

# Exercise 3

**Purpose:** *Articulate an explanation and defense for your research*

<u>DIRECTIONS</u>

Role-play your appearance before the research committee in a health care agency. The purpose of the committee hearing is twofold: first to explain what you will study and how you will study it and second, to request permission to conduct the study in this agency.

The class should assume the role of committee members who seek further information and clarification about your study. They should conclude the role play by making a judgment about whether or not you should be given permission to conduct the study in their agency.

# Exercise 4

**Purpose:** *Gain insight into the interrelatedness of the components of the research process*

<u>DIRECTIONS</u>

The entire class should select one broad area of interest for research, such as access to health care, client satisfaction, or culturally appropriate nursing care. Consider both quantitative and qualitative research approaches. Once the research topic is agreed upon, then the class should divide into small groups.

Each group is responsible for developing only one component of the research study. For example, one group should identify the research problem, another group should state the research question or hypothesis, another group develop the theoretical framework, another group create the design, and another group should identify the data collection methods and instruments. Each group works independently and does not engage in intergroup collaboration. Each group selects a recorder who writes down the group response and a spokesperson who presents a report to the larger class.

After each group has completed its task, the members should rejoin the larger class. The spokesperson for each group should present the group's response to the entire class. After each presentation has been made, discuss the following:

1. Did the components fit together into a smooth, cohesive research study? Why or why not?

2. What did you learn about the interrelatedness of the components of the research process?

3. Would any nursing research journal print this study? Why or why not?

4. How could you improve the research study?

## Exercise 5

**Purpose:** *Refine your ability to evaluate nursing research*

### DIRECTIONS

Each member of the class should evaluate the same research report using the format presented in this chapter. Each student's evaluation should be done individually, without consultation with other members of the class.

When each student has completed the evaluation, discuss the findings as a class. Conduct the discussion following the categories listed in the format to evaluate evidence derived from qualitative research. Compare and contrast everyone's analyses. Discuss more fully those categories in which students evaluated the study differently and came to different conclusions. What were the reasons for these differences? For example, was the difference in opinion a result of different interpretations of the data, a lack of understanding of a procedure, or some other reason?

## Exercise 6

**Purposes:** *Integrate knowledge about quantitative and qualitative research*
*Create a quantitative and qualitative research study*

### DIRECTIONS

Form groups of individuals who currently share the same clinical practice assignments (i.e., work in the same clinical subject area or work on the same clinical unit). This exercise has several activities that each take time.

Reflect on the clients with whom you are working. Describe their obvious characteristics such as age, gender, ethnicity, and apparent socioeconomic and educational levels. Describe the most common health problems experienced by these clients.

Generate some researchable questions by asking what else you would like to know about these clients. Identify at least 10 questions that could be answered through a research study. Describe how you would select the sample. Describe what data should be collected, how you would collect it, and how you would analyze it.

Now, assume that you have answers to the questions you posed. You may create these answers to make the activity more interesting and challenging. Based on these answers, identify at least 10 questions that could be answered through research study. Set up the research design for one of the questions. Describe how you would select the sample. Describe what data should be collected, how you would collect it, and how you would analyze it.

Examine the many variables that you have identified in this exercise. Do you suspect that some variables may be statistically related to one another? On which ones would you do a correlational study? Why? What other statistical procedures would you use?

# Exercise 7

**Purpose:** *Evaluate evidence derived from clients*

<u>DIRECTIONS</u>

Reflect on the following questions. You may respond to them individually or in small groups.

1. What evidence did you observe in a client for whom you have recently cared?

2. How did you interpret the client's subjective and objective data; that is, what meaning did this evidence have for you?

3. What conclusions did you draw from the evidence? Did you establish a nursing diagnosis?

4. What nursing actions did you take based on the evidence you observed? Provide a rationale for your nursing actions.

5. Were your nursing actions effective? What evidence do you have to support your answer?

# Exercise 8

**Purpose:** *Record your thoughts and insights*

<u>DIRECTIONS</u>

Write in your journal about the following questions:

1. What does it mean to be a consumer of research?

2. What role would you like to have related to nursing research?

3. How can you apply the information in Chapters 6 and 7 to your practice of nursing?

4. Why is research in nursing important?

5. How will research benefit you in your role as a nurse?

6. How will research benefit the clients for whom you care?

## REFERENCES

Brockopp, D.Y., and Hastings-Tolsma, M.T. (1995). Fundamentals of nursing research (2nd ed.). Boston: Jones and Bartlett.

Browne, M.N., and Keeley, S.M. (1994). *Asking the right questions* (4th ed). Englewood Cliffs, N.J.: Prentice Hall.

Carter, M.A. (1985). The philosophical dimensions of qualitative nursing science research. In M.M. Leininger (Ed.), *Qualitative research methods in nursing* (pp. 27-32). Orlando, Fla.: Grune and Stratton.

Coward, D.D. (1990). The lived experience of self-transcendence in women with advanced breast cancer. *Nursing Science Quarterly, 3*(4), 162-169.

Davis, A.T. (1991). America's first school of nursing: The New England Hospital for Women and Children. *Journal of Nursing Education, 30*(4), 158-161.

Davis, M.L.E. (1995, January). Personal communication.

Dzurec, L.C. (1994). Schizophrenic clients' experiences of power: Using hermeneutic analysis. *IMAGE: Journal of Nursing Scholarship, 26*(2), 155-159.

Fairman, J. (1992). Watchful vigilance: Nursing care, technology, and the development of intensive care units. *Nursing Research, 41*(1), 56-58.

Jones, P.S., and Martinson, I.M. (1992). The experience of bereavement in caregivers of family members with Alzheimer's disease. *Image, 24*(3), 172-176.

Kauffman, K.S. (1994). The insider/outsider dilemma: Field experience of a white researcher "getting in" a poor black community. *Nursing Research, 43*(3), 179-183.

Kondora, L.L. (1993). A Heideggerian hermeneutical analysis of survivors of incest. *IMAGE: Journal of Nursing Scholarship, 25*(1), 11-16.

Kruman, M.W. (1985). Historical method: Implications for nursing research. In M.M. Leininger (Ed.), *Qualitative research methods in nursing* (pp. 109-118). Orlando, Fla.: Grune and Stratton.

Leininger, M.M. (1992). Current issues, problems, and trends to advance qualitative paradigmatic research methods for the future. *Qualitative Health Research, 2*(4), 392-415.

————. (1985a). Ethnography and ethnonursing: Models and modes of qualitative data analysis. In M.M Leininger (Ed.), *Qualitative research methods in nursing* (pp. 33-71). Orlando, Fla.: Grune and Stratton.

————. (1985b). Nature, rationale, and importance of qualitative research methods in nursing. In M.M. Leininger (Ed.), *Qualitative research methods in nursing* (pp. 1-25). Orlando, Fla.: Grune and Stratton.

————. (1985c). Southern rural black and white American lifeways with focus on care and health promo-tion. In M.M. Leininger (Ed.), *Qualitative research methods in nursing* (pp. 195-216). Orlando, Fla.: Grune and Stratton.

Liehr, P.R., and Marcus, M.T. (1994). Qualitative approaches to research. In G. LoBiondo-Wood and J. Haber (Eds.), *Nursing research: Methods, critical appraisal, and utilization* (3rd ed., pp. 253-285). St Louis: Mosby.

Miller, M.P. (1991). Factors promoting wellness in the aged person: An ethnographic study. *Advances in Nursing Science, 13*(4), 38-51.

Neufeldt, V. (1991). *Webster's new world dictionary* (3rd ed.). New York: Webster's New World.

Nightingale, F. (1992). *Notes on nursing.* Philadelphia: J.B. Lippincott.

Ragsdale, D., Kotarba, J.A., and Morrow, J.R. (1992). Quality of life of hospitalized persons with AIDS. *Image, 24*(4), 259-265.

Ray, M.A. (1985). A philosophical method to study nursing phenomena. In M.M. Leininger (Ed.), *Qualitative research methods in nursing* (pp. 81-92). Orlando, Fla.: Grune and Stratton.

Swanson, K.M. (1990). Providing care in the NICU: Sometimes an act of love. *Advances in Nursing Science, 13*(1), 60-73.

Tanner, C.A., Imle, M., and Stewart, B. (1989). Guidelines for evaluation of research for use in practice. In C.A. Tanner and Lindeman, C.A. (Eds.)., *Using nursing research* (pp. 35-60). New York: National League for Nursing.

Uphall, M.J. (1992). Nursing perceptions of collaboration with indigenous healers in Swaziland. *International Journal of Nursing Studies, 29*(1), 27-36.

Wilson, H.S. (1993). *Introducing research in nursing* (2nd ed.). New York: Addison-Wesley.

# *Reasoning*

Chapter **8**

## OVERVIEW

Chapter 8 introduces you to the two major forms of argument, deductive and inductive, which are used in reasoning. Reasoning also is applied to problem solving and to the examination of controversial issues.

Understanding deductive and inductive arguments is essential to critical thinking. Chapter 8 defines argument, differentiates between arguments and nonarguments, and discusses the nature of deductive and inductive arguments. It examines the structure of categorical propositions and some of the logical relations among them. The chapter discusses immediate inferences, disjunctive syllogisms, and hypothetical syllogisms as forms of deductive reasoning. The chapter examines three forms of inductive reasoning: reasoning by analogy, causal reasoning, and empirical generalizations. It then explains how reasoning is used to solve problems and to analyze controversial issues.

Arriving at a conclusion is the end result of the arguing process. Each conclusion may result in an action, or it may sustain or discount a belief, all of which have implications. Implications are the consequences of our actions and beliefs.

## REASONING APPLIED TO ARGUMENTS

We use language to express many things such as feelings, opinions, and observations. We ask questions, tell stories, make announcements, give illustrations, bestow praise, complain, explain, apologize, and so on. None of these actions, however, are arguments. Disputes or quarrels that are used in daily conversation also are not arguments. Argument is a form of reasoning that has two basic elements: a conclusion supported by one or more reasons (premises). The conclusion is the statement being supported. The reasons, also known as premises, are statements that support the conclusion. Logic is the examination of arguments, or the relationship between the reasons and the conclusions (Chaffee, 1994). Kurfiss (1988) describes arguments as a train of reasoning in which claims and supporting reasons are linked to support and justify a position. Thus, the basic structure of arguments is *this, because of that* (Browne and Keeley, 1994).

## Arguments and Nonarguments

How do you distinguish arguments from statements that are not arguments? Consider the following examples:

1. "You should get substantial pain relief from this medication. Let me know how effectively it works for you." These statements do not constitute an argument. The first is a prediction about the medication's anticipated effect. What follows is not, however, a reason for thinking this is true; instead, it is only a request for feedback from the client about its effectiveness.

2. "The client has pale skin. This is probably due to a weak heart." These statements also do not constitute an argument. The second statement explains why the client has pale skin; it does not give a reason to believe the client does have pale skin. Explanations assume statements are true and give reasons why they are true.

3. "Nurses should be present in all discussions about downsizing in health care facilities. Nurses are more concerned than others about both quality and safety issues surrounding client care. Nurses also are the largest group of health care providers." These statements constitute an argument because they contain a conclusion supported by premises. The conclusion is that nurses should be present in all discussions about downsizing in health care facilities. It is supported by two premises designed to establish the conclusion's truth.

4. "I felt sad when the client died. I did everything I knew to do, but it just wasn't enough. What else should I have done?" This is not an argument; it is an expression of emotion coupled with a question.

5. "If you do not drink milk, you will have a calcium deficiency." This sentence is not an argument, but instead a conditional statement. It does not conclude that you will have a calcium deficiency; it says this will happen *if* you do not drink milk.

***Arguments and Explanations.***    Explanations are not arguments. Explanations may appear to be arguments, but they are different. They have the same structure (*this, because of that*), but their goals are different. The goal of an argument is to show *that* some proposition is true, whereas the goal of an explanation is to show *why* some proposition is true (Kelley, 1994). The following statements illustrate the difference:

1. Ralph will make a good committee chairperson because he has a lot of experience and knows hospital politics.

2. Ralph resigned from his staff nursing position because he intends to move to another part of the country.

Both statements make a claim and offer a reason as indicated by the word *because*. The first statement is an argument. It claims that Ralph will be successful and seeks to establish the truth of the claim based on the premises that he has a lot of experience and knows hospital politics. The reasoning moves forward from the premises to the conclusion. It attempts to answer the question, "Is it true?"

The second statement is an explanation. The conclusion that Ralph resigned from his staff nursing position is not in doubt; it is a known fact. An explanation for that fact is that Ralph intends to move to another part of the country. An explanation assumes that the statement is true and gives a reason why it is true. The reasoning moves backward from a fact to the cause or reason for that fact. It answers the question, "Why is it true?"

**Arguments and Conditionals.**    Conditional statements, such as "If you do not drink milk, you will have a calcium deficiency," are not arguments. They are similar to arguments because they express a line of reasoning, from the condition that if you do not drink milk, to the statement that you will have a calcium deficiency. But this statement is not really concluded, because genuine conclusions are asserted as true. In accepting an argument, the listener assents to the truth of the premises and draws the conclusion, thus coming to believe it also. To accept the conditional statement above, however, you do not have to believe that in fact you do not drink milk, only that *if* you do not, you will have a calcium deficiency. It can become an argument by rephrasing it as "You do not drink milk; therefore, you will have a calcium deficiency." To accept this, you must believe the premise and use the line of reasoning to come to believe the conclusion.

## Uses of Argument

The goal of any argument is to provide support for a statement previously in doubt. Thus, arguments are used to decide, predict, and persuade (Chaffee, 1994).

**Arguments to Decide.**    You may use an argument to make a decision about an issue. Concerned individuals present reasons, supported by evidence, for their positions. Debate is an example of an argument to decide; it is commonly used in the discussion of controversial issues. A debate may occur between individuals or it may occur at the community, state, and national levels. Health care reform is an example of a controversial issue that is generating considerable debate throughout the United States. Proponents present their views, which are then countered by the views of their opponents. Through the debate process, the public becomes better informed and, optimistically, a plan for reform becomes further refined.

Debating the merits of having one centralized city hospital versus having the city hospital plus strategically placed neighborhood health clinics is an example of a controversial issue on a local level. Consider the hypothetical situation of health care providers who were against a neighborhood clinic because they were already insufficiently staffed at the city hospital and did not believe they could adequately staff another facility. Furthermore, they did not believe the city had the financial resources to support a neighborhood clinic. They also were concerned that care might be compromised without immediate and direct access to the resources of the city hospital. The residents felt differently and wanted a health clinic in their neighborhood. They believed they were not getting adequate care from the overburdened services at city hospital. Many of the residents were place bound and did not have transportation to get to the city hospital. They believed the city council could afford to support the clinic by readjusting the budget. They reasoned that they were not getting proper health care under the current system and a neighborhood clinic would improve health care for them. This argument may be diagramed as follows:

### Health Care Providers' Position:

**Reason:**      Insufficient providers are available to staff a neighborhood health clinic.

**Reason:**      Health care would be compromised.

**Reason:**      The city does not have financial resources.

**Conclusion:**  The centralized city hospital would provide the best health care.

### Neighborhood Citizens' Position:

**Reason:**      Health care is inadequate at the overburdened city hospital.

**Reason:**      Lack of transportation keeps residents from using the city hospital.

**Reason:**      Financial resources could be available by readjusting the city's budget.

**Conclusion:**  Health care would improve with a neighborhood health clinic.

Many other reasons could be offered by both sides in support of their positions. Do the reasons make sense to you? Do they address the conclusion? What other reasons might each side give? The pros and cons of this issue should be discussed and weighed carefully before an informed decision is made.

*Arguments to Predict.*    Another kind of truth to establish deals with a future event that can be supported by past experience. Thus, an argument may be used to predict something that will occur. For example, many factors affect our health such as eating nutritiously and judiciously from the Food Guide Pyramid, exercising regularly, and dealing effectively with life stressors. People who practice these behaviors do so anticipating that the effect will be a long life that also is relatively free from illness.

**Reason:**      I eat nutritiously and judiciously from the Food Guide Pyramid.

**Reason:**      I exercise regularly.

**Reason:**      I deal effectively with life stressors.

**Conclusion:**  I will live a long life that is relatively free from illness.

Create an argument to predict something and diagram it as shown in the example above.

*Arguments to Persuade.*    An argument may be used to persuade others about the truth of something such as the merits of a belief, plan, decision, or a course of action. For example, how do nurses get a reluctant client with arthritis to ambulate and exercise more? They may persuade the client by presenting reasons why ambulation and exercise are good health practices. This argument may be diagrammed as follows:

**Reason:**      Regular exercise improves circulation, muscle tone, and bone density.

**Reason:**      Regular exercise will reduce pain and stiffness.

**Conclusion:**    You should exercise regularly to improve circulation, muscle tone, bone density, and reduce pain and stiffness.

Consider the example of a pharmaceutical representative who tried to persuade the nurses that his dressing tray was more cost effective than another brand. The representative displayed the product in the best possible light and presented reasons why the nurses should choose his product. Imagine the reasons the representative might have given and diagram the argument.

## DISTINCTION BETWEEN DEDUCTION AND INDUCTION

The conclusion of deductive arguments should *necessarily* follow from the premises (reasons). The conclusion of inductive arguments should *likely* follow from the premises; that is, it should follow only *with probability* (Chaffee, 1994; Missimer, 1990). Bandman and Bandman (1995) describe the distinction between deductive and inductive arguments as:

> The premises of a deductive argument provide complete evidence for the conclusion, whereas an inductive argument provides only some evidence for its conclusion. Deductive arguments are certain; inductive arguments are uncertain, and are at most probable or likely (p. 172).

This distinction describes good deductive and good inductive arguments and will be illustrated in the discussion that follows.

## DEDUCTIVE REASONING

A good deductive argument claims to provide complete evidence for the conclusion. This section discusses immediate inferences (containing one premise), and syllogisms (containing two premises), and looks at the application of these to nursing.

Premises form the foundation for an argument. If the premises are not true or if the conclusion does not follow from them, then you are not justified in believing the conclusion based on the strength of the argument. When you evaluate an argument, ask if the premises are true and assess whether or not the conclusion follows from them.

All arguments are based on the assumption that the premises are true. Deductive arguments are special in the amount of support that the premises are supposed to provide for the conclusion. A deductive argument claims that the conclusion *must* be true because the premises are. If the conclusion follows from the premises the structure is *valid*. It is impossible for the premises to be true and the structure valid and the conclusion false. Notice that an argument can be valid and still have false premises. When a completely successful deductive argument has all true premises and is valid, it is called *sound*.

### Categorical Propositions

Understanding propositions is an important skill in reasoning. The categorical proposition is the simplest type of proposition. It is the type of proposition found in the simplest forms of deduction, namely immediate inference and categorical syllogism.

Arguments are composed of two or more propositions, the conclusion and the premises. A proposition is a statement made in the form of a declarative sentence that contains a subject and a predicate. The subject of the proposition is the part that identifies what is being talked about. The predicate indicates what is being said about this. The declarative sentence asserts that something is a fact. It is always either true or false, although its truth or falsity may not be known (Kelley, 1994).

The categorical proposition makes an assertion about the relations among categories or classes. All categorical propositions contain a subject and a predicate. For example:

No health care providers are vegetarians.
All nurses are health care providers.
Therefore, no nurses are vegetarians.

Because both the premises and conclusion are categorical propositions, they are about classes (i.e., all health care providers, all vegetarians, or all nurses). A class is a collection of all objects that have a common characteristic (Copi and Cohen, 1994).

Classes may be related to each other in various ways. The second premise states that all nurses are members of another class (i.e., health care providers). Perhaps some, but not all members of one class, are members of another. For example, some members of the class of health care providers and some members of the class of nurses may be vegetarians and some may not be. The subject and predicate are linked by the copula, the "are" or "are not" component of the propositions in this example. The copula is a form of the verb "to be," which can be affirmative or negative.

The four standard forms of categorical propositions and their symbolic representation follow (Copi and Cohen, 1994; Kelley, 1994). $S$ represents the subject and $P$ represents the predicate terms in the propositions.

All nurses are vegetarians.
    (All $S$ is $P$.)
No nurses are vegetarians.
    (No $S$ is $P$.)
Some nurses are vegetarians.
    (Some $S$ is $P$.)
Some nurses are not vegetarians.
    (Some $S$ is not $P$.)

The first statement, "All nurses are vegetarians," is called a universal affirmative proposition. The proposition has two classes (i.e., the class of all nurses and the class of all vegetarians). The proposition means that every member of the first class is also a member of the second class. All is universal; that is, it includes *every* member of a class. The proposition is written symbolically as "All $S$ is $P$."

The second statement, "no nurses are vegetarians," is called a universal negative proposition. The proposition has two classes (i.e., all nurses and all vegetarians). It wholly excludes all members of the class of nurses from the class of vegetarians. The proposition is written symbolically as "No $S$ is $P$."

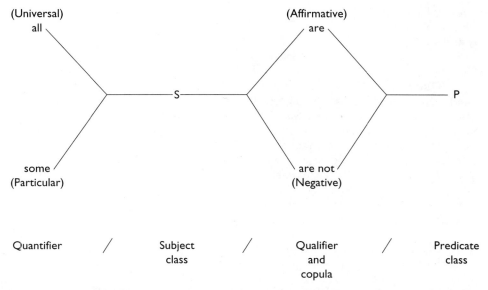

**Fig. 8-1**  The categorical proposition includes a quantifier (universal or particular), a subject class (*S*), a qualifier and copula (affirmative or negative), and a predicate class (*P*).

From Benson S: Philosophy 111: Logic, language, and persuasion (class handouts), Denver, 1991, Metropolitan State College of Denver.

The third statement, "some nurses are vegetarians," is called a particular affirmative proposition. The proposition affirms that some members of the class of all nurses are also members of the class of all vegetarians. It neither affirms nor denies that *all* nurses are vegetarians. *Some* is an indefinite term that means at least one. It affirms that at least one member of the class of nurses is also a member of the class of vegetarians. The proposition is written symbolically as "Some *S* is *P*."

The fourth statement, "Some nurses are not vegetarians," is called a particular negative proposition. This proposition refers to some members of the class of nurses; it is particular. It affirms that at least one member of the class of nurses is excluded from the whole class of vegetarians. It is written symbolically as "Some *S* is not *P*."

Fig. 8-1 illustrates the categorical proposition symbolically. Fig. 8-1 shows the components of the categorical proposition. *All* means universal, and *some* means at least one. The words *all* and *some* quantify the subject class (*S*). *Are* means affirmative and *are not* means negative in reference to a class. They qualify the predicate class (*P*).

Because only two qualities (affirmative or negative) and two quantities (universal or particular) are possible, only four standard logical forms for categorical propositions—regardless of the complexity of the subject and predicate terms—exist. The standard form for these categorical propositions have traditional labels, the letters *A, E, I,* and *O.*

**A:**    All *S* is *P.*
**E:**    No *S* is *P.*
**I:**    Some *S* is *P.*
**O:**    Some *S* is not *P.*

***Quantity and Quality.***    Quantity refers to the "all," "no," and "some" that precede the subject in each categorical proposition. Quantity answers the question of how many of the subject class are said to be contained or excluded from the predicate class. Quality refers to the affirmative or negative character of a proposition. It pertains to whether those members of the subject class are said to be included or excluded from the predicate class. An *A* proposition is universal affirmative; *E* is universal negative; *I* is particular affirmative; and *O* is particular negative. Each categorical proposition has both a quantity and a quality. Taken together, quantity and quality determine the logical form of a proposition, and the subject and predicate determine its content (Bandman and Bandman, 1995; Kelley, 1994).

***Distribution.***    Distribution is important to understand because it is a prelude for distinguishing valid from invalid arguments. Distribution refers to the way terms *S* or *P* occur in standard form categorical propositions. They are designated as distributed or undistributed. For example, the *A* proposition states that "All *S* is *P*" (i.e., each and every *S* is *P*). The proposition does not say anything about all *P*s. *S* is accordingly distributed, and *P* is not. The proposition "All registered nurses are licensed practitioners" places every registered nurse in the class of licensed practitioners, but it does not make a claim about all licensed practitioners. We know that the class of licensed practitioners includes many other practitioners such as physicians, engineers, and occupational therapists who are not stated in the proposition. The proposition makes a claim about all registered nurses but does not do so about the class of licensed practitioners. In this example also, the *S* is distributed, and *P* is undistributed. Distribution refers to the claim a proposition makes about the entire class of both the subject and the predicate. This concept of distribution also applies to the terms in the other categorical propositions, *E, I,* and *O.* Table 8-1 illustrates distribution.

The subject term is distributed if the proposition is universal and undistributed if the proposition is particular. That is, "All *S*s" makes a claim about all *S*s in a class

    Table 8-1    **Distribution in Categorical Propositions***

| PROPOSITION | SUBJECT (S) | PREDICATE (P) |
| --- | --- | --- |
| *A:* All *S* is *P.* | Distributed | Undistributed |
| *E:* No *S* is *P.* | Distributed | Distributed |
| *I:* Some *S* is *P.* | Undistributed | Undistributed |
| *O:* Some *S* is not *P.* | Undistributed | Distributed |

▌ *Modified from Kelley D: The art of reasoning (2nd expanded ed.), New York, 1994, W.W. Norton and Co.

(distributed), and "Some *S*s" do not make such a claim (undistributed). For the subject term, what matters in distribution is quantity, not quality (Kelley, 1994).

The predicate term in propositions *A* (All *S* is *P*) and *I* (Some *S* is *P*) is undistributed because no claim is made about all the members of the class *P*. We do not know if all *P*s belong to the class of *S*s or if some are excluded. In both of these propositions, the predicate term is undistributed.

Let us look at the predicate term in the *E* proposition (No *S* is *P*) and use the example, "No nurses are U.S. presidents." The *E* proposition completely separates nurses as a class from U.S. presidents as a class. The proposition states that no nurses are U.S. presidents. This proposition also says something about every member of the class of U.S. presidents. It implies that no member is identical with any member of the class of nurses. In general, "No *S* is *P*" is the same as "No *P* is *S*." In this case, *P* is distributed.

This same reasoning applies to the *O* proposition (Some *S* is not *P*). Some members of class *S* are excluded from the class of *P*s. For example, in the proposition, "Some nurses are not caring," let us identify nurse X as not caring. The proposition states that nurse X is not identical with anyone in the class of caring people. The proposition implies that no one in the class of caring people is identical with nurse X. Thus, the predicate of the proposition is distributed.

Quality, not quantity, is what matters for the predicate. If the proposition is negative (*E* or *O*), the predicate term is distributed. If the proposition is affirmative (*A* or *I*), the predicate is undistributed (Kelley, 1994).

## Immediate Inference

Recall that every argument has two basic elements: a conclusion supported by one or more premises. Some conclusions are made from a single premise; that is, the inference is drawn directly from one premise without the mediation of any other premise. These inferences are called immediate inferences. Conversion and obversion are two kinds of immediate inferences (Copi and Cohen, 1994; Kelley, 1994).

***Converse.***   Converse is an immediate inference, which also is called conversion, or taking the converse. The converse of a standard form categorical proposition results when we switch the subject and predicate terms and determine if the proposition follows. For example, inferring the converse of an *A* proposition is not legitimate. The converse of "All registered nurses are licensed people" is "All licensed people are registered nurses." The first proposition is true, but its converse does not logically follow. "All *S* is *P*" does not mean that "All *P* is *S*." The most that we can conclude from the proposition is that some *P* is *S*; that is, some licensed people are registered nurses. This is called taking the converse by limitation. We limit our claim and infer only that some *P* is *S*.

For the converse of an *E* proposition, if the first proposition is true, the second must be true also. For example, the converse of "No nurses are astronauts," is "No astronauts are nurses." The converse follows logically from the first proposition.

For the *I* proposition, the converse of "Some nurses are hospital employees," is "Some hospital employees are nurses." If some nurses are hospital employees, it follows logically that some hospital employees are nurses.

The *O* proposition and its converse are often both true. For example, "Some nurses are not caring people" and "Some caring people are not nurses." However, the converse does not logically follow from the *O* proposition. For example, from "Some humans beings are not nurses," it does not follow that "Some nurses are not human beings."

To summarize, the converse of only E and I propositions is legitimate. Note that the converse logically follows only when the subject and predicate terms are identical in their distribution value. Observe that both the subject and predicate are distributed in the *E* proposition and both the subject and predicate are undistributed in the *I* proposition (see Table 8-1).

Note that the converse does not logically follow when the subject and predicate in the original proposition are not identical in their distribution value. In proposition *A*, the subject is distributed and the predicate is undistributed. In proposition *O*, the subject is undistributed and the predicate is distributed. To take the converse in propositions *A* and *O* is to move a term that was undistributed into a position where it is distributed. The result is a claim that is not valid. For example, the predicate in the proposition *A* (All *S* is *P*) is undistributed. The proposition is making a statement about all *S*s, not about all *P*s. Its converse (All *P* is *S*) changes the distribution of *P* from undistributed to distributed. It then makes a claim about all *P*s.

**Obverse.**    Obversion is another type of immediate inference. Obversion is about classes. Recall that a class is the collection of all objects having a common characteristic. For example, all humans belong to a class as do all right-handed people and all people who have heart disease. A class can be more complex, such as all men age 55 and older who have heart disease and live in Japan.

Every class, *C*, has a complementary class, or complement, which is a collection of all things that do not belong to the original class. Thus, the complement to the class of all humans contains no people but would contain everything else such as houses, cars, fruits, trees, and so forth. It is called the class of nonhumans. The complement to the class, *C*, is usually labeled as "non-*C*." The complement to the class of right-handed people is the class of all things that are not people who are right-handed, including people who are left-handed, but also stones, numbers, and so forth. The complement to the class of people who have heart disease is the class of all things that are not people who have heart disease including people who do not have heart disease but also trees, stones, and so forth.

The obverse of a proposition makes two changes. First, we replace the predicate term with its complement. Second, we change the quality of the proposition from affirmative to negative or from negative to affirmative. The obverse of each proposition follows logically. The obverse of an *A* proposition (All *S* is *P*) is an *E* proposition (No *S* is non-*P*). For example, the obverse of "All registered nurses are licensed" is "No registered nurses are nonlicensed (or unlicensed)."

The obverse of an *E* proposition (No *S* is *P*) is an *A* proposition (All *S* is non-*P*). For example, the obverse of "No nurses are astronauts" is "All nurses are nonastronauts."

The obverse of an *I* proposition (Some *S* is *P*) is an *O* proposition (Some *S* is not non-*P*). For example, the obverse of "Some nurses are caring" is "Some nurses are not uncaring."

The obverse of an *O* proposition (Some *S* is not *P*) is an *I* proposition (Some *S* is non-*P*). For example, the obverse of "Some medicines are not addictive" is "Some medicines are nonaddictive."

Note that in each obversion the subject term and the quantity remain the same. If the predicate already has the non-*P* form, then it is changed to its complement, which is *P*. The two changes (replacing the predicate term *P* with its complement non-P and changing the quality from affirmative to negative or from negative to affirmative) cancel each other. Hence, the obverse really conveys the same information.

A term and its complement divide the entire universe into two mutually exclusive classes. Terms that are opposed should not be mistaken for complementary terms. For example, the complement of winner is not loser; instead, it is nonwinner. Not everyone is either a winner or loser, but everyone is either a winner or a nonwinner. Winner and loser are opposites, not complements. The complement of conscious is not comatose; instead, it is nonconscious. Not everyone is either conscious or comatose, but everyone is either conscious or nonconscious.

## Categorical Syllogisms

The word *syllogism* comes from two Greek words: *syn*, meaning "together," and *logizesthai,* meaning "to reason." Aristotle, who was the first person to study and systematize syllogistic arguments, coined the word (Engel, 1994). A categorical syllogism is a deductive argument consisting of two premises, from which a conclusion is inferred. The argument contains exactly three terms, each of which occurs twice in different propositions. The categorical syllogism must not have more or less than three terms. Categorical syllogisms have a standard form when the premises and conclusion are arranged in a specific order (Copi and Cohen, 1994). Consider this kind of pattern:

**Premise:**      All *M* are *P*.
**Premise:**      Some *S* are *M*.
**Conclusion:**   Therefore, some *S* are *P*.

The major term of the syllogism is the term that occurs as the predicate (*P*) of the conclusion. The minor term is the subject (*S*) term of the conclusion. The middle term is symbolized by the letter *M*. Both premises must overlap as described so there is common ground for a conclusion; otherwise, a conclusion cannot be supported.

The first premise is called the major premise, not because it is listed first, but because it contains the major term. The second premise is called the minor premise, not because it is listed second, but because it contains the minor term. Both premises are assumed to be true. Consider the following classic Aristotelian syllogism:

**Premise:**      All men are mortal.
**Premise:**      Socrates is a man.
**Conclusion:**   Socrates is mortal.

In this example, if you accept as true that all men as a class are mortal and that Socrates belongs to the class of men, then it necessarily follows that Socrates is mortal. Adding the symbols, the argument would look like this:

**Premise:**      All men (*M*) are mortal (*P*).
**Premise:**      Socrates (*S*) is a man (*M*).
**Conclusion:**   Therefore, Socrates (*S*) is mortal (*P*).

Consider another example:

**Premise:**      All registered nurses must pass a licensing examination.
**Premise:**      Stacey is a registered nurse.
**Conclusion:**   Therefore, Stacey passed a licensing examination.

The syllogism contains two premises and one conclusion. In this example, the meaning of the word *term* as used in syllogisms is enlarged. A term can be more than just a single word; it also can be a larger expression. The three terms used in this example are "registered nurses," "Stacey," and "pass a licensing examination." Each refers to a different class, and each is used exactly twice within the whole argument. Write in the symbols, *S*, *P*, and *M* where they belong. "Stacey" is the subject (*S*), "pass a licensing examination" is the predicate (*P*) and "registered nurse" is the middle (*M*) term. Suppose that the premises are true, that all registered nurses must pass a licensing examination to be able to use that title and that Stacey is a registered nurse. Does the conclusion follow from the premises? Yes, and therefore the argument is valid. Even if the premises were not true, the structure still makes it valid. If the premises also are in fact true, then it is a sound argument.

To construct a categorical syllogistic argument use no more than three terms, *S*, *P* and *M*, and state the terms consistently so that a definitive relationship can be established and judged. Without this structure, the argument makes little sense. For example:

All nurses are registered.
Stacey is a nurse.
Therefore, Stacey has been to Europe.

The example is invalid; no conclusion is justified from the statements when four terms are used. When constructing a syllogistic argument, you must be sure to adhere to the correct structure.

Let us look at another example:

**Premise:**      All pediatric clients with persistent diarrhea should be seen by a health care provider.
**Premise:**      Annie Lou is a pediatric client who has persistent diarrhea.
**Conclusion:**   Therefore, Annie Lou should be seen by a health care provider.

In this example, the two premises and one conclusion contain three terms: "all pediatric clients with persistent diarrhea," "should be seen by a health care provider," and

"Annie Lou." Each proposition contains two different terms, referring to two different classes. For example, Annie Lou is a member of the class of "all pediatric clients with persistent diarrhea." "Annie Lou" refers to that class that contains just Annie Lou. Write in the symbols, *S, P,* and *M,* where they belong. "Annie Lou" is the subject (*S*) of the conclusion; "should be seen by a health care provider" is the predicate (*P*) of the conclusion; and "all pediatric clients with persistent diarrhea" is the middle term (*M*).

Suppose that the premises that all pediatric clients with persistent diarrhea should be seen by a health care provider and Annie Lou is a pediatric client who has persistent diarrhea are true. Does the conclusion follow from the premises? If Annie Lou is a member of the class of "all pediatric clients with persistent diarrhea," it follows that Annie Lou should be seen by a health care provider. The conclusion is logically inferred from what we assume to be true premises; therefore, it is valid. If the premises really are true, it is a sound argument.

## Evaluation of Deductive Arguments

For a deductive argument to be sound, it must meet two standards: (1) the premises must be true and (2) the structure must be valid. If the premises are true and the structure is valid, then the argument is said to be sound. *Truth, validity,* and *soundness* are the words used to evaluate deductive arguments (Engel, 1994).

***Premises Must Be True.***    Truth of the premises is the first standard by which to evaluate deductive arguments. Whether the premises are true or false is a characteristic of the premises themselves, not of the process of reasoning. Ask if the premises are true. For example:

**Premise:**      All people who are kind and softhearted make good nurses.
**Premise:**      Jane is kind and softhearted.
**Conclusion:**   Therefore, Jane will make a good nurse.

Do you concur that the premises are true? Do all people who are kind and softhearted make good nurses? We doubt that you will agree with this statement or accept it as true.

Does the conclusion follow from the premises? Write in the symbols, *S, P,* and *M* and evaluate the basic structure of the argument. The conclusion does follow from the premises. The argument is logically valid, but this does not make the conclusion true or the argument sound. Jane may or may not make a good nurse. When the conclusion follows from the premises logically, the argument is valid. Validity and invalidity refer to the process of reasoning used to infer the conclusion. Truth refers to the accuracy of the premises.

***Structure Must Be Valid.***    Validity is the second standard by which to evaluate deductive arguments. In a valid deductive argument, we must necessarily accept the conclusion of an argument if we accept the premises as true. Ask if the conclusion follows from the premises. To tell whether it does, look to the structure. For example, change the structure of the classic syllogism so that the conclusion does not follow from the premises.

**Premise:**          All men are mortal.
**Premise:**          Socrates is a man.
**Conclusion:**     Therefore, all men are Socrates.

This syllogism has the requisite three propositions and the three terms: *men, Socrates,* and *mortal*. However, each term does not appear exactly twice in the different propositions. Mortal appears only once and men/man appears three times, which changes the structure. With little analysis, you know the conclusion of this syllogism does not follow. The structure of the syllogism is faulty. The premises are true but the conclusion does not logically follow from them.

Now consider this argument:

**Premise:**          All frogs are planets.
**Premise:**          Freddy is a frog.
**Conclusion:**     Therefore, Freddy is a planet.

This syllogism has the same structure as the original argument about Socrates and is therefore valid. If the premises were true, the conclusion would have to be true. Because deductive arguments are valid due to their structure, even if we change all the terms of a valid argument, the result will be valid so long as the same structure is preserved.

Let us look at another example:

**Premise:**          Some men are mortal.
**Premise:**          Socrates is a man.
**Conclusion:**     Therefore, Socrates is mortal.

This argument has the same terms in the same pattern as the original example, but it does not have the same structure. Changing "all" to "some" in the major premise changes the quantity of the proposition and therefore its logical form. Thus, the whole structure of the argument is changed, and, in fact, this new structure is not valid. Compare this argument with the following:

**Premise:**          Some nurses are men.
**Premise:**          Stacey is a nurse.
**Conclusion:**     Therefore, Stacey is a man.

Both examples have this structure:

**Premise:**          Some $M$ are $P$.
**Premise:**          All $S$ are $M$.
**Conclusion:**     Therefore, all $S$ are $P$.

The second example of this pattern shows how this structure allows cases of true premises with a false conclusion and therefore is not a valid structure. This means that all arguments of this structure are not valid, including the first example.

**Soundness.**　The soundness of an argument refers to the truthfulness of the premises and the validity or invalidity of the reasoning. If the premises are true and the reasoning is valid, the argument is sound. If the premises are true and the reasoning invalid, the argument is unsound. If any one of the premises is false and the reasoning is valid, the argument is unsound. If any one of the premises is false and the reasoning is invalid, the argument is unsound. Table 8-2 illustrates these relationships.

The following arguments illustrate each of these relationships.

**Premise:**　　All children should be immunized.
**Premise:**　　Danny is a child.
**Conclusion:**　Therefore, Danny should be immunized.

The premises are true and the structure is valid; therefore, the argument is sound.

**Premise:**　　No one taking medicine X should take medicine Y.
**Premise:**　　Todd is taking medicine X.
**Conclusion:**　Therefore, Todd also should take medicine Y.

In this example, the premises are assumed to be true but the conclusion does not follow from them. It is an invalid structure and therefore an unsound argument.

**Premise:**　　All old people will eventually live in a nursing home.
**Premise:**　　Mr. Garcia is an old person.
**Conclusion:**　Therefore, Mr. Garcia will eventually live in a nursing home.

In this example, our reasoning is valid. The conclusion necessarily follows from the premises. However, is the first premise true? Do all old people eventually live in a nursing home? No, only about 5% of those aged 65 and older live in nursing homes

 Table 8-2　**Evaluation of Categorical Syllogistic Arguments**[*]

| PREMISES | STRUCTURE | ARGUMENT |
|---|---|---|
| True | Valid | Sound |
| True | Invalid | Unsound |
| False | Valid | Unsound |
| False | Invalid | Unsound |

[*]Categorical syllogistic arguments are evaluated as sound or unsound according to the characteristics of the premises and structure of each argument.

at any given time. The rest of those aged 65 and older live as follows: 44% with their spouse, 31% alone, and 25% with other people, both relatives and nonrelatives (U.S. Senate Special Committee on Aging, et al., 1991). The structure is valid, but the major premise is false; therefore, the argument is unsound.

| | |
|---|---|
| **Premise:** | All hospitalized clients can care for themselves to some degree. |
| **Premise:** | Mr. Taylor is a client. |
| **Conclusion:** | Therefore, Mr. Taylor can do his own oral hygiene. |

In this example, our premises are false because some clients are unconscious and unable to care for themselves. The structure of the argument is invalid. It is an unsound argument.

## Other Kinds of Syllogisms

Some propositions are more complex and require a different kind of reasoning than the classic *A, E, I,* and *O* form. This accounts for the fact that there are other kinds of syllogisms besides the categorical syllogism. These other kinds of syllogisms use propositions and logical connectives that take us beyond the limitations of the classical forms. For example, some propositions come in the *either . . . or* form and the *if . . . then* form. Because reasoning in these forms is common in nursing, we should examine the relevant structure (Kelley, 1994; Bandman and Bandman, 1995; Copi and Cohen, 1994).

Syllogisms take their names from the kinds of propositions they contain. Disjunctive and hypothetical syllogisms are two such examples. Their form is different from categorical syllogisms where the categorical form, subject, and predicate terms are the focus of analysis. Disjunctive syllogisms have the structure of *p or q,* and hypothetical syllogisms have the structure of *if p . . . then q.*

The single lowercase letters like *p, q, r,* and *s* represent the components in the propositions, which are themselves whole propositions, perhaps categorical ones. The distinctive feature of these complex propositions is that they assert a certain relationship exists between the components. This relationship is the focus of analysis.

## Disjunctive Syllogism

The disjunctive syllogism is a valid argument form. It gets its name from a kind of premise that has the connective *or* between two or more components. The components are called disjuncts and are labeled *p* and *q*; the whole component (or statement) is called a disjunction. For example, James is in either the x-ray department or James is in the physical therapy unit. The proposition is a disjunction with two components (disjuncts): "James is in the x-ray department" (label *p*) and "James is in the physical therapy unit" (label *q*).

The disjunctive proposition, or disjunction, does not actually state that *p* is true or that *q* is true, but it does assert that one or the other of them is true and it allows for the possibility that both may be true. Suppose we know that one of the disjuncts is not true (James is not in the x-ray department), we could then infer that the other must be true (James is in the physical therapy unit). The disjunctive syllogism looks like this:

James is in either the x-ray department or the physical therapy unit.
James is not in the x-ray department.
Therefore, James is in the physical therapy unit.

Using the labels $p$ and $q$, the structure of the disjunctive syllogism is:

Either $p$ or $q$
$-p$

___

$q$

The negative symbol in front of $p$ ($-p$) means not $p$. $p$ and $-p$ are contradictory propositions; if one is true the other is false. Assuming the premises are true, the conclusion also must be true. If we have a disjunction and the denial of one of the disjuncts, then we can validly infer that the other disjunct is true. Any argument in this form is a disjunctive syllogism and is valid.

The syllogism would still be valid if the negative symbol were in front of $q$ because we could have first checked the physical therapy unit to locate James. The syllogism would then look like this:

Either $p$ or $q$
$-q$

___

$p$

The reasoning would be either $p$ or $q$, but $-q$, therefore $p$.

By extending this form, we can allow any number of disjuncts. For example, the reasoning with four disjuncts would look like this (Kelley, 1994):

Either $p$ or ($q$ or $r$ or $s$)
$-p$

___

Either $q$ or $r$ or $s$

    Either $q$ or ($r$ or $s$)

    $-q$

    ___

    Either $r$ or $s$

Either *r* or *s*

–*r*

––––

*s*

Additional disjuncts are given different letters as shown by the use of *r* and *s*. The reasoning illustrated is a process of eliminating disjuncts until we have one that must be true, assuming the disjunctive premise is true.

> ***Inclusion and Exclusion.***    The connective *or* has two uses, inclusion and exclusion, both of which are found in nursing practice. The inclusive sense means "*p* or *q* or both." The exclusive sense means "*p* or *q* but not both." The following illustrates the inclusive use: "The nurse fed the toddler either peaches *or* pears." The inclusive use means that the nurse could have fed one or both foods to the toddler. The statement is true in either case.

The following illustrates the exclusive use of the connective *or*: "The nurse fed the toddler either peaches or pears, but not both." The exclusive use of *or* means choosing one of the disjuncts but not both. One action totally excludes the other action.

The exclusive use of *or* facilitates decision making when the choices are limited to two. For example, to reduce swelling within the first 24 hours after an athletic injury to a knee, the nurse should apply either heat or cold, but not both. The nurse knows that heat raises tissue temperature, causes vasodilation, and increases local circulation. The nurse also knows that cold stimulates vasoconstriction, inhibits local circulation, relieves inflammation, and prevents edema. Thus, the nurse reasons that he or she should apply either heat (*p*) or cold (*q*), but not both. It is not heat (–*p*); therefore, it is cold (*q*).

A common mistake in using disjunctions is not to examine options that should be examined. For example, 90-year-old Edna will be discharged from the hospital tomorrow. An erroneous use of *or* states that either Edna can be discharged to a nursing home or she can be discharged to her apartment. By failing to consider further alternatives, if one option is eliminated, the other option is chosen. Thus, acceptance of the disjunction has erroneously limited our options in this example. Suppose Edna has the following options:

▼  She could live with a family member.
▼  She could move in with a friend.
▼  She could have her friend move in with her.
▼  She could move to a retirement community.

The erroneous use of the connective *or* may cause us to ignore these other options. This erroneous use is called the fallacy of false alternatives, also known as the false dilemma fallacy. The fallacy occurs when we rely on a disjunctive premise that does not identify all of the possible alternatives.

***Validity and Invalidity.***   An argument that denies a disjunct and derives the other disjunct as the conclusion is valid in both inclusion (*p* or *q* or both) and exclusion (*p* or *q* but not both). An argument that affirms a disjunct is valid only if the connective *or* is used in the exclusive sense. A problem occurs when we do not know which meaning, inclusion or exclusion, is intended. When this occurs, we must rely on the context to determine the intended meaning. Unless otherwise indicated, we assume the inclusive meaning of the connective *or*. This is a more cautious interpretation, because it allows the possibility that both disjuncts are true.

Because not all disjunctions are exclusive, to affirm a disjunct is, in general, invalid. To illustrate this, review the inclusion example about the nurse feeding the toddler either peaches *or* pears.

The nurse fed the toddler either peaches *or* pears.
The nurse fed the toddler peaches.
Therefore, the nurse did not feed the toddler pears.

The second statement affirms one disjunct. But affirming this disjunct does not mean the nurse did not feed the toddler pears. Therefore, the reasoning is invalid, or fallacious. Consistent with the first statement, the nurse may have fed the toddler peaches and pears. The truth of one action does not imply the falsehood of the other action because both of them can be true.

## Hypothetical Syllogisms

Hypothetical syllogisms have conditional propositions of the *if . . . then* form. *p* and *q* represent the two component propositions. The form of the proposition is "*If p . . . then q.*" The component proposition that follows *if* is called the antecedent; the component proposition that follows *then* is called the consequent. For example, if Amy is exposed to the influenza virus and she has not been previously vaccinated against it (antecedent), then she may get the flu (consequent).

Hypothetical propositions are used in everyday nursing practice and in living to assess the interrelatedness among facts, events, and possibilities. For example, if the electrical equipment is not grounded, then it should be fixed before a fire occurs. If the client has a communicable disease, then the client should be placed in isolation. If the budget for a nursing project is overspent, then no more supplies can be purchased.

The truth of *p* or *q* in a hypothetical proposition is not actually asserted. Instead, it asserts that the truth of *p* would be sufficient for the truth of *q*. For example, we do not assert the truth of the statement "The electrical equipment is not grounded." Instead, the truth of the statement is sufficient for the truth of the following statement; "It should be fixed before a fire occurs." Hypothetical syllogisms have pure and mixed forms.

***Pure Hypothetical Syllogism.***   The pure hypothetical syllogism contains conditional propositions exclusively. It looks like this:

If *p* . . . then *q*.
If *q* . . . then *r*.

———

If *p* . . . then *r*.

The role of *q* in this syllogism is the same as role of the middle term in categorical syllogisms. It links *p* and *r* together in the conclusion. An argument in this form is valid. The pure hypothetical syllogism is commonly used to link events in a chain where each event causes the next. The following example illustrates the link:

> If children are not immunized against childhood illnesses, an increased incidence of these diseases will occur. And if an increase in these diseases occurs, an increase in morbidity and mortality rates will occur. Therefore, if children are not immunized against childhood illnesses, more disease and death will result.

The reasoning in this example is purely hypothetical. The premises and the conclusion are all conditional statements. In this type of syllogism, we make no assertion that the component propositions are actually true; only the conditional statements themselves are asserted.

*Mixed Hypothetical Syllogism.*    Mixed hypothetical syllogism has one conditional premise and one categorical premise. The mixed hypothetical syllogism comes in two valid forms: the modus ponens and the modus tollens. The modus ponens affirms the antecedent, and the modus tollens denies the consequence. Both forms are valid.

**Modus Ponens.**    Modus ponens is a valid argument form that affirms the antecedent. The first premise is conditional (the *if . . . then* statement) and the second premise affirms the antecedent of the conditional statement. The argument uses the *if . . . then* premise and the second premise to affirm the consequent of the *if . . . then* premise. It has the following structure:

If *p*, then *q*
*p*

———

*q*

For example:

If you stop arterial bleeding, then you will increase client survival rates.
You stopped arterial bleeding.
Therefore, you increased client survival rates.

Consider the case of Mr. Norman:

*If* Mr. Norman had a myocardial infarction, *then* the nurse would assess him for acute anxiety; persistent crushing substernal pain that may radiate to the left arm, jaw, neck, or shoulder blades; shortness of breath; nausea; vomiting; diaphoresis; and cool, pale skin.

Mr. Norman had a myocardial infarction. Therefore, the nurse assesses him for acute anxiety; persistent crushing substernal pain that may radiate to the left arm, jaw, neck, or shoulder blades; shortness of breath; nausea; vomiting; diaphoresis; and cool, pale skin.

This argument form is valid regardless of the terms that are used. As noted previously with other valid argument forms, the conclusion is true if the premises are true.

**Modus Tollens.**    Modus tollens is the second valid form of the mixed hypothetical syllogism. Modus tollens denies the consequent. The first premise is conditional (the *if . . . then* statement), and the second premise denies the consequent of the conditional premise. The third statement (the conclusion) denies its antecedent. It has the following structure:

If $p$ . . . then $q$
$-q$
___
$-p$

For example:

If Betsy has an infection, then she has painful and frequent urination.
Betsy does not have painful and frequent urination.
Therefore, Betsy does not have a urinary tract infection.

**Invalid Forms.**    Two fallacious forms of argument that resemble modus ponens and modus tollens are the fallacy of affirming the consequent and the fallacy of denying the antecedent. The fallacy of affirming the consequent has the following structure:

If $p$ . . . then $q$
$q$
___
$p$

For example:

If Tony exercises daily, then he will gain strength.
Tony gained strength.
Therefore, Tony exercised daily.

This argument is not valid although the premises may be true. Tony may have gained strength by resting and eating well.

The fallacy of denying the antecedent has the following structure:

If *p* . . . *then q*

−*p*

⎯⎯

−*q*

For example:

If Bob has an injury, then he is incapacitated.
Bob does not have an injury.
Therefore, Bob is not incapacitated.

This argument is not valid even if we assume the premises are true. Bob may be incapacitated for reasons completely unrelated to an injury.

Other types of deductive reasoning not discussed in this chapter exist. You should continue learning about deductive reasoning by seeking out additional sources of information.

## INDUCTIVE REASONING

Inductive reasoning is the second kind of reasoning. In good inductive arguments, the conclusion is *likely* to follow from the premises; that is, it follows only with *probability*. The conclusion is uncertain. The following example illustrates the difference between deductive and inductive reasoning:

**Deductive:**
All the syringes in that box are 2 cc syringes.
All these syringes in my hand are from that box.
All these syringes in my hand are therefore 2 cc syringes.

**Inductive:**
All these syringes in my hand are from that box.
All these syringes in my hand are 2 cc syringes.
All the syringes in that box are probably 2 cc syringes.

In the deductive example, the conclusion *necessarily* follows from the premises; it follows with certainty. In the inductive example, the conclusion follows only with *probability*. We do not know with certainty that all the syringes in that box are 2 cc syringes. We know only that they are probably 2 cc syringes. Perhaps 10 cc syringes are in the box, and we did not reach far or deep enough into the box to find them. We do not know with certainty that the box contains only 2 cc syringes, only that it probably does.

In the deductive argument, the premises contain all the information of the conclusion. To arrive at a conclusion, we do not need to refer to anything outside the premises. In contrast, the conclusion of an inductive argument goes beyond the information found in the premises. Therefore, the conclusion of an inductive argument is less certain, but it can have a high probability of being true. Engel (1994) uses this classic example to illustrates this probability:

The sun has risen every morning since time immemorial.
Therefore, the sun will rise tomorrow.

It is highly probable that the sun will rise tomorrow, but we cannot say with absolute certainty that it will.

## Evaluation of Inductive Arguments

Inductive arguments are evaluated differently than deductive arguments. Inductive arguments are evaluated as either good or bad, strong or weak, based on the degree of support the premises provide for the conclusion. Truth continues as a standard for evaluation of the premises; however, the truth of the premises does not guarantee the truth of the conclusion. It is true that the sun has risen every morning since time immemorial, but we do not know with absolute certainty that it will tomorrow. Nevertheless, what has happened in the past is a likely indicator of what will occur in the future. Because the conclusion is based on probability and not on necessity, we cannot be absolutely certain that the conclusion is supported by the premises. The greater the probability that the premises confer on the conclusion, the greater the merit of the argument (Copi and Cohen, 1994; Engel, 1994). With inductive arguments, if new information becomes available, the conclusion may no longer follow. Bandman and Bandman (1995) illustrate this as:

Registered Nurse 1 is female.
Registered Nurse 2 is female.
Registered Nurse 3 is female.
Registered Nurse 4 is female.
Therefore, all registered nurses are female.

Because all of the individual cases examined were female, it appears accurate to conclude that all registered nurses are female. However, this conclusion is not true because 2% to 4% are male. Once this new information is added to the premises, the conclusion no longer follows. This is distinctive of inductive arguments. By contrast, if a deductive argument is valid, no additional information can be added to the premises that causes the conclusion not to follow. This is because the original premises themselves guarantee the truth of the conclusion.

Reasoning by analogy, causal reasoning, and empirical generalization are three forms of inductive reasoning.

## Reasoning by Analogy

An analogy points out the similarity in some respect that is shared between things that might otherwise be unlike. It is the likening of one thing to another on the basis of this similarity (Neufeldt, 1991). Analogies are used to explain and describe things to make them more easily understandable. For example, children learn that their bodies are similar to a machine such as a car. Both require input (food, water, gasoline), have functional processes by which to use the input (activities of daily living and vehicle operation), and output (gastrointestinal, kidneys, and exhaust). Both must be cared for to stay in peak condition. Analogies help us think on a conceptual level and to find meaning in our observations.

Nursing students learn that the heart lung machine and dialysis equipment are analogous to the function of the respective bodily organs. Nurses find similarities among clients who have the same health problem such as heart disease and cancer. These examples are analogies that serve to explain and describe instances.

Analogies also can be used to provide support for a conclusion in an argument. For example, Pam, a maternity nurse, has many years experience working with clients in labor and delivery. She instructs Jen, a nursing student, to observe grand multiparous mothers closely for postpartum hemorrhage. To make her point, Pam likens the uterus of grand multiparous mothers to an overextended rubber band. Both have reduced recoil ability. The uterus of grand multiparous mothers has been stretched, has diminished muscle tone, and is prone to muscle relaxation. As a result, the uterus may not clamp down on the placental site sufficiently, resulting in hemorrhaging (Olds, London, and Ladewig, 1992). Using this analogy, Pam persuades Jen to conclude that she should watch the grand multiparous mothers closely.

When an analogy is used in argument, you must analyze and evaluate it before you agree that it supports the conclusion. Copi and Cohen (1994) provide useful criteria for this purpose. The first criterion to evaluate analogical arguments is to identify the number of instances of one thing being like another. For example, if a colleague advised you against using brand X dressing because it is not very absorbent, based on this one experience, you may wonder if your colleague had arrived at a premature conclusion. However, if your colleague stated that he had used brand X dressings on a dozen clients and found that it was not very absorbent, the conclusion that brand X is not very absorbent has a higher probability of being true. Suppose further that you discussed brand X dressing with other colleagues, several of whom agree that brand X dressing is not very absorbent. You now have more instances to support the conclusion about the absorbency of brand X dressing. Although the increasing number of instances adds support for the argument, no simple numerical ratio between the number of instances and the probability of the conclusion exists.

The second criterion to evaluate analogical arguments is the number of respects in which the things involved are said to be analogous. For example, when you and your colleagues reflect on your experiences with brand X dressings, think about other aspects of the analogy. Were all of the dressings brand X? Were they all manufactured by the same company? Were they in the same production lot? Were the dressings used in a similar way for all clients? Were the clients in similar physical conditions? If the answer to these questions is yes, then a greater support for the conclusion exists.

The third criterion to evaluate analogical arguments is the number of points of difference between the instances. For example, suppose you learn that the dressings did not come from the same production lot, that some of the dressings were manufactured in the United States and some in another country, and that some clients had a lot of bleeding while others had very little. These points of difference weaken the support for the conclusion that brand X dressing is not very absorbent.

The fourth criterion to evaluate analogical arguments looks at the number of diverse types of problems an item has affected positively. Suppose that you found brand X dressing to be exceptionally absorbent. The dressing was used on a number of clients who had very different kinds of health problems. Some clients were the first day after surgery, some were several days after surgery, some were in the emergency room, some were in critical care, and some were in maternity. In each instance, brand X dressing was found to be exceptionally absorbent. The diversity of the different uses of the dressing supports the conclusion that brand X dressing is exceptionally absorbent.

The fifth criterion to evaluate analogical arguments is the relevance of the reasons cited in the premises to the conclusion. Relevance is the most important criterion, because it underlies all of the other criteria. For example, the reasons why you identify brand X dressing as not very absorbent must be relevant to the conclusion. If you examine the use of the dressings and the conditions of the clients, you have selected relevant reasons. Suppose, however, that you examine the age range of the clients  (20 to 30 years old), their educational level (all high school graduates), and their ethnicity (one ethnic group) and use this information to support the conclusion that brand X dressing is not very absorbent. The latter reasons would be irrelevant to support the conclusion. A correlation between each of these factors and the conclusion may exist. For example, suppose all clients were high school graduates. However, you have enough background knowledge about level of education and the absorbency of dressings to know that this is just a coincidence.

Reasoning by analogy is common activity in daily living and in nursing practice. If you allow your curiosity to further ponder similarities between instances, you might want to look at causal connections, and perhaps even engage in formal research.

## Causal Reasoning

Causal reasoning is a type of inductive reasoning whereby a claim is made that one event or set of events is caused by another event or set of events (Chaffee, 1994). Causal reasoning is a natural thinking process in nursing and in everyday living. For example, when your computer does not work properly, you engage in causal reasoning. What is wrong? Is it a software or hardware problem? When your client states he has pain, you wonder what is the cause of the pain. Is it related to a treatment the client received? Is it caused by a new or unknown health problem? Is it related to something the client did (e.g., eat or exercise) or did not do (e.g., take the pain medicine as prescribed)? A client may wonder if his disease is due to psychological stress, inadequate diet, or exposure to environmental contaminants.

Nursing diagnoses are based on the assumption that each client problem has a cause or causes and that once identified, the nurse can alter the course of the cause and return the client to the previous state of health. Medical diagnoses are based on a similar assumption: for each disease, there is a cause. Without making these assumptions, there is no need to engage in diagnostic reasoning and to use the nursing and medical diagnostic categories. Nurses have more power to solve problems and physicians have more power over diseases when the causes are known. When nurses administer a treatment, give a medication, and teach a client, they anticipate a specific effect. Nurses engage in causal reasoning on a daily basis in the practice of nursing.

Two approaches are useful to establish causality. One is a general purpose technique to identify and analyze causal relationships of any type. The technique is based on understanding the distinction between necessary and sufficient conditions. The other approach is the methods to establish causality developed by John Stuart Mill, a nineteenth-century noted philosopher (Bandman and Bandman, 1995; Kelley, 1994).

### Necessary and Sufficient Conditions.

*Necessary and Sufficient Conditions.*   Understanding the distinction between necessary and sufficient conditions is essential to understanding causal reasoning. Copi and Cohen (1994) define and illustrate necessary and sufficient conditions as follows:

> A **necessary condition** for the occurrence of a specified event is a circumstance in whose absence the event cannot occur.
> A **sufficient condition** for the occurrence of an event is a circumstance in whose presence the event must occur (p. 480).

For example, the presence of oxygen is a necessary condition for combustion to occur. If it occurs, then oxygen must have been present because it cannot occur in the absence of oxygen.

Although the presence of oxygen is a necessary condition for combustion to occur, it is not a sufficient condition for combustion because oxygen can be present without combustion occurring. For combustion to occur, other conditions must be present. The substance must be within the temperature range for combustion to occur and an ignition source must be present.

Necessary conditions for human life are a beating heart, food, water, and shelter, without which life cannot be sustained. A sufficient condition to life would be being awake and engaged with others and the surrounding environment. If one is awake and engaged with others, one is surely alive.

In causal reasoning, "cause" may sometimes be used in the sense of necessary conditions and sometimes in the sense of sufficient conditions. It most commonly refers to necessary conditions when the problem is to eliminate some undesirable phenomenon. In this case, we must find some condition that is necessary to the existence of the undesirable phenomenon and then eliminate that condition (Copi and Cohen, 1994). For example, researchers seek to discover the cause of human immunodeficiency virus (HIV) infection to find a cure for it. The HIV virus is the cause of the disease in the sense of a necessary condition for it, because in absence of the HIV virus, the disease cannot occur. To date, researchers have been unsuccessful in finding a drug that eliminates the HIV virus. But if they do find such a drug, it will be said to eliminate "the cause" of AIDS.

"Cause" is commonly used in the sense of sufficient conditions when the concern is to produce something desirable rather than eliminate some undesirable phenomenon (Copi and Cohen, 1994). For example, in working with families living in poverty, you most likely will not be able to eliminate the undesirable phenomenon (poor living conditions), but you may be able to teach the parents to use their creativity to stimulate their children's curiosity and intellectual and physical development. You also can teach parents how to make the best food choices while living within their budget. Increased abilities and better food choices are causes of happiness in the sense that their presence is sufficient to increase happiness.

Chapters 6 and 7 discuss many examples of causal reasoning. The application of the scientific method to the study of nursing and health problems is the most structured and systematic way available to establish cause-and-effect relationships. As you may have observed, the most carefully controlled experimental studies often cannot establish with certainty the complex relationship between an event and its cause(s). When looking for the cause of something, look for conditions that are both necessary and sufficient.

**Mill's Methods.**   John Stuart Mill gave us several methods to establish evidence of causal connections. His methods are called the methods of agreement, difference, concomitant variations, and residues (Kelley, 1994) To apply the method of agreement and difference, you first look at the individual instances or cases to determine in what respects they agree (method of agreement). For example, reflect on the clinical experiences you have had to date. Which ones have you liked the best? How were these experiences alike? Was it the age of the clients? The health problem(s)? The instructor who guided you in the experience? The staff nurses with whom you worked? The nature of the clinical service area such as pediatrics or surgery? The sense of satisfaction of truly helping clients? Suppose the common link among these experiences was the latter, the sense of satisfaction you got from helping your clients. The next step is to test your conclusion. Next, you examine those clinical experiences in which you did not have this sense of satisfaction to see if you did not enjoy them. By doing this you remove the sense of satisfaction as a factor and see if the effect still occurs (method of difference).

The method of agreement looks for commonalities across cases. The method of difference requires that we hold the circumstances constant, remove the factor, and see if the effect still occurs. The process of quantitative research using the experimental research design illustrates this. Recall that in this design, the experimental group receives a treatment and the control group receives the placebo. The groups are selected in such a way that they are alike in certain respects (random selection and random assignment) except for the factor(s) being investigated. The difference between the two groups is then attributed to this factor(s). The method of difference is a process of elimination.

When looking for the cause of something, use both the methods of agreement and of differences. The method of agreement provides evidence that the common factor is sufficient for the event in question, and the method of difference provides evidence that it is necessary.

The methods of agreement and of difference were used to investigate the cause of an outbreak of Type A hepatitis in a large metropolitan community. The physicians were required by law to report the individual cases of the disease to the state health department. Public health officials then interviewed all clients who contracted the disease to identify the commonalities across all of the cases. Prior knowledge about Type A hepatitis guided the officials in their investigation. They knew that the disease is highly contagious and is usually transmitted by the fecal-oral route. The most common cause is ingestion of contaminated food, water, or milk. With this background knowledge, the officials looked for a common source of the virus (i.e., a commonality across all individual cases). All of the clients had ingested food from a particular catering service within the previous 45 days. With further investigation, they concluded the outbreak was caused by a food handler who was the only carrier of the virus who worked at the catering service. The food handler did not wash his hands properly. When this food handler was reassigned to other responsibilities not associated with food preparation, the outbreak was eliminated. A careful investigation provided very strong evidence for this conclusion.

In this example, the method of agreement provided evidence that the sufficient condition was that all clients ate food supplied by a common catering service. The method of difference provided evidence that the necessary condition was the food handler who was the only carrier of the virus.

Although the methods of agreement and difference may appear to be a straightforward process, in real life establishing cause-and-effect relationships is more complex (Kelley, 1994). For example, causal relationships exist at many different levels. A disease can be investigated by looking at its effects on cells, on an organ, on the interaction of organs (whole body), on the behavior of the person, on the community, and even on the nation. What an investigation reveals depends on the level at which it is examined.

Causal relationships are conceptualized in different ways. For example, nurses, physicians, chemists, biologists, psychologists, sociologists, and anthropologists all have different ways of looking at and explaining life events. It is the concept of frame of reference applied to a discipline or body of knowledge. The researcher selects a conceptual approach and, in the process of investigation, may discover other ways in which to classify that which she or he observes.

The direction of causality is difficult to determine. Which is the cause and which is the effect in events? Events occur continuously and simultaneously in an interactive, interrelated fashion according to established patterns such as the laws of nature. Isolating these events is an arduous task for researchers. The level on which events are examined, how events are conceptualized, and the difficulty in separating cause from effect are all factors that add to the complexity of understanding causal relationships.

Mill's method of concomitant variations pertains to a quantitative variation in the factors that cause an event. Concomitant variation is concerned with the degree in which both the cause and the effect are present. It is not concerned about whether the effect is present or absent when the cause is present. For example, by increasing (or decreasing) the amount of daily exercise, a person's resting heart rate will correspondingly decrease (or increase). This correlation between the amount of exercise and one's resting heart rate is established by varying the amount of exercise and seeing a corresponding variation in the resting heart rate. Unlike the method of agreement or difference, we do not entirely remove the cause or the effect; some level of activity and some heart rate will always occur. But we can see differences in the amounts of these, and when we see that changing the amount of one is attended by a corresponding change in the amount of the other, we have good evidence that a causal relationship exists between them.

Mill's method of residues also requires the quantification of the effect. This method looks at the factors (*a, b,* and *c*) that are known usually to cause an event (*E*). In a particular case, certain factors (*a* and *b*) are known to be responsible for part, but not all, of the effect. By eliminating what is known (*a* and *b*), we create a "residue" and conclude that the effect must be caused by (*c*). The method uses only a single case and relies on prior knowledge about the effects of known factors (*a* and *b*). The role of *c* is inferred by subtracting the known effects of the other factors.

For example, a client is experiencing edema in her ankles. She has not minimized her intake of table salt or restricted high sodium foods from her diet. Both of these factors are known to cause edema. Nevertheless, the edema is so severe that even taking these measures could not eliminate it entirely. There must, therefore, be some additional cause for her edema—perhaps a medication (e.g., estrogen) that she takes. By eliminating from consideration the amount of effect from the known causes (the table salt and high sodium foods), we infer from the fact that some effect would remain, that there is a residual cause.

When you express causal relationships, unless you are certain, it is more accurate to say, "based on my experience," or "from what I have learned so far," or "from the four research studies I have read." Making accurate statements and warranted generalizations are essential characteristics of critical thinkers.

## Empirical Generalization

An empirical generalization is a form of inductive reasoning. It is a generalization about an entire group based on the observation of a sample of the group (Chaffee, 1994). Empirical refers to observation that results from experiment or common experience. Let us examine the following statements:

1. Research revealed that less than 1% of nurse practitioners and less than 6% of nurse-midwives were sued for malpractice.

2. Multiple research studies with nurse practitioners have shown they are more cost-effective than physicians in delivering primary care

3. Survival rates for codes (cardiac resuscitation) range from 5% to 15%.

All three statements are about a sample population. An inductive argument is made when, based on these findings, an inference is made that these findings are true of a larger population (i.e., the target population). It is in the generalization that you must evaluate whether or not the inference is warranted. As a critical thinker you will learn to evaluate generalizations and not accept them at face value.

When evaluating a generalization, you need to know more about the sample from which it was made. Specifically, you need to know the sample size, the sample breadth (i.e., whether the diversity in the sample supports the conclusions), and whether the sample is representative (if it were randomly drawn). How strong or how weak an inductive argument is depends upon these characteristics of the sample (Browne and Keeley, 1994).

Review the first statement, "Research revealed that less than 1% of nurse practitioners and less than 6% of nurse-midwives were sued for malpractice." Would this statement be stronger if you knew that all nurse practitioners and nurse-midwives in the United States participated in the research study? Or if all nurse practitioners and nurse-midwives in California participated in the study? How would you evaluate the information if you learned that the sample population was derived primarily from nurse practitioners and very few nurse-midwives in one large metropolitan area who volunteered to participate in the study? As you read the statement, evaluate whether or not the generalization about the target population is warranted based on what you know about the sample that was studied.

Review the second statement, "Multiple research studies with nurse practitioners have shown they are more cost-effective than physicians in delivering primary care." What does "multiple research studies" mean? If you knew that it referred to approximately 100 studies over the past 10 years, would you have more confidence in it than if it were based on five studies over the past year? How would you evaluate the information if nurse practitioners in 20 states participated and physicians in 5 states participated? What else would you want to know about those studies? You should know how the nurse practitioners were selected, if the sample were representative (randomly drawn), how the physician population was selected, and the basis upon which the nurse practitioners and physicians were compared.

Review the third statement, "Survival rates for codes (cardiac resuscitation) range from 5% to 15%." You need to know more about the sample before you believe that the survival rates for codes represent an accurate picture of the target population. You must know the sample size of the quoted studies, the sample breadth, and whether the sample items were representative (randomly drawn).

Next, ask how the characteristic of interest, or the variable, was measured. In the first statement, how did the researchers determine the percentages of nurse practitioners and nurse-midwives sued for malpractice? Did they ask the nurses? Did they ask insurance companies who insure the nurses? Did they go through court documents and count the number of cases?

In the second statement, the characteristic of interest is cost-effectiveness. Ask how was cost-effectiveness was defined. How were the data gathered? How did the researchers determine that nurse practitioners were more cost effective than physicians? Were clients interviewed? Was a measurement instrument used? If so, is the instrument reliable and valid?

In the third statement, the characteristic of interest was survival rates. How were the data gathered? Was a chart study done? If so, what years were examined? Was a survey used?

Chapters 6 and 7 discuss reasoning as it applies to the scientific method. These chapters enrich the meaning of the concepts of sample size, sample breadth, and sample representativeness as they apply to nursing research.

### Differentiate between Warranted and Unwarranted Inferences

To differentiate between warranted and unwarranted inferences is to summarize the discussion about the evaluation of deductive and inductive arguments. A good argument is one that establishes the truth of its conclusion. With deductive arguments, the premises must be true and the conclusion must follow validly from the premises. When these standards are met, the conclusion is warranted. When these standards are not met, the conclusion is unwarranted. With inductive arguments, the claim about the truth of the conclusion is based on the degree of support the premises provide for it. The stronger the support, the greater the merit of an inductive argument (Copi and Cohen, 1994).

One final comment about all forms of deductive and inductive arguments: If you find yourself in disagreement with others, do not argue about the conclusion; instead, focus on the premises. Explicate and examine them. It is disagreement about the premises—whether they are true or whether they would, if true, support the conclusion—that often creates disagreement about the conclusion.

## REASONING APPLIED TO PROBLEM SOLVING

Problem solving is a process by which nurses, clients, families, colleagues, and administrators search for a course of action to correct a situation that is unacceptable (Ruggiero, 1991). It is driven by a need to correct something that is a problem; the goal is to solve it. Once the situation is corrected, it no longer generates the time and attention that it once did. Arguments also are used in problem solving.

The most common problem-solving process used in nursing is the nursing process. It involves five phases: (1) assessment (gathering data), (2) diagnosis (stating the problem), (3) solution planning, (4) solution implementing, and (5) solution evaluating. Wilkinson (1992) identified some critical thinking skills that nurses use during each of these phases. For example, during the assessment phases, nurses observe clients and events, distinguish between relevant and irrelevant data, distinguish between important and unimportant data, validate data, organize data, and categorize data. During the diagnosis phase, nurses find patterns and relationships in the data they observe, make inferences, state the problem, and suspend judgment. During the planning phase, nurses generalize based on their past experience and previous knowledge, transfer knowledge from one situation to another, develop evaluative criteria, and hypothesize. During the implementation phase, nurses apply their knowledge and test their hypotheses. During the evaluation phase, nurses decide whether or not the hypotheses are correct and make criterion-based evaluations.

Reflect on your nursing care of one of your more challenging clients. Describe your thinking while you were assessing, diagnosing, planning, implementing, and evaluating the nursing care. What examples of critical thinking can you identify? How do your examples fit with those Wilkinson identifies?

## REASONING APPLIED TO CONTROVERSIAL ISSUES

An examination of controversial issues is different from problem solving. Controversial issues are matters about which intelligent, informed people disagree even after careful, reasoned effort. To resolve a controversial issue means to decide what belief or viewpoint is the most reasonable (Ruggiero, 1991). Argument is also used in the discussion and resolution of controversial issues. Many controversial issues confront us daily, such as health care reform, capital punishment, AIDS, gun control, right to die, right to life, educational reform, welfare reform, domestic violence, and the federal budget. Using the knowledge in this text, you can think through these issues and arrive at your own conclusions without being unduly influenced by how others view them.

When you engage in a dialogue, ask yourself what the speaker wants you to do or believe. When you address an issue, seek the most reasonable belief to embrace. When you address a problem, search for the best action to take (Ruggiero, 1991). How do you construct an argument so that it is sound and persuasive? How do you evaluate the arguments of others? As a critical thinker, you should consider issues carefully before you take a position. When you do take a position, you should state why you believe as you do. You should support your position with reasons and evidence.

The three components to analyze in controversial issues are: (1) a statement of the issue, (2) the conclusion, and (3) the reasons given in support of the conclusion. When you analyze an issue, identify the issue and the conclusion, and evaluate the reasons given in support of the conclusion. However, for the purpose of discussing these components in this chapter, they are presented in this order: issues, reasons, and conclusions.

## Issues

When thinking critically about controversial issues, you must focus the discussion. The Critical Thinking Skills Applied to Nursing: Focus box below lists four skills that are important to focusing a discussion.

***Distinguish between the Central Issue or Problem and the Peripheral Issues or Problems.*** Your first task is to distinguish between issues and problems. Issues are stated as questions and begin with the words *is, does,* or *should.* Problem statements typically begin with the word *how.* Issue questions are about which beliefs to embrace; problem statements are about which action to take. Issue questions should capture the central element of an issue (Ruggiero, 1991). Examine these issue questions about health care:

▼ Is health care a right or privilege?
▼ Do taxpayers have sufficient say in determining Medicare benefits?

---

**Critical Thinking Skills Applied to Nursing: Focus**

▼ Distinguish between the central issue or problem and the peripheral issues or problems
▼ Clarify the central issue or problem
▼ State the central issue or problem

---

▼ Should all citizens have a right to organ transplants regardless of their chosen lifestyles?

▼ Is universal health care coverage a critical aspect of health care reform?

▼ Does the insurance industry have a right to determine who will and will not be insured?

▼ Should we have a national system for rationing health care?

Problem statements, by contrast, change the focus of the discussion from what is believed to how the problem can be solved. Consider how the meaning changes if these same issue questions begin with the word *how.*

▼ How can we make health care a right for all?

▼ How can taxpayers have sufficient say in determining medicare benefits?

▼ How should we determine who will receive an organ transplant?

▼ How can universal health care coverage be implemented?

▼ How can we ensure that the insurance industry does not determine who will and will not be insured?

▼ How can we develop a national system for rationing health care?

Expressing a statement in the "how" form changes the meaning entirely. What was once an issue question becomes a problem statement. With problem statements, the focus is on finding a workable solution. With issue questions, the focus is on deciding what to believe. Problem statements direct us to find a mutually evolved solution. Issue questions create a dividing line, moving us to choose a side to take.

***Clarify the Central Issue or Problem.*** To clarify the central issue in any discussion about controversial issues is important. By nature controversial issues have multiple aspects. By agreeing ahead of time on the issue, you can focus the discussion and present your views.

When you clarify the central issue or problem, you help all participants involved in the discussion focus on the same issue or problem. Many times participants discuss different aspects of a particular issue or problem without realizing they are not focused on the same aspect or problem. Consider, for example, the multiple issues that surround third-party reimbursement for registered nurses:

▼ Should registered nurses be included as qualified providers in health insurance plans?

▼ Should third-party reimbursement be limited to advanced practice nurses?

▼ Should the definition of advanced nursing practice include all nurses? nurse practitioners? clinical nurse specialists? nurse-midwives? nurse anesthetists? all nurses with 5 or more years of experience?

▼ Should all registered nurses in independent practice be reimbursed regardless of their label (e.g., nurse practitioner or clinical nurse specialists)?

▼ Should all registered nurses be considered independent contractors?

Before you engage in a lively discussion about third-party reimbursement for registered nurses, be sure you have identified which aspect of this issue you will focus on.

Sometimes the central issue is not stated obviously, and you must ferret it out from what is said or read. Read the following editorial, (Stewart, 1993, adapted with permission):

> All hospital staff nurses worry about codes (resuscitation). When an arrest is discovered, staff nurses are trained to call codes, do basic CPR, and perform a few other peripheral tasks, but they rely on critical care nurses to provide the definitive treatment. Unfortunately critical care nurses usually arrive too late. Survival rates range from 5–15%. One factor in this procedure could be controlled and that is the time delay between discovery of the arrest and its definitive treatment. This delay could be reduced if staff nurses were taught to provide definitive treatment. Training large numbers of nurses as ACLS providers is not feasible because the scope of ACLS courses is simply too great; however, staff nurses could be taught to use defibrillators. The majority of lives saved, both in and out of hospitals, results from the simple act of giving a shock to a heart in ventricular fibrillation. After all, if emergency services personnel serving a community use trained first responders to defibrillate before ACLS trained paramedics arrive, why shouldn't nurses be taught to use them in the hospital? Defibrillators are found on most units today. Furthermore, American Heart Association ACLS guidelines state that all personnel who are required to perform basic CPR should also know how to use defibrillators. Checking the carotid pulse is the main assessment skill required. The skills required in using a defibrillator are less complex than those for basic CPR. The staff nurse does not need a general knowledge of dysrhythmia analysis, rather just the ability to distinguish between ventricular fibrillation and organized rhythms on a cardiac monitor. The option of using automated external defibrillators, which make the distinction automatically, is also available. Also, there have been no documented cases of death or disability to a client or caregiver attributed to improper defibrillation. To save lives, it follows that staff nurses should be taught to defibrillate.

What is the central issue in this passage? What are peripheral issues? The central issue is, "Should nurses be taught to defibrillate?" Some peripheral issues include the following:

▼ Should hospital code procedures be revised?
▼ Should all nurses be ACLS certified?
▼ Is the delay in definitive treatment the only controllable factor?

**State the Central Issue or Problem.**   State the issue, both verbally and in writing. Writing down the statement helps you clarify the issue. When you write, you externalize the issue, further examine it, and clarify and refine your wording. Many times people think they are discussing the same issue when they are actually taking turns expressing views on different aspects of a related issue.

## Reasons

The next component of a controversial issue to develop and analyze is the reasons given in support of the conclusion. This requires you to examine your thoughts carefully. What are your reasons for believing as you do? What evidence do you have

**Critical Thinking Skills Applied to Nursing: Reasoning**

▼  Evaluate deductive and inductive arguments
▼  Differentiate between warranted and unwarranted inferences
▼  Distinguish among issues, reasons, and conclusions
▼  Evaluate pertinence of the reasons
▼  Assess for errors in reasoning

to support your reasons? The Critical Thinking Skills Applied to Nursing: Reasoning box above lists the critical thinking skills associated with reasoning.

**Distinguish among Issues, Reasons, and Conclusions.**   As you listen or read, certain words will help you distinguish between reasons and conclusions. Cue words that identify reasons are (Browne and Keeley, 1994; Chaffee, 1994; Engel, 1994):

| | |
|---|---|
| since | in view of |
| for | first, second |
| because | in the first (second) place |
| as shown by | may be inferred from |
| as indicated by | may be deduced from |
| given that | may be derived from |
| assuming that | for the reason that |
| for one thing | is supported by |
| for example | inasmuch as |
| also | on the grounds that |

The conclusion is usually found at the beginning or the end of a written essay, but sometimes it may be obscure. For clarity, some writers may put it at both the beginning and the ending. Certain cue words indicate a conclusion will follow; however, they are not always present (Chaffee, 1994; Engel, 1994; Missimer, 1990). Some cue words are:

| | |
|---|---|
| therefore | consequently |
| thus | it follows that |
| hence | thereby showing |
| so | demonstrates that |
| then | we may infer that |
| which shows that | we may conclude that |
| which proves that | you see that |
| implies that | leads me to believe that |
| as a result | allows us to deduce that |

Although cue words help to identify reasons and conclusions, they do not automatically signal the presence of an argument. An argument is comprised of a conclusion supported by one or more reasons.

Let us look at an example that integrates what has been discussed to this point. Read the following paragraph and identify the issue, reasons, and conclusion.

> The delivery of health care is one of the most important issues facing the United States and certainly is a very important one for the nursing profession. For one thing, nurses are highly skilled professionals with strong educational preparation and experiential backgrounds. Also, the nurse is the only health care professional who enjoys the highest level of confidence and credibility with the public. Multiple research studies with nurse practitioners have shown they are more cost effective than physicians in delivering primary care. It follows then, that nurses should have a greater role in the delivery of primary health care.

The first step in analyzing a controversial issue is to identify the conclusion. What is the main point? What does the writer want you to believe or accept? What cue words identify the conclusion? Once you have identified the conclusion, then identify the reasons given in support of the conclusion. What cue words identified the reasons?

Dissect the written passage. Underline the conclusion and place the letter *C* by it. Put parentheses around each reason and identify each as "R1," "R2," etc. When you are finished, your paragraph should look like this:

> The delivery of health care is one of the most important issues facing the United States and certainly is a very important one for the nursing profession. For one thing, (nurses are highly skilled professionals with strong educational preparation and experiential backgrounds).[R1] Also, (the nurse is the only health care professional who enjoys the highest level of confidence and credibility with the public).[R2] (Multiple research studies with nurse practitioners have shown they are more cost effective than physicians in delivering primary care).[R3] It follows then, that <u>nurses should have a greater role in the delivery of primary health care.</u>[C]

Now, go back and review the paragraph discussing staff nurses and defibrillation. Dissect the written passage as shown above. What is the writer's conclusion? What are the reasons? List all of them. Compare your list with your classmates. Are they the same?

***Evaluate Pertinence of the Reasons.***     Pertinence means having some connection with the matter at hand (Neufeldt, 1991). To evaluate the pertinence of the reasons, ask if the reasons are pertinent to the conclusion.

Let us enrich an earlier example. Residents in a low-income neighborhood want a health clinic because they have many medical emergencies during the night. They also believe the clinic would show that the city council cares about them as much as it does the high-income neighborhoods.

What do you think about these reasons? On the surface, they may appear sensible. Think about them again. Review the first reason, *the neighborhood has many medical emergencies during the night*. What kinds of health problems constitute "medical emergencies" in this neighborhood? Neighborhood health clinics are usually health maintenance and health promotion facilities and do not routinely treat medical emergencies. Most large communities have established regional centers where medical emergencies are best handled.

Review the second reason, *to show the neighborhood residents the city council cares about them.* Establishing a neighborhood health clinic is an expensive, complex way to show the residents that the city council cares about them. If the goal is to show caring to the residents, there are other effective, less costly ways to achieve this. What other reasons can you think of that would be more pertinent to the conclusion?

**Assess for Errors in Reasoning.**    Arguments may be evaluated using one of two approaches: the criterial approach and the fallacies approach. Chapter 9 discusses both approaches in depth.

## Conclusions

The last component of a controversial issue to analyze is the conclusion. A conclusion is what you want another person to believe or do or what someone else wants you to believe or do. The Critical Thinking Skills Applied to Nursing: Conclusions box below contains the critical thinking skills that are important in arriving at a conclusion.

**Support Conclusions and Beliefs with Relevant Reasons.**    Evaluating the relevance of the reasons was discussed under the previous section entitled "Reasons." It is reinforced here because of its importance in arriving at conclusions that are sound and supported by strong evidence. We draw your attention to beliefs because we do not always examine them in a logical, rational way. As children we acquired some beliefs that we have probably not put through the rigorous process of logical examination.

Beliefs are statements we accept as true such as creeds, doctrines, or tenets. They are statements in which we trust and have confidence although absolute certainty may be absent (Neufeldt, 1991). Because we believe something is true does not mean it is necessarily true. We may have many beliefs that are not true; we are just unaware of them. To arrive at a conclusion based on untrue beliefs is an error in reasoning (Kelley, 1994).

Our beliefs may unwittingly interfere with our reasoning process; that is, we may abandon the rules of good reasoning in favor of our personal beliefs. For example, college students were asked if the following syllogism was valid:

**Premise:**      All things that are smoked are good for the health.
**Premise:**      Cigarettes are smoked.
**Conclusion:**   Therefore, cigarettes are good for the health.

## Critical Thinking Skills Applied to Nursing: Conclusions

▼  Support conclusions and beliefs with relevant reasons
▼  Evaluate deductive and inductive arguments
▼  Evaluate the strength of the evidence supporting conclusions and beliefs

What is your answer? The argument is valid because the conclusion follows logically from the premises. The major premise, however, is not true. Many students stated that it was not valid because they disagreed with the major premise. When nonsense words like *ramadians* were substituted for *cigarettes,* the errors in logic were markedly reduced. This phenomenon is known as the belief bias effect. What the students believed about the harmful effects of smoking interfered with their ability to think logically (Markovitz and Nantel, 1989). The belief bias effect allowed the students to ignore evidence that did not fit with what they believed.

Many of our beliefs are so ingrained that they are neither questioned nor examined. When you rapidly move to a conclusion, or automatically rule out a statement or position, or think you already know the answer, you may need to examine your basic beliefs about the issue or problem. You are not likely to do this unless the issue is of concern to you or you are confronted with two opposing positions when you must choose one.

***Evaluate Deductive and Inductive Arguments.***    For deductive arguments to be sound, the conclusions must logically follow from the premises (validity) and the premises must be true. Inductive arguments are evaluated as good or bad, strong or weak, based on the truth and strength of the premises supporting the conclusion. The greater the support, the greater the merit of the argument. The evaluation of deductive and inductive arguments is reinforced here because of its importance in reasoning. Such evaluation will help you clarify your thinking and make better choices about what to believe or do.

***Evaluate the Strength of the Evidence Supporting Conclusions and Beliefs.***    To evaluate the strength of the evidence supporting your conclusions and beliefs, review this chapter and the previous chapters on evaluating quantitative, qualitative, and other evidence. The greater the strength of the evidence to support your conclusions and beliefs, the stronger the argument.

You should examine your beliefs as carefully as you examine evidence. For example, many high-rise hotels skip thirteen as a floor number because some people persist in believing it to be an unlucky number. Some believe that ingesting shark cartilage is preferable to surgery in the treatment of some types of cancer. Some believe in the efficacy of therapeutic touch to relieve congestion in the energy field and to promote healing. The evidence supporting your conclusions and beliefs should undergo careful examination; you should have good reasons for your conclusions and beliefs.

When you communicate about a claim of support, you should be accurate in your choice of words. For example, if a claim enjoys the support of research-based evidence, then you may make statements such as, "Jones' study showed . . ." and "the latest issue of *Nursing Research* has an article about . . ." If the claim enjoys the status of theory, you may say, "Rogers theorizes that . . ." and "Levine proposed a theory of nursing that . . ." If the claim is something you assume to be common knowledge, you may say, "It is my understanding that . . ." And if the claim is something you believe but have no evidence for, you may say, "It is my belief that . . ."

**Critical Thinking Skills Applied to Nursing: Implications**

▼ Identify implications of conclusions and beliefs
▼ Evaluate desirability of the implications
▼ Anticipate consequences

## IMPLICATIONS

Other aspects of reasoning are important to analyze. The Critical Thinking Skills Applied to Nursing: Implications box above lists the critical thinking skills associated with anticipating implications and consequences.

### Identify Implications of Conclusions and Beliefs

Implications are the consequences that result when an issue is resolved, a problem is solved, and an action is taken. Implications extend beyond what is immediately apparent. All of our beliefs and actions have implications, some of which are more significant than others. To anticipate consequences, reflect on the implications of a decision and begin by identifying all the alternative possibilities you see (Hughes, 1992). You might want to ask trusted colleagues what they see. It also might help to list them, leaving room to add the consequences that may occur with each alternative. Earlier in the text this was referred to as consequential thinking.

The following passage discusses the implications of the present fee-for-service basis of the health delivery system (Moccia, 1988, used with permission).

Organization of the health care system on a fee-for-service basis has implications for nursing and for nursing education. The procession of educated men has led us to a profit-driven biomedical enterprise that now finds itself without the expertise or skills necessary to meet the health care needs of a population that is increasingly aged, chronically ill, and without access to health services.

There are several significant problems with this approach to structuring health care. First, sicker patients will continue to suffer, since it is more profitable to the provider to serve healthier patients who need less service. Second, the more than 40 million Americans who have no insurance simply will get no care. Third, a profit-driven fee-for-service system is unable to exert sufficient control over costs, because as long as providers control the number of services in order to increase their profits, the aggregate costs to the payers in the health care system will continue to be difficult to control. Finally, and perhaps most profoundly, the process of determining and attaching a fee for service necessarily distorts the humanity of both providers and patients. When the health care system attempts to isolate services and fees, people's complex health needs are separated into discrete units, by design. This separation, which is necessitated by the fee-for-service approach, is untrue to the reality of the patient's experience. In addition, since life and death are subject to the same market conditions that any commodity is, people are reduced to object status, and interpersonal relations become avenues of commerce. As a result, the isolation and dehumanization of the larger society are reinforced and sustained by the health care system.

Consequently, though fee-for-service is seemingly a financial and economic issue, the choice between it and some other form of reimbursement is actually a choice to reinforce and legitimize one understanding of human phenomena rather than another and to adopt one philosophy of interpersonal relations rather than another (pp. 57-58).

State the issue to which Moccia is responding. What is her position? What does Moccia believe has been the impact of the fee-for-service system in the United States? Do you agree with the implications she has identified? Why or why not? Do you see implications that she does not mention?

## Evaluate Desirability of the Implications

To evaluate the desirability of the implications, add the consequences of each alternative to your list of alternatives as shown in Fig. 8-2. Examine each alternative. What would happen with each course of action? Because you may not be able to identify all of the consequences, you should discuss the situation with trusted colleagues. After studying each alternative, ask which alternative best achieves the goal. Which produces the most desirable and undesirable results? What are the long-term consequences? What are the indirect consequences? What effect will this have on other

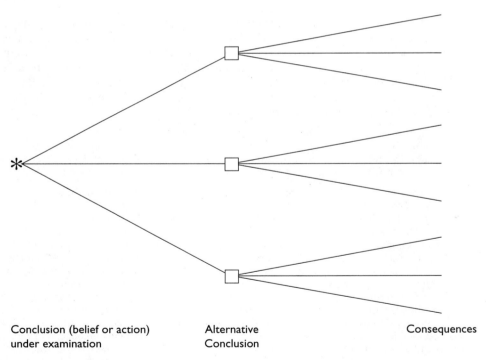

Conclusion (belief or action)          Alternative          Consequences
under examination                      Conclusion

**Fig. 8-2**  Decision/Implications Tree.

people? What would the world (i.e., home, my life, work, community) look like with each alternative? Be consistent when you identify the consequences of each alternative. For example, if cost is a consequence, then specify cost for each alternative. Other consequences may be time and energy.

Implications can be subtle and very important. Consider the impact on viewers about how nurses are portrayed in a television sitcom. How nurses are portrayed provides the context, or backdrop, for the main plot. It sends one message if nurses are portrayed as independent professionals on the health care team and another if nurses are portrayed as handmaidens to physicians.

Review the passage by Moccia. What would the health delivery system look like if the United States did not have a fee-for-service structure? What do you think would happen if the payment structure would change? Compare your view of what would happen with others in your class.

### Anticipate Consequences

Based on your answers to the desirability of each alternative, you are now ready to select the one with the most preferred consequences. Once you arrive at a conclusion, you must then deal with both anticipated and unanticipated consequences as they arise. Consequential thinking is very important whenever the results of deliberations will be followed by any kind of action.

Consider a woman in group therapy who was confronted about her negative attitude toward her employer. When quizzed, she admitted she had steady work, good benefits, and good hours. As treatment progressed, she realized that she received positive reinforcement from certain individuals for grousing about her employer. When she started speaking more favorably about her employer, she experienced unexpected and unanticipated consequences: they started turning on her. Eventually she quit associating with these individuals and made new friends.

## CONSTRUCTING ARGUMENTS

Now it is time to construct an argument of your choosing. How will you go about it? The following format will help you through this process.

### Focus the Issue

Begin with an issue about which you are concerned. For example, what bothers you most about nursing? The delivery of nursing care in hospitals? In homes? The nature of collaborative relationships among nurses as colleagues? Between nurses and other health care provider colleagues? The nature of a specific nursing role, such as advocate, care giver, or teacher? The care of children? The elderly? The nature of a specific nursing intervention, such as therapeutic communication, medication administration, or client education? Write it down, think it through, and refine your statement. Have others critique it. What do others think you mean?

▼ Distinguish the central issue from peripheral issues
▼ Clarify the central issue
▼ State the central issue

## State the Reasons

State your conclusion before you begin to address the points associated with reasons. What is your position on the issue?

▼ List your reasons
▼ Evaluate relevance of your reasons
▼ Use sound deductive reasoning and inductive reasoning based on strong evidence
▼ Make warranted inferences
▼ Assess for errors in reasoning

Write down your reasons. Putting them on paper helps clarify and objectify your thinking process. If you are having a hard time expressing your reasons, you may have not fully formulated them; that is, you know what your position is but you do not know why. To identify and clarify your reasons can be a difficult task. Critical thinking is hard work. You may think you know why, but when it comes to expressing your reasons you may consider them silly or trite. If you evaluate your reasons this way, you must learn to get beyond that notion and realize that your voice is as important as that of others. It will take repeated effort and practice, but it will come.

Once you have identified your reasons, think about how you will present them—how you will build your case so that you will persuade listeners to believe (or accept) your position. Present your reasons in a persuasive sequence. Decide which reason should be presented first, second, and so forth. Similar reasons should be grouped together so that your listeners will have an easier time following your line of reasoning. The sequence you choose, however, may vary depending upon whom you are trying to persuade. You may want to present your most persuasive reason first or save it for the last. It is your choice.

Once you determine the order in which you will present your reasons, be sure you fully develop each reason before you move on to develop the next one. If you identify something as a reason, do not brush it off lightly with a mere mention. Discuss the reason in sufficient depth so that others will understand it. Look at your list of reasons and ask if you have omitted any really important ones. Ask a colleague for help.

When you have completed this phase, take the opposite position on the issue. What objection(s) might others have? If you cannot see them, give your paper to someone else and ask that person to play the devil's advocate. To be persuasive, you should anticipate the objections your listeners may have and prepare a response to each one. This process helps you get outside your own frame of reference and examine the issue from another person's perspective.

### State a Conclusion

Does your conclusion make sense in light of your reasons? Is your reasoning deductive or inductive? Complete the following:

▼ Support your conclusions and beliefs with relevant reasons.
▼ Evaluate the soundness of deductive arguments.
▼ Evaluate the strength of the evidence supporting your conclusions and beliefs.

Many times the conclusion is given at the outset of an essay or oral presentation; either way is acceptable. Just be sure that the listeners know where you stand and why.

Appendix D, Guidelines for Writing an Issue Paper, summarizes the important points made in this section and will guide you if you choose to write an issue paper.

## SUMMARY

Two kinds of reasoning are deductive and inductive. Argument is a form of reasoning that has a conclusion supported by one or more premises. Argument may be deductive or inductive. Deductive arguments are evaluated according to the standards of truth and validity. Inductive arguments are evaluated as good or bad, weak or strong, based on the standards of truth and the strength of the evidence the premises provide for the conclusion. The stronger the support, the greater the merit of the argument.

Reasoning is used in deductive and inductive arguments, problem solving, and controversial issues. In controversial issues, three components were analyzed: issue, reasons, and conclusion. With each conclusion (i.e., a belief or an action), implications must be taken into account. Implications, or the consequences of our beliefs and actions, are the end products of thinking. They can be anywhere on a continuum from negligible to profound and from desirable to undesirable.

Critical thinking is hard work. It is more than a popular buzz word. It is an ongoing commitment to self-examination and to the analysis of others' thinking, whether it be in spoken or written form. With continual awareness of one's own thinking and consistent practice, thinking critically can become a way of living that is progressively refined with the passage of time.

# EXERCISES

## Exercise 1

**Purpose:** *Create arguments*

### DIRECTIONS

Construct one argument for each of the following purposes of argument: to decide, predict, and persuade. Create one or more reasons for each. Use the following format:

**Reason:**
**Reason:**
**Conclusion:**

## Exercise 2

**Purpose:** *Distinguish between arguments and nonarguments*

### DIRECTIONS

Review the following statements and determine which ones are arguments and which ones are nonarguments. If you determine that it is an argument, then specify if it is an argument to decide, predict, or persuade. If you determine that it is a nonargument, then create an argument from it.

1. What do you think of the latest plan to reorganize the nursing unit? I think it is just another way to accomplish the same goals, but it does cut back on the numbers of nursing staff needed.

2. Your medication should be taken with your meals. It will cause less gastric irritation.

3. Nurses should be the leaders in the movement to reform health care. They are the largest group of health care providers and can wield tremendous clout if they choose to.

4. The emergency room gets a lot of interesting cases but it surely is stressful. The surgical floor might be a better place to work.

5. If the toddler Zachary does not go to bed early, then he will be fussy the next day.

6. The client is nauseated. It is probably due to the general anesthesia she had earlier.

7. This hospital should develop a library of pamphlets and other information for clients. No such resource is presently available for clients in this community. Many clients ask for information about their health problems.

8. Before you choose a place of employment, examine the employer's philosophy of nursing, evaluate the workplace environment, and interview the nursing staff. You will save time and money in the long run. You will have a greater probability of achieving professional satisfaction and success.

## Exercise 3

**Purpose:** *Analyze categorical propositions*

### DIRECTIONS

Read the following categorical propositions and do the following:

1. Specify the form of the proposition (A, E, I, O)
2. Bracket and label the subject and predicate terms.
3. Circle the term that is distributed and underline the term that is undistributed.

- ▼ All critical care nurses are certified in basic life support.
- ▼ Some medications have untoward side effects.
- ▼ No clients should be in pain.
- ▼ All administrators are educated.
- ▼ Some clients do not have family support systems.
- ▼ No medications are completely safe.
- ▼ Some charts are computerized.
- ▼ Some nurses have baccalaureate degrees.

For example: All [ (critical care nurses) ] are [certified in basic life support.]

                         Subject                          Predicate

A: All *S* is *P*

## Exercise 4

**Purpose:** *Create and evaluate standard form categorical syllogisms*

### DIRECTIONS

Create a standard form categorical syllogism from each categorical proposition in Exercise 3. For example:

All critical care nurses are certified in basic life support.

Sally is a critical care nurse.

Therefore, Sally is certified in basic life support.

## Exercise 5

**Purpose:** *Analyze categorical syllogisms*

### DIRECTIONS

Read the following arguments and determine if the premises are true and the conclusion follows from them; that is, determine if the argument is sound or unsound. Explain why.

**Premise:** All clients undergoing major surgery should have nothing by mouth (NPO) after midnight the night before.

**Premise:** Matt is a client who will undergo major surgery.

**Conclusion:** Therefore, Matt should have nothing by mouth (NPO) after midnight the night before.

**Premise:** All clients whose weight is in the normal range have fewer adverse complications from surgery.

**Premise:** Mildred is underweight and will have surgery.

**Conclusion:** Therefore, Mildred should gain weight to avoid adverse complications from surgery.

## Exercise 6

**Purpose:** *Construct and evaluate arguments*

### DIRECTIONS

Read the following statements and create sound, strong arguments using the statement to stimulate your creative thinking. The premises must provide support for the conclusion.

1. Angela got the only A on the last test. She must be a real brain.

   For example: Angela got the only A on the last test. She studies at least 3 hours everyday and has a GPA of 3.78. She applies herself and earns good grades.

2. Did you hear that most of the nurses at Community Hospital voted to become a collective bargaining unit? Linda works there. She is probably a supporter of unions and all that goes with them.

3. Environmentalists do not care about the ordinary person who has to earn a living. They just want to protect the earth regardless of the cost.

4. Mr. Wu has developed a rash all over his left arm. He takes about a dozen different medications. Someone ought to teach him about the side effects of medications.

5. I read that 70% of physicians prefer to prescribe acetaminophen to aspirin for their clients. Acetaminophen must be more effective than aspirin.

6. The doctor was really nice to my client. She must be a very competent surgeon.

7. It looks like the job market for nurses is really tightening up. Jose was out looking for a job and could not find one.

8. Everybody should be required to wear a seat belt. The state patrol officer said George would be alive today had he worn one.

9. That is the fourth time today she has requested a pain medication. She must be addicted.

10. Look at poor little Eric whimper. He has been here for a week. I feel so sorry for him. He is only 5 years old, and his parents have only been in to see him twice. They must not care very much about him.

## Exercise 7

**Purpose:** *Analyze disjunctive propositions*

### DIRECTIONS

Determine if the inclusive or exclusive use of *or* is intended in the following disjunctive propositions. If the use is exclusive, identify those propositions that commit the false dilemma fallacy.

1. Either you or Gerta must admit the new client.

2. The client in cardiac arrest due to ventricular fibrillation must receive either manual cardiopulmonary resuscitation or electroshock treatment.

3. The client in cardiac arrest must be either resuscitated or he will die.

4. The baby is crying because it is either hungry or in pain.

5. The nurse should either fill out the medication error form or call the nursing supervisor and physician.

## Exercise 8

**Purpose:** *Analyze conditional propositions*

### DIRECTIONS

Analyze the following conditional propositions of mixed hypothetical syllogisms. Label the antecedent and the consequent of the proposition. Determine if the structure is valid or invalid. If valid, specify the form: modus ponens or modus tollens. If invalid, specify which fallacy it commits: fallacy of affirming the consequent or fallacy of denying the antecedent. Explain your answers.

1. If the client has AIDS, then the nurse uses universal precautions.
   The client does not have AIDS.
   Therefore, the nurse does not use universal precautions.

2. If the client has gastrointestinal bleeding, then the nurse would look for black, tarry stools.
   The client has gastrointestinal bleeding.
   Therefore, the nurse looks for black, tarry stools.

3. If the nurse is sick, then she cannot go to work.
   The nurse cannot go to work.
   Therefore, the nurse is sick.

4. If the client has an acute asthma attack, then he has dyspnea, wheezing, a hacking cough, and pallor.
   The client does not have dyspnea, wheezing, a hacking cough, and pallor.
   Therefore, he does not have an acute asthma attack.

## Exercise 9

**Purpose:**  *Reason by analogy*

### DIRECTIONS

Read the following statements and construct an argument using an analogy.

1. A 4-year-old child is to undergo tonsillectomy tomorrow morning. Your goal is to prepare him so he will be cooperative.

2. You observe a classmate give an incorrect medication and fail to report it. You find time to talk to your classmate about it to persuade your classmate to report it.

3. Describe your typical workday to your supervisor and make a case for additional professional nursing staff.

## Exercise 10

**Purpose:**  *Distinguish issue statements from problem statements*

### DIRECTIONS

Read the following paragraphs to stimulate your thinking and then create as many issue and problem statements as you can.

1. Nursing students should be allowed to make their own client care assignments. Each student could then select the clients who would provide the best learning experience. After all, who best to know what an individual student needs to learn than the student himself or herself?

2. Clients should have a greater say in their care. They should be able to state a preference for a nurse caretaker and have that request honored. They also should help formulate their own nursing care plan. By doing so, they will better understand their nursing care and medical treatment. They also will be more likely to comply with any health education requirements after they are discharged.

# Exercise 11

**Purpose:** *Identify the issue, reasons, and conclusion*

<u>DIRECTIONS</u>

Identify the issue, reasons, and conclusion of the following passage:

> The harmful effects of cigarette smoking are well known. The federal government spends billions of dollars every year in treating tobacco-related diseases, so it should take a more active role in discouraging consumption. A higher excise tax on tobacco products has many international precedents: Canada and most European countries tax tobacco at rates five to ten times that of the United States. Therefore, taxes should be increased on cigarettes and the money raised should go toward paying health care costs.

# Exercise 12

**Purpose:** *Identify the components of a controversial issue*

<u>DIRECTIONS</u>

Read the following paragraph that summarizes Mallison's (1992) appeal to the president (adapted with permission). Distinguish among the central issue, reasons, and conclusion.

> Health care reform is one of the most important issues facing our nation and the nursing profession. Nurses should be in charge of primary care as they will save money, improve quality and improve access to health care. Three-quarters of adult primary care, up to nine-tenths of pediatric primary care, and at least three-quarters of all prenatal care and delivery of babies could be provided by nurse practitioners and certified nurse-midwives who are much less costly than physicians. Furthermore, nurses focus on prevention and maintenance of wellness. Multiple research studies with nurse practitioners and certified mid-wives have shown they are more cost effective than physicians in delivering primary care. Compared to physicians, nurse practitioners prescribe fewer drugs, use fewer tests and select lower-tech options for clients' care. Nurse-midwives reduce the number of C-sections and reduce the need for costly intensive care for neonates. Nurses provide more education and empower clients to take control of their own health. Finally, less than 1% of nurse practitioners and less than 6% of nurse-midwives are sued for malpractice. This is considerably less than the one-third of all physicians and four-fifths of all obstetricians. It follows then, that nurses should be in charge of primary health care delivery.

## Exercise 13

**Purposes:**    *Distinguish the central issue from the peripheral issues*
*Distinguish the reasons from the conclusions*
*Construct a counterargument*

### DIRECTIONS

Read the following passage. What is the central issue? What are peripheral issues? What are the reasons? What is the conclusion? Do you agree? What are your objections? Construct a counterargument.

> Legalizing marijuana for medicinal reasons would do more harm than good. The number of clients who would benefit from its use are limited to clients undergoing chemotherapy and those who seek relief from nausea, vomiting, and pain. We already have drugs available that are safe and non-addicting that provide relief from these symptoms. Besides, no credible research study has ever shown smoking marijuana to be beneficial. Anecdotal cases reporting benefit do not constitute carefully controlled research that is credible with scientists. Furthermore, the legalization of marijuana would increase public acceptance of it; that would eventually lead to wide-spread use. It does not make sense to add one more addicting drug to those already legalized such as caffeine, nicotine and alcohol.

## Exercise 14

**Purpose:**    *Refine your reasoning skills*

### DIRECTIONS

1. Select an issue that interests you, preferably a nursing issue being debated at the state or national level.

2. Identify your position on the issue.

3. State your reasons in support of your position.

4. Anticipate objections to your reasons and respond to them.

Present your issue to the class. Did your reasons make sense to the listeners? Were your arguments sound? Did you have strong research-based evidence to support your reasons? Did you anticipate your classmates' objections to your position and reasons? What objections did you not anticipate? Why?

# Exercise 15

**Purpose:** *Reflect on your reasoning*

<u>DIRECTIONS</u>

Write in your journal about the following questions:

1. Reasoning critically is a lot of work. Why do it?

2. What were the primary messages in this chapter?

3. Can you think of a place or time when you might have used a thinking structure described in this chapter to your advantage? Describe it. If not, imagine a time and situation when you could use it.

4. Think of a situation in which your ideas were not taken seriously. Why? Redo the transaction and write a dialogue that is more satisfying for you.

# REFERENCES

Bandman, E.L., and Bandman, B. (1995). *Critical thinking in nursing* (2nd ed.). Norwalk, Conn.: Appleton and Lange.

Benson, S. (1991). *Philosophy I I I: Logic, language and persuasion* (class handouts). Denver: Metropolitan State College of Denver.

Browne, M.N., and Keeley, S.M. (1994). *Asking the right questions* (4th ed.). Englewood Cliffs, N.J.: Prentice Hall.

Chaffee, J. (1994). *Thinking critically* (4th ed.). Boston: Houghton Mifflin.

Copi, I.M., and Cohen, C. (1994). *Introduction to logic* (9th ed.). New York: Macmillan.

Engel, S.M. (1994). *With good reason: An introduction to informal fallacies* (5th ed.). New York: St. Martin's Press.

Hughes, W. (1992). *Critical thinking.* Lewiston, N.Y.: Broadview.

Kelley, D. (1994). *The art of reasoning* (2nd expanded edition). New York: W.W. Norton.

Kurfiss, J.G. (1988). *Critical thinking: Theory, research, practice, and possibilities* (ASHE-ERIC Higher Education Report No. 2). Washington, D.C.: Association for the Study of Higher Education.

Mallison, M.B. (1992). Dear Mr. President . . . *American Journal of Nursing, 92*(11), 7.

Markovits, H., and Nantel, G. (1989). The belief-bias effect in the production and evaluation of logical conclusions. *Memory and Cognition, 17,* 11–17.

Missimer, C.A. (1990). *Good arguments: An introduction to critical thinking* (2nd ed.). Englewood Cliffs, N.J.: Prentice Hall.

Moccia, P. (1988). Curriculum revolution: An agenda for change. In National League for Nursing, *Curriculum revolution: Mandate for change* (pp. 53–64). New York: Author.

Neufeldt, V. (1991). *Webster's new world dictionary* (3rd ed.). New York: Webster's New World.

Olds, S., London, M., and Ladewig, P. (1992). *Maternal Newborn Nursing* (4th ed.). Redwood City, Calif.: Addison-Wesley.

Ruggiero, V.R. (1991). *The art of thinking* (3rd ed.). New York: Harper Collins.

Stewart, J.A. (1993). Why not let staff nurses defibrillate? *American Journal of Nursing, 93*(12), 7.

U.S. Senate Special Committee on Aging, the American Association of Retired Persons, the Federal Council on the Aging, and the U.S. Administration on Aging. (1991). *Aging America trends and projections.* Washington, D.C.: Author.

Wilkinson, J.M. (1992). *Nursing process in action: A critical thinking approach.* Redwood City, Calif.: Addison-Wesley Nursing.

# *Evaluating Arguments*

Chapter 9

## OVERVIEW

Chapter 9 discusses how to evaluate both your own and other people's arguments. The chapter begins by focusing on the fundamental skill of listening, because listening allows us to develop understanding and find meaning in our interactions with others. The chapter introduces two approaches to the evaluation of arguments: criterial and fallacies. The criterial approach refers to the standards for assessing arguments; the fallacies approach refers to a search for errors in the content of reasoning. The chapter offers guidelines for using the criterial approach and detecting some common fallacies in reasoning.

## THE IMPORTANCE OF LISTENING

To evaluate arguments you must be able to grasp the meaning that the sender wishes to convey. Communication theory has much to offer us in pursuit of accurate listening. Communication is the exchange of thoughts, messages, and the like through speech, signals, or writing (Neufeldt, 1991). This chapter focuses on spoken communication.

Communication is dynamic and cyclical. It is a living and open system. The sender has a purpose and provides input. Communication is a process during which a message is encoded, sent, and decoded. The system has an output: the message that the receiver decodes. Feedback is provided by the receiver who feeds back to the sender another message, based on the message she or he received (Fig. 9-1). The cycle repeats until either member of the communication system leaves the field.

### The Process

Communication is a complicated process with numerous steps. Consider both sides of the paradigm: the sender and the receiver. An important aspect of communicating is hearing the position of your communication partner.

The sender gathers his or her thoughts together. These thoughts are colored by the sender's physical, psychosocial, cultural, and spiritual health, as well as everything else that he or she has learned. The sender's communication methods also are influenced by lifetime experiences with communicating, experience with previous

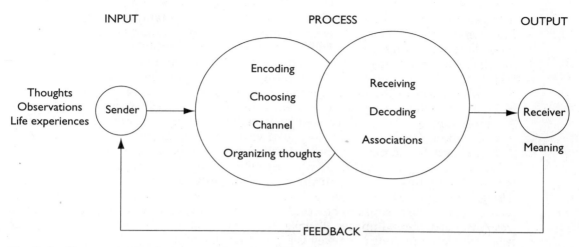

**Fig. 9-1** Communication is two way, dynamic, and cyclical.

attempts to communicate, his or her purpose for communicating, and the message he or she wishes to convey.

The sender encodes thoughts into utterances or makes notes on paper. The sender then sends the message through some channel to the receiver. The channel may be auditory (sound waves), visual (pictures, words, sketches), kinesthetic (bodily contact, braille, a sculpture), or some combination of the above such as in a television show, a motion picture, a speech, a recorded speech, a book, a letter, or a telephone conversation. Other options include a person-to-person encounter or an encounter aided by a microphone and other audiovisual aids, such as an overhead projector and slides.

During the communication transaction, an atmosphere exists through which the message is conveyed. This atmosphere is both physical and psychological. If a telephone or microphone is used, the quality of electronic equipment will affect the clarity of the message (a physical variable). The familiarity of the speaker with the equipment will affect the speaker's psychological condition. The speaker's attitude toward the listener also will affect the speaker's ability to speak effectively. For example, if the speaker expects to be ridiculed or have his or her message rebuffed, he or she may speak differently. If the speaker expects the message to be received warmly and openly, he or she may speak differently. If anxious or relaxed, the speaker may act differently. Listeners are more likely to comprehend the message if the speaker organizes his or her ideas into an intelligible arrangement. Chapter 10 provides more information on effective presentation.

## Meaning

The meaning of words to both the sender and the receiver is so important that it has been mentioned throughout the text. But the word *meaning* itself is ambiguous.

Often we are concerned with the literal interpretation of a word, i.e., just the information conveyed about what the word symbolizes. Cultural differences can change the literal meaning of words even among people who assume that they speak the same language. In the United States "Let us *table* that motion" means "Let us take it off the table, or put it aside from discussion at this time." In England, the same phrase means "Let us put it on the table, or bring it up for discussion" (Satir, 1967, p. 64).

In addition to the literal interpretations, words evoke connotations. Connotations are the affective associations, ideas, and life experiences associated with a word. Connotations can be either positive or negative. They are meant to create an emotional response in others by calling up a visual image (Wassman and Rinsky, 1993). When a mother told her neighbor that her daughter intended to shop at a local thrift store, the neighbor thought she was just being cheap, whereas the mother thought she was being frugal. Reflect on the mental images that occur with the words *thrift, cheap,* and *frugal.* The literal meanings of the three words are similar (i.e., not to be wasteful and to live simply); however, each word brings to mind different emotional responses and mental images. To take for granted that the receiver gets the message that the sender intends to convey is a very risky assumption.

Metacommunication is the communication process during which we communicate on the nature of the communication itself. This process may be conscious, unconscious, spoken, or unspoken. In the conversation between the mother and neighbor, the neighbor is assuming that the daughter has the financial means to shop elsewhere. Example of other more conscious metacommunication comments include: "I wonder if we both mean the same thing by the same word." "Wait a minute. You are responding in a different way than what I was suggesting. Let us start over."

## Listening

What occurs when you are receiving in the listener role? Your ability to receive the message depends on many things, including your attitude toward a speaker. You are more likely to have a positive attitude toward a speaker who is fluent and in command of the subject matter, and who has done his or her homework in preparing a well thought out and easy to follow line of reasoning. When you like the speaker and when the speaker or the subject is important to you, you can listen easily. When the speaker presents an idea that fits your frame of reference and when the message makes sense to you, you also are more likely to listen. It is easy to hear what you expect and want to hear (Babcock and Miller, 1994).

When the above conditions are absent, you may have difficulty hearing the message, especially if the speaker is a person whom you dislike or do not respect. To hear a message with which you disagree also presents problems. Your first response may be to disagree with the message before you finish listening to the person's utterances.

You may disagree with the statement aloud (e.g., a shouting match in which neither you nor the other person listen), or you may continue to look at the other person (who thinks you are still listening) while quietly planning your counterattack. In such a circumstance you actually have lost out on the rest of the other person's message, and the other person is not even aware that communication ceased some time ago.

Listening is a challenge and essential in dialogue. It consists of attitudes, mental discipline, and skills. Openness and a willingness to consider other points of view must be accompanied by a desire to understand another's point of view and the genuine humility to assume that you might learn something from this person—however simple the lesson might be.

## Establishing the Goal

Establishing your goal is important. It will help you listen better and focus on what you need to find out from the other person. As a listener you need to consider why you are engaged in this encounter. Do you feel obliged to listen because this person has power over you? Does this person have information you want? Are you interested in proving this person wrong? Are you interested in persuading this person to do something different? Do you wish to convince this person that you are right? Are you interested in searching for the truth, or coming closer to the truth, with this person?

You might listen to the nurse manager and the doctor because they have the power to affect your job. You may listen to the nursing assistant who has information you want. You may want to prove to an administrator that there is a better way to do something within the institution. You may want to convince the client that she should submit to a procedure or eat differently. You may want to listen to a client to investigate his knowledge of asepsis. You may want to get this client to listen to you and change the way he is doing a procedure. You may want to work out with a client a pattern of care and rehabilitation that fits in with his health beliefs and that you believe will accomplish the main goals as you see them.

Accurate listening is an important step in communication. You are most likely to select the strategy that will best help you reach your goal when you have heard the other person's complete message. To get into the proper mind-set, do something to relax yourself and to make yourself properly receptive. You can give yourself a pep talk, saying "I am more apt to respond wisely if I comprehend the other person's point of view. We both want the same goal: recovery, a cost-effective and high quality product."

After you have gotten yourself into a receptive set of mind, present a relaxed, open, and alert acceptance with your body language. Listen as carefully as you can; pay attention to the words *and* the thoughts that you believe the sender is attempting to convey. Notice any gaps in the sender's presentation. Note what is clear to you and what is fuzzy.

## Feedback

The next communication step is to give feedback. The purpose of feedback at this point in the dialogue is to indicate to the sender that you understand the message. To clarify the message as the sender intended to convey it and as you received it, you may paraphrase the message and ask further questions. You may summarize in your own words what you heard the sender say, and add "Is that right?" "Did I get your point?"

This will give the sender an opportunity to pick up any misperceptions or connotations that may have crept into your transaction. The sender then has a chance to clarify the message before you both proceed. At this point the sender may indicate that you did indeed get the point, or correct your misunderstanding.

Another way is to ask for additional information that invites the sender to elaborate on what he or she said. Your intention thus conveys the metacommunication that you heard the sender and that you really want to understand his or her position more thoroughly. Depending on the sender's perception, your quizzing may feel like deep interest, confrontation, or interrogation.

Your line of questioning should be designed to detect the assumptions on which the sender is basing his or her argument. This is a crucial effort. This is, in fact, the heart of the issue in argument. You must establish the sender's and your own assumptions to find out if you share any common ground. Until you find some common ground, your efforts to proceed further are unlikely to be fruitful.

Questioning helps clarify the meaning between the sender and you the receiver. As the receiver, you might ask the following:

"What do you mean when you say that we are overstaffed?"
"What is the client doing that makes him look worse to you?"
"Do you mean *all* administrators, or just the ones you have met?"
"What have I done that is not acceptable? What in particular?"
"Do you mean that by making the 'right' decision we will decide to do it your way?"

If the sender is a good communicator, she or he at this point will try to clarify with statements such as:

"Let me restate that."
"His color is poor. He looks gray. He is gasping for breath."
"I will give some examples to clarify my position."
"I may be giving my opinion. It looks so clear to me. You may not share my view. How do you see it?"

Both the sender and the receiver are responsible for ensuring the message is clear before proceeding to the next step. After you have clarified the message that the sender intended to convey, you are ready to examine carefully the sender's argument and your evaluation of the sender's remarks.

When you are ready to respond, keep in mind that the sender will have an easier time understanding you if you use metaphors that are intelligible to him or her. The sender also will find it easier to listen if you emphasize your common ground. Stressing the benefits to the other person of following your line of reasoning also will make your message more palatable.

## EVALUATING ARGUMENTS

As you listen to the reasons and the evidence given in support of a position or conclusion, you will need some criteria by which to evaluate them. Philosophers have developed two approaches to the evaluation of argument, criterial and fallacies. The criterial approach is a new approach whereby an argument is measured against criteria (standards) for a good argument. If an argument meets the criteria, it is considered a good argument; if it does not, it is considered a bad argument. The fallacies approach is the traditional approach whereby an argument is examined to determine if any errors (fallacies) in reasoning have been made that detract from its soundness. A good argument has no fallacies, whereas fallacious arguments are bad. The criterial approach is positive because it establishes the criteria for a good argument. In contrast, the fallacies approach is negative because it focuses on detecting errors in reasoning (Hughes, 1992). This chapter discusses both approaches, beginning with the criterial approach.

## EVALUATING ARGUMENTS: CRITERIAL APPROACH

The Criterial Approach to Argument Evaluation box below lists the elements of the criterial approach to argument evaluation. Recall that in the previous chapter we discussed how to evaluate deductive and inductive arguments. We now expand on that discussion about the evaluation of arguments by providing additional criteria.

### Premises Must Be Acceptable

Recall from previous information that true premises are essential for a sound argument. If a premise is false, even if the argument is logically valid, the argument is unsound. What if a premise is probably true, but you are not absolutely certain it is true? What if there is no feasible way to determine if the premise is certainly true? To encompass these situations, Hughes (1992) expands the scope of sound arguments to include premises that are acceptable as well as certainly true. Hughes notes that many times we do not know with absolute certainty if a premise is true; good reasons may exist to accept a premise, although we do not know for sure if it is true.

For example, we know that there is compelling evidence that establishes a causal link between cigarette smoking and lung cancer, although we cannot prove this link with certainty. The present evidence is based on causal-comparative research (ex post facto research) that explores the causal relationship among variables that cannot be manipulated experimentally. The purpose of this method is to discover possible

 **Criterial Approach to Argument Evaluation**

- ▼ Premises must be acceptable
- ▼ Premises must be adequate
- ▼ Reference to authorities must be appropriate
- ▼ Sources of information must be credible
- ▼ Missing information must be weighed
- ▼ Personal experience must be cited appropriately
- ▼ Self-interest needs must be weighed

causes by comparing subjects in whom a pattern is present with subjects in whom a pattern is absent or present to a lesser degree. The causes are studied after they have presumably exerted their effect. Thus, two populations are studied that are comparable in all respects except for the critical variable: one group smokes cigarettes and the other does not. Using accepted statistical procedures, the significance of the findings can be determined with a high degree of accuracy. This research method tells us if a relationship exists between two variables, but we cannot infer that one causes the other (Borg and Gall, 1989).

To generate stronger evidence that cigarette smoking causes lung cancer would require a large scale, experimental study with two groups, one that receives the experimental treatment and one that serves as a control. The experimental group would have to receive consistent exposure to cigarette smoking over an extended period of time after which statistical procedures would be conducted to determine the significance of the findings. Such a study is offensive to contemplate and would violate the codes of ethics and human rights guidelines of professional researchers. Thus, it is justifiable to accept the present evidence that establishes a causal link between cigarette smoking and lung cancer. Therefore, when using this standard to evaluate the premises, ask if you are justified in accepting them.

## Premises Must Be Adequate

To meet the criterion of adequacy, examine the degree of strength the premises provide for the conclusion, and make a judgment about it (Hughes, 1992). The critical question to ask is: Do the premises provide sufficient support for the conclusion? The premises may provide no, very little, some, quite a lot, or a great deal of support for the conclusion. The argument violates this criterion if it provides no support. It also violates the criterion if it provides some, but not enough, support to justify accepting the conclusion. Recall that for deductive arguments, the issue is whether the argument is valid or invalid. In these arguments, the structure determines if the premises provide full support or none at all. In inductive arguments, however, the support comes in degrees. In either case, we must judge whether the premises are adequate in the sense that, if they are true, they show that the conclusion is at least *likely* to be true.

You may ask questions to determine if the premises are adequate. Where did the evidence come from? How was it compiled? Is the evidence biased? Is there another way to interpret the evidence? Is the evidence from an empirical study? If a generalization is made from an empirical study, is the generalization from the sample to the target population appropriate? If a generalization is made from an empirical study, are the size, breadth, and representativeness of the study population appropriate and adequate? What is the meaning of the statistical findings? See Chapters 6 and 7 for a more thorough discussion of evidence.

When we rely on premises that are weak or inadequate to support a conclusion, we call it "jumping to conclusions" or reaching a "hasty conclusion." An argument is more likely to violate the criterion of adequacy if it claims to prove its conclusion; it is less likely to violate the criterion if it is stated tentatively.

## Reference to Authorities Must Be Appropriate

To hear someone refer to an authority figure as evidence of support for an argument is common. By doing so, the speaker brings the weight of an expert to bolster her or his position. Examples of authority figures are a parent, a judge, a nurse, a leader, and a health care administrator.

When a reference to authority is made, note who the expert is, if she or he is recognized as a expert by others, and the background that qualifies the person to be an authority on that particular subject. Verify if the authority figure has been quoted accurately, if possible. The Evaluation of Authorities box below lists the criteria for assessing an authority (Hughes, 1992).

**Authorities Must Be Identified.**   The authority must be identified by name. You cannot assess an authority if you do not know his or her identity.

**Authorities Must Be Recognized as Expert in the Field.**   The authority must be generally recognized as an expert in his or her field. Authorities in different fields have to meet certain standards to be recognized as experts. For example, nurses and physicians must meet certain licensing requirements. If licensing is not required, then degrees, certification, and diplomas indicate a level of educational achievement. Because licensing and education do not ensure expertness, you must determine if the authority is recognized as such by others in the field.

**Authorities Must Confine Claims to the Area of Expertise.**   The authority should make claims only within his or her area of expertise and should not comment beyond that. It is reasonable to expect lawyers to know more about the law than educators, nurses to know more about nursing care than salespersons, and carpenters to know more about construction than airline pilots.

**Authorities Must Have Expertise in a Recognized Field of Knowledge.**   The field must be one in which genuine knowledge exists. Genuine knowledge means that there is a systematically ordered body of facts and principles that are objective in

---

 **Evaluation of Authorities**

Authorities must:
- ▼ Be identified
- ▼ Be recognized as expert in the field
- ▼ Confine claims to the area of expertise
- ▼ Have expertise in a genuine field of knowledge
- ▼ Have consensus in the field of knowledge
- ▼ Be unbiased
- ▼ Have life experience in the area of expertise

nature. If none exists, then there is no basis upon which a person can claim to be an authority. For example, smoking as an effective means of weight control is not a recognized field of knowledge. Neither are the many "wonder cures" for illness that are based on testimonials rather than scientific knowledge.

***Authorities Have Consensus in the Field of Knowledge.***    A consensus among the experts in the field regarding the particular matter in support of which the authority is cited must exist. Controversial issues exist in every field of knowledge. Where controversial issues exist, it indicates that there is insufficient knowledge about these issues even though the field itself may have a strong knowledge base. Be cautious when authorities disagree among themselves.

***Authorities Must Be Unbiased.***    Assess if there is any reason to suspect that the authority is biased. Move cautiously if the authority has something to gain such as financial reward. For example, some physicians consult with lawyers and testify that silicone breast implants are safe, while other physicians testify that they make women sick. They all agree, however, that the money for offering these opinions is excellent. Fees range from $300 to $600 per hour. This raises at least the appearance that money might influence a physician's opinion (Implant, 1995).

***Authorities Must Have Life Experience in the Area of Expertise.***    Assess what real life experience the authority has had in his or her area of expertise. Experience that is theoretical and lacks any practical or lived component should be evaluated carefully. For example, a child psychologist who has raised children has more expertise than one who has not and whose knowledge base is theoretical.

## Sources of Information Must Be Credible

What is the source of the information? How reliable and credible is the source? Recall the argument about staff nurses learning to defibrillate clients in Chapter 8. To bolster the strength of his argument, the writer indicated that the source of his information was the American Heart Association (AHA). Does this add credibility to his arguments? Yes, it does; the AHA is widely recognized as a credible and reliable source. If he had quoted the local newspaper, would it have had the same impact? No. With professional health care providers, information from the AHA is more credible than information from the local newspaper. AHA recommendations are made by a panel of recognized experts in this field.

## Missing Information Must Be Weighed

What information is missing? Information may be incomplete for a variety of reasons (Browne and Keeley, 1994). First, information may be incomplete because it is not possible to organize it or to include all the information that we may like. We are limited in the amount of time we can devote to an argument. Second, we have a limited attention span and get bored when messages are too long. Third, we do not have complete knowledge when we present an argument. We use the best information that we have that is available to us. Fourth, information may be missing because of an outright attempt to deceive. We may omit information that would weaken our arguments. Finally, our values, beliefs, and attitudes may be different from those who are trying to persuade us. Thus, they bring a different set of assumptions to the argument. When you reflect on an argument, consider what information has been omitted.

## Personal Experience Must Be Cited Appropriately

If the reasons are based on an individual's personal experience, inquire about the circumstances surrounding the experience. Have distortions or mistakes in perception been made? Have others had similar or conflicting experiences? Are there other explanations for the experience? Some common errors in relying on personal experience are selection bias, unwarranted generalizations, faulty memory, and oversimplification (Browne and Keeley, 1986).

*Selection Bias.*   Selection bias is paying attention only to experience that favors a belief and ignoring instances that contradict the belief. For example, a nurse made three errors in one evaluation period. At his next evaluation conference he received an evaluation with "room for improvement." The nurse felt badly and felt he would never again be a "good nurse." In this nurse's mind, the evaluation experience canceled all of the good things he had done.

*Unwarranted Generalization.*   Unwarranted generalization is generalizing from only a few experiences. Our experiences bias us as we tend to generalize from whatever experiences we have had. We may use the word *all* when *some* is indicated. For example, a nursing student had clinical experiences in a state home for the mentally retarded where she cared for several children with Down syndrome. She concluded that all children with Down syndrome must be institutionalized without realizing that many continue to live at home or in group homes.

*Faulty Memory.*   Faulty memory is failing to keep track of events, to count, and to control. Memory is faulty and selective. Careful documentation is needed. Consider the nurse who worked in the emergency department of a large city hospital. She saw many homeless clients, many of whom were alcoholics. She mistakenly concluded that most of the homeless who came to the emergency department were alcoholics. Reading the institution's year-end report, she learned that homeless clients comprised a very small percentage of the total clients seen by the department; and of those homeless clients, an even smaller percent were treated for alcoholism. She worked the evening shift and had assumed that her perceptions were representative of homeless clients served on all shifts.

*Oversimplification.*   Oversimplification is failing to notice all of the important variables and contributing factors to a situation. Consider the possibility that there may be other explanations for the behavior you have observed. For example, a client came to the emergency room with "indigestion." He had experienced it in the past but ignored it because it was short-lived and never severe. He did not like to seek help and did not want to appear to be in poor health. He concluded that he ate too much the previous evening and blamed the "indigestion" on the sausage that he ate. He sought help when the "indigestion" did not go away. When the physicians and nurses completed their evaluation of the client, they determined that he had a mild myocardial infarction.

### Self-interest Needs Must Be Weighed

When you listen and read, consider the self-interest needs and biases of the speaker or writer. What is at stake? What does the person stand to gain if you and others yield to his or her influence? For example, to allow everyone who has any type of training in nursing to use the title "registered nurse" would be against the self-interests of registered nurses. To allow nonphysician health care providers to serve as the gatekeepers to the health care system would be against the self-interests of physicians. To see beyond our self-interest needs and make a sacrifice for the greater good of the profession and community are very difficult.

If you determine that the speaker or writer does indeed have a stake in the issue, you still should evaluate the argument on its own merits. Just because the person has a stake in the issue is neither a sufficient basis to discredit the argument nor sufficient reason to determine it has no merit. Evaluate it as you would other arguments.

## EVALUATING ARGUMENTS: FALLACY APPROACH

The purpose of an argument is to prove the truth of the conclusion. An argument can lead to an incorrect conclusion in two ways. First, the premises may be false, thereby leading to an incorrect conclusion. Second, the conclusion may not follow logically from the premises, in which case the reasoning is said to be erroneous or fallacious. A fallacy is an argument of the second kind; although the premises are true, they do not support the conclusion at all. The argument may appear to be correct but it is, in fact, not correct. Thus, the fallacy approach to evaluating arguments means to examine them for one or more errors in reasoning (Copi and Cohen, 1994).

A fallacy may be either formal or informal. A formal fallacy occurs when a deductive argument has an invalid structure or "form." Two formal fallacies were illustrated in the discussion of modus ponens and modus tollens in Chapter 8 (the fallacy of affirming the consequent and the fallacy of denying the antecedent).

Informal fallacies are different from formal fallacies. Informal fallacies are errors in reasoning commonly found in ordinary discourse. The premises appear to provide support for the conclusion, but upon closer examination, they fail to do so. Studying fallacies is important because they can be detected and avoided once you understand them. Aristotle was the first person to classify fallacious arguments. He was followed by other medieval logicians who identified and labeled many other fallacies (Kelley, 1994).

There are different types of informal fallacies and different ways to classify them. The following section covers some of the most common informal fallacies, ones that

## Fallacy Approach to Argument Evaluation

**FALLACIES OF RELEVANCE**
- ▼ Appeal to authority
- ▼ Appeal to emotion
- ▼ Appeal to ignorance
- ▼ Personal attack
- ▼ Appeal to majority

**FALLACIES OF PRESUMPTION**
- ▼ Hasty generalization
- ▼ Sweeping generalization
- ▼ False dilemma

**FALLACIES OF CAUSAL REASONING**
- ▼ False cause
- ▼ Post hoc ergo propter hoc
- ▼ Slippery slope

you are likely to encounter in your daily personal and professional life. Three categories of informal fallacies will be addressed: (1) fallacies of relevance, (2) fallacies of presumption, and (3) fallacies of causal reasoning. The Fallacy Approach to Argument Evaluation box above outlines these three categories and the specific fallacies within them.

## Fallacies of Relevance

Fallacies of relevance introduce some piece of irrelevance that tends to confuse. These fallacies contain irrelevant information that can—but not necessarily always—arouse emotions and thus obscure the real issue. When emotions become a factor in argument, a conclusion not supported by the premises might be accepted that would otherwise be rejected (Engel, 1994). Table 9-1 summarizes the fallacies of relevance.

***Appeal to Authority.*** Appeal to authority is referring to someone who has expertise in some area of knowledge and whose word carries special weight. It is not necessarily fallacious to resort to authority because many arguments are bolstered by the testimony of experts. According to Kelley (1994) an argument becomes fallacious when we rely on an authority who testifies outside his or her area of knowledge and who does not meet the two conditions of credibility: competence and objectivity.

To meet the first condition of credibility, the alleged authority must be competent in the field in question, confine her or his remarks to this field, and not presume to be an authority outside of it. As we discussed under the criterial approach, you

Table 9-1   **Fallacies of Relevance**\*

| FALLACY | DEFINITION |
| --- | --- |
| Appeal to authority | Cites experts or tradition |
| Appeal to emotion | Arouses emotions such as pity, fear, guilt, and outrage |
| Appeal to ignorance | Opponent is challenged to disprove the argument |
| Personal attack | Attack on a person's credibility |
| Appeal to majority | Cites the fact that a large number of people support the conclusion |

\*Fallacies of relevance seek to persuade, not by reliance on good reasoning supported by evidence, but rather by reliance on an appeal to authority, emotion, ignorance, personal attack, and majority.

would expect properly credentialed registered nurses to be experts in the nursing care of clients, not in matters of criminal law, and properly credentialed physicians who specialize in oncology to be experts in treating clients with cancer, not in matters of civil engineering. When an authority speaks outside his or her area of expertise, his or her opinions rank along with those of laypersons, and an argument based simply on an appeal to this person's supposed expertise is fallacious.

What if the experts disagree? For example, nurse A recommends a hot application and nurse B recommends cold. Physician C recommends surgery and physician D recommends chemotherapy. This is a difficult dilemma for knowledgeable professionals in the field. It is even more difficult for people with little knowledge about the field. When you are confronted with this dilemma, first verify that each person who claims to be an expert is indeed a genuine, recognized authority rather than a self-proclaimed one. If you have verified that each person is indeed a recognized authority in the subject matter, then you must listen carefully to both sides, become as informed as you have the time and energy to do, and make your own judgment about the issue.

To meet the condition of objectivity, the alleged authority must not have any emotional commitment or vested interest in the issue. For example, a well-accepted maxim is that a surgeon should not operate on a member of her or his family, nor should a lawyer represent himself or herself in court. When a person has a vested interest in an issue, he or she has compromised the condition of objectivity. For example, if a person is paid to represent a special interest group, such as a lobbyist, or is paid to endorse or sell a product, or is representing an employer, objectivity is lost. No one can be expected to be unbiased under these circumstances. Objectivity may be difficult to assess, but we should make every effort to do so. Kelley (1994) noted that with enough imagination and cynicism, we can find a reason to impugn anyone's objectivity. He recommends that we presume an authority is objective unless we have good reason to believe otherwise.

Engel (1994) adds an important dimension to this fallacy: reliance on tradition as authority. A person using this appeal may seek to persuade by citing tradition as authority rather than providing evidence. "We have always done it this way" is an example of reliance on tradition.

***Appeal to Emotion.*** Appeal to emotion occurs when a person attempts to persuade others about a conclusion by appealing to emotion rather than relying on good reasons supported by evidence. The speaker attempts to arouse emotions such as pity, fear, guilt, and outrage that, as reasons, are irrelevant to the conclusion. If the listener responds as the speaker hopes, it is the listener who then commits this fallacy. Emotions, per se, are not the problem; rather, the substitution of emotions for good reasons and evidence makes this argument fallacious. There is nothing wrong in arousing emotions when the reasons support a conclusion. In fact, many speakers and writers strive to achieve this effect. The problem occurs when we are moved to act on emotion rather than rational judgment (Kelley, 1994).

As with the appeal to authority, to appeal to emotion is acceptable when it is directly related to the issue (Missimer, 1990). For example, the sad plight of hungry, poorly nourished, and disease-ridden people fleeing Rwanda appealed to our pity and deserved our efforts to alleviate their suffering. That we should assist them out of pity is a relevant reason because they are, in fact, suffering.

An appeal to pity is fallacious when it is not relevant to the issue. Consider the appeal to pity made by a nurse who was consistently late to work and sometimes absent. She explained that she had to prepare breakfast for her husband every morning and prepare her young child for day care. Her transportation was unreliable, and she often overslept simply from sheer exhaustion. Her neighbor's children were frequently at her home because their parents were gone most of the time. In addition to all of this, the family pet died and everyone was upset. All of these reasons may be true, and they may evoke our pity, but they are irrelevant to the issue of meeting her employment responsibilities.

An argument may appeal to scare tactics and arouse fear (Moore and Parker, 1992). For example, nurses at two health care institutions were asked to forego pay raises while the institutions merged to form one large health care center. The nurses were told that their sacrifice would ensure the financial strength and profitability of the new institution. The nurses accepted this only to learn that the chief executive officer and members of the board of directors celebrated the merger by compensating themselves handsomely with bonuses. When several nurses complained to a supervisor, they were reminded that some nurses were laid off because of the merger and they should consider themselves fortunate that this was not their fate. The message was clear: complain and you may lose your job. The message evoked fear among these nurses. The threat of job loss was real. At this point there is no error of reasoning. Suppose, however, that under the fear caused by this threat, they changed their minds and really came to believe that it was good that they got no raises, then they have committed the fallacy of appeal to emotion.

***Appeal to Ignorance.*** Appeal to ignorance occurs when a person emphasizes the lack of evidence against a position—not the evidence for a position; that is, one person presents a conclusion and challenges the opponent to disprove it. The opponent's ignorance and inability to refute the conclusion become the evidence in support of it. The burden of proof is thus shifted to the opponent (Engel, 1994). Consider this example:

> Before Jay's serious illness, he was under a lot of pressure at work. The pressure was continuous over the past year, and it weakened his immune system. If you can prove this is not so, you will have my attention; otherwise, you will have to acknowledge that my conclusion is correct.

In this example, the burden of proof shifted from the person stating the argument to the listener. When the listener could not provide the reasons and evidence, the person stating the argument used this ignorance as proof of the conclusion. In any argument, the burden of proof always rests with the person who presents the argument. An argument is irrelevant and fallacious when the burden of proof is shifted away from the person who proposed it  and onto another person (Chaffee, 1994).

**Personal Attack.**    Personal attack occurs when the credibility of the source is brought into question. This common fallacy is also known as the ad hominem argument. It literally means "against the man" and is essentially name-calling (Missimer, 1990). It is a personal attack on the credibility of the person who presents the argument instead of a focus on the reasons, evidence, and conclusion he or she purports. Consider the example provided by Engel (1994):

> This theory about a new cure for cancer has been introduced by a woman known for her Marxist sympathies. I don't see why we should extend her the courtesy of our attention (p. 200).

A variation of the ad hominem fallacy is the genetic fallacy. It exists when a person attempts to prove a conclusion is false by condemning its source (i.e., genesis) (Engel, 1994; Kim, 1994). Consider this example:

> "Why should we keep this community elder day care center open? It was formed 10 years ago in response to political pressure by local citizens. The politicians caved in to the pressures applied by a few vocal proponents."

The genesis of an event may be interesting and enlightening information, but it is irrelevant to the merits of the argument. The decision about whether to keep the day care center open should depend on other factors such as current usage instead of how it originated.

**Appeal to Majority.**    The appeal to majority, also called the appeal to belief, occurs when a proponent of an argument offers as a reason the fact that a large number (not necessarily a majority) of people support the conclusion. Believing and supporting a conclusion simply because a large number of people do so is irrelevant to the merits of it (Kelley, 1994; Moore and Parker 1992). Recall that at one time most people believed the world was flat and the earth was the center of the universe. Believing that something is true does not make it true. Consider this example:

> "Jennifer, you should support Joel as the new president of the Nurses' Club. Are you aware that most of our colleagues in the nursing school support him?"

Although many nursing students may support Joel, this is an insufficient reason for Jennifer to support him. If Jennifer chooses to support Joel, she should choose so on the merits of his candidacy for the position, not because many nursing students support him. This fallacy, then, is committed whenever someone accepts a conclusion just because a large number of people accept it.

## Fallacies of Presumption

Fallacies of presumption are associated with how we identify common qualities or formulate general principles from particulars. Making presumptions and generalizations is common human experience. It also is related to the process of inductive reasoning, which was discussed in Chapter 8. Recall that an inductive argument involves reasoning from specific facts and empirical data to a generalization about a target population. The conclusion follows the premises with probability because it is a generalization about the target population based on a sample taken from the target population. Examples of fallacies of presumption are hasty generalization, sweeping generalization, and false dilemma. Table 9-2 summarizes fallacies of presumption.

***Hasty Generalization.*** The fallacy of hasty generalization is committed when a person draws a conclusion that, because the samples are a certain way, all will be that way. It could be true in which case there is no error in reasoning. It also could be coincidental. Committing this fallacy is often a matter of not having enough samples. Consider these examples:

The two elderly people I cared for this morning both had senile dementia. It must be that everyone will develop senile dementia if they live long enough.

I have cared for several clients with diabetes mellitus who must inject insulin to control their disease. This experience leads me to conclude that all clients with diabetes mellitus must take insulin injections.

In both of these examples, the nurse made an incorrect conclusion based on experience with two people in the first example and several persons in the second. The sample size, breadth, and representativeness were inadequate to justify drawing these conclusions and the result is an incorrect conclusion. The nurse was hasty in making these generalizations.

Table 9-2  **Fallacies of Presumption***

| FALLACY | DEFINITION |
| --- | --- |
| Hasty generalization | Draws conclusion based on insufficient evidence |
| Sweeping generalization | Applies a generalization that is usually true inappropriately |
| False dilemma | Confines the number of options to two |

▌ *Fallacies of false generalization misrepresent facts in the premises.

The following example is taken from a research study about the most effective media for delivering health education to three different cultural groups (Corell, 1984):

> A study of white, black and Mexican Americans found that television was the primary source of information for all three groups. Following television, whites turned to magazines, then to family members for information. Blacks turned to physicians, then to pamphlets. Mexican Americans turned to magazines and then to radio.

This example provides a somewhat stronger case for supporting some generalizations than did the dementia or diabetes mellitus examples. The sample population in this study was 64 residents of Galveston, Texas. The sample was stratified by ethnicity; it included 24 whites, 20 blacks, and 20 Mexican Americans. The households were selected from census tracts with at least 60% of the residents from each ethnic group. Blocks within the selected tracts were randomly chosen; all households were contacted. Although this example provides a stronger basis for making generalizations than the previous examples, the basis is still weak. What do you think about the sample size, breadth, and representativeness? To what extent can generalizations be made about these three groups outside of Galveston? To all of Texas? To all of the United States? What effect would a larger sample size have on the strength of the argument?

***Sweeping Generalization.***   The fallacy of sweeping generalization is related to difficulties in interpreting information. Chaffee (1994) provides the following example:

> Vigorous exercise contributes to overall good health. Therefore vigorous exercise should be practiced by recent heart attack victims, people who are out of shape, and women who are about to give birth (p. 591).

In this instance, the speaker has taken a generally accepted tenet for maintaining good health and applied it to situations where it is inappropriate. A person who commits the fallacy of sweeping generalization takes a valid idea and applies it to an exceptional case without giving due consideration to the peculiarities of the case (Engel, 1994). Let us look at another example:

> All children need good nutrition. Milk provides many nutrients, including protein, calcium, and vitamin D. Therefore, all children should drink milk.

This sounds like a perfectly good health practice; however, the majority of Mexican Americans, African Blacks, African Americans, Native Americans, and Asians are lactose intolerant. Whites of northern European descent have the lowest level of intolerance at 5% to 15% (Giger and Davidhizar, 1995). Lactose intolerance is a condition in which the body is lactase deficient. Lactase is an enzyme that breaks down the lactose that is found in milk. This argument is sound for children who are lactose tolerant but erroneous if we refer to all children.

***False Dilemma.***   The person who commits the false dilemma fallacy believes that only two alternatives exist: either it is this way or it is that way. There is no middle ground, no other alternatives (Ruggiero, 1991). False dilemma is also known as the black-and-white fallacy, the either/or fallacy, and the fallacy of false alternatives.

Recall that we discussed this fallacy under the latter name in Chapter 8 in our discussion about disjunctive syllogisms (Edna's choice was erroneously limited to being discharged either to a nursing home or to her apartment). Consider this example:

> A client, Mrs. Bee, is not complying with the instructions on proper foot care. Either she does not understand what she should do or she does not care about her health.

The two reasons given for Mrs. Bee's noncompliance may have nothing to do with why she is not taking care of her feet. Why must the "real" reason be either of these statements? To avoid committing the fallacy in this example, ask Mrs. Bee to explain her foot care regimen—what she is doing and how she is doing it. Perhaps Mrs. Bee is complying with all of the instructions and her physical condition continues to deteriorate in spite of her actions. The false dilemma fallacy provides an opportunity for the nurse to reassess Mrs. Bee's situation and adapt the care to the client's circumstances.

The false dilemma fallacy is a common way to back ourselves into a corner. When we see only two options, we unnecessarily restrict our imagination. When you think in either/or terms, describe the situation to trusted colleagues and ask what options and alternatives they see. This may spur your thinking beyond the either/or dilemma.

## Fallacies of Causal Reasoning

Causal reasoning is an attempt to find a relationship between and among phenomena. Seeking causal relationships is a way for us to have some understanding and control over our lives. For example, when you discover a car tire is flat, you wonder what caused it. Did you drive over a nail? Did you drive around a construction area? Did the tire wear out? Kelley (1994) challenges us to imagine a world without causality. In such a world you would turn the wheel of the car and it would not respond. You would step on the brakes and nothing would happen. You would lose control of the car. Now imagine this loss of control on a wider scale where you would have no impact at all. It is both scary and difficult to imagine.

Disease and wellness states of health are fertile topics for speculation about causal relationships. When something goes wrong or a significant event occurs, we look for the cause. For example:

Why did Brian oversleep?

- ▼ Was he that tired?
- ▼ Did the alarm fail to go off?
- ▼ Was he out too late?

Why did the client develop cancer? heart disease? AIDS? tuberculosis?

- ▼ Was it related to lifestyle choices such as diet and exercise?
- ▼ Was it genetic?
- ▼ Was it environmental?

Why did the intravenous line stop running?

▼   Is there a clot in the needle?

▼   Is the tubing blocked?

▼   Did the vein collapse?

Quackery is a multimillion dollar business in the United States (Hales, 1994). It thrives because the peddlers prey on suffering clients by promising relief and holding out the hope of a cure. These people, who are very effective communicators, promote for profit worthless and unproven health products and services. They are experts at implying and getting the consumer to believe that there is a causal relationship between their products and relief or cure. Because it is the nature of many diseases to wax and wane, it is easy for clients to infer that a particular treatment resulted in the relief of their symptoms.

Disease has such a profound impact on people's lives that the purpose of most medical research is to establish cause-and-effect relationships and find effective cures. Through scientific inquiry we can study causal relationships and make inferences based on statistical reasoning, assigning mathematical probabilities to these inferences. Much of what the nurse does is associated with solving problems, finding the cause of a problem, and fixing it. When we erroneously make the inferential leap between cause and effect, we commit a fallacy in this category.

In the category of fallacies of causal reasoning, we discuss the fallacies of false cause; post hoc ergo propter hoc; and slippery slope. Table 9-3 summarizes fallacies of causal reasoning.

***False Cause.***   The fallacy of false cause is committed when a person infers that two events are causally related when the causal connection has not been established (Engel, 1994). The fact that two events occur together or in sequence is not sufficient evidence to prove that one caused the other. Many things occur together in time that are merely coincidental. Neither one caused the other.

For example, Kirk visited his sick friend who had gastroenteritis. His friend has just returned from a 2-week vacation on the West Coast. The next day Kirk developed

Table 9-3   **Fallacies of Causal Reasoning***

| FALLACY | DEFINITION |
| --- | --- |
| False cause | Infers that two events are causally related when the causal relationship has not been established |
| Post hoc ergo propter hoc | Infers that what follows an event was caused by it |
| Slippery slope | Infers that one action will set off a chain of undesirable and uncontrollable events |

❚ *Fallacies of causal reasoning seek to establish a false relationships between events.

nausea, vomiting, diarrhea, and abdominal cramping (symptoms of gastroenteritis). He was concerned that during his visit he had unwittingly exposed himself to the "bug" that caused his friend's problem. Because Kirk did not eat the same foods as his friend during his visit, he assumed the "bug" must have been airborne. Later Kirk learned he had contracted salmonella, a food poisoning bacteria, from a local restaurant. Kirk's illness and his friend's illness were coincidental and not causally related. Kirk erroneously thought a causal relationship existed and inferred that the "bug" must have been airborne.

Notice that Mill's methods, which were discussed in Chapter 8, are designed to collect enough data so that the correlation in question appears not to be coincidental. If Kirk had found instead that his friend had been exposed to several other people and all of them got the same illness, he would be applying in effect Mill's method of agreement. It could be coincidental (remember that inductive arguments are always uncertain); but with more and more of the data collected by Mill's methods, this appears even more unlikely. And this means that the data constitute evidence of not merely a correlation but a causal relationship.

***Post Hoc Ergo Propter Hoc.***    In Latin, this phrase literally means "after this, therefore because of this." Post hoc ergo propter hoc is a variation of the false cause fallacy. It occurs when a person observes an event and concludes that what follows was caused by it (Engel, 1994; Missimer, 1990). Consider this example:

> Maria, a 23-year-old Hispanic woman, gave birth by cesarean section to her second child. She subsequently developed kidney failure and was treated with peritoneal dialysis. On her fifth day of treatment, she asked what the doctor had left in her body that the nurses were trying to wash out.

Maria assumed that the doctor had left something in her abdomen and that "something" was now the cause of her kidney failure. Although this incident is a somewhat dramatic example of the post hoc ergo propter hoc fallacy, the fallacy is common. Let us look at another example:

> When Bob died of a heart attack at age 50 while jogging, his wife concluded that his daily jogging routine was the cause. Bob had an extensive family history of cardiac disease. Many family members had relatively short life spans. She believed that with his family history, Bob should not have exercised so much and so vigorously.

Although these two events, jogging and death, occurred together, one may not have caused the other. We do not know that to be a fact, regardless of what the wife believes to be true. Given Bob's family history, his exercise routine may have prolonged his life beyond what it would have been had he not exercised so regularly.

***Slippery Slope.***    The slippery slope fallacy occurs when a person assumes that one action will set off to a chain of undesirable and uncontrollable events (Engel, 1994). Consider the following:

> Drinking alcohol is just the first step to a life of drug abuse and degradation. It begins with an occasional glass of wine and leads to an unquenchable addiction and daily dependence on alcohol. You will lose your family, friends, and money and end up homeless.

And this example:

> If nurse practitioners receive direct reimbursement for services not only from Medicare but also from insurance companies, then all the other health care providers will pressure Congress for this privilege. When all these providers have their hands in the till, the costs for health care will soar and it will bankrupt the nation.

And this humorous advice given to college freshmen (Green, 1938):

> Do not leave your room messy. Your roommate will talk about you. If she does that, folks will brand her as a nasty gossiper. If she gossips, she will lie. If she lies, she will steal. If she steals, she will do anything. Save your roommate's reputation and clean the room.

In each of the above examples the speaker claims that one event will surely lead to others that are even more undesirable and more uncontrollable, resulting in utter degradation and unthinkable chaos. The reasoning is fallacious because although the following events could occur, they are not likely; and when they are strung out, the unlikelihood that all will occur increases.

## ASSESSING ARGUMENTS

When you assess arguments, you may find the following summary useful. They bring together what we have discussed throughout the book.

1. Diagram the argument, and identify the conclusion and premises.

2. Identify the assumptions.

3. Evaluate the evidence.

4. Evaluate the argument using the standards, criterial, and fallacy approaches.

5. Anticipate the implications of the conclusions.

## SUMMARY

Evaluating your arguments and those of others requires listening skills and critical and reflective thought. The criterial and fallacies approaches are frameworks through which you may evaluate arguments. Each approach provides a unique, thorough perspective to the examination of one's own arguments and those of others. You think critically about arguments when you evaluate them according to recognized standards. And through this process, you refine your ability to construct sound arguments supported by strong evidence.

# EXERCISES

## Exercise 1

**Purpose:** *Enhance listening skills*

### DIRECTIONS

1. a. Arrange yourselves in triads. Decide who is Sender, who is Receiver, and who is Recorder. Sender and Receiver: sit facing each other. Recorder: notice if Sender allows the Receiver to do the task, and if Receiver's feedback is accurate. Notice body language between the other two.

   b. Sender: state your position on some issue (your choice or teacher-selected choice). State your position, one sentence at a time. Pause a bit between each sentence.

   c. Receiver: repeat verbatim after each sentence what the Sender says, without passing judgment. Try to repeat as accurately as possible what you hear. Say it softly enough not to interfere with Sender's flow of thoughts.

   d. Recorder: note whether or not Receiver pays close attention to Sender, and whether or not Receiver accurately repeats Sender's words.

2. a. After 15 minutes, proceed to this next exercise.

   b. Sender: continue with issue or choose another. Change your flow of speech to *short* paragraphs. Pause after each paragraph to give Receiver a moment to restate what you said. You do not have to listen at this point. Stay with your thoughts.

   c. Receiver: paraphrase softly what Sender said after each paragraph.

   d. Reporter: note whether or not Receiver is accurately paraphrasing Sender.

3. Switch roles until each individual has had an opportunity to play each role. Discuss these activities and share your observations acquired in each role with each other.

4. a. Sender: continue with above issue or choose another as instructed by the teacher. Receiver: paraphrase what Sender says, so that Sender can hear you. Sender: speak in short paragraphs. Stop after each paragraph and listen to Receiver's interpretation of what you said. If it is incorrect, correct it and have Receiver restate it until you are satisfied that Receiver got your message accurately.

   b. Receiver: work with Sender to paraphrase Sender's message to Sender's satisfaction.

   c. Recorder: note what methods they use to clarify their transactions.

5. a. Sender: continue with explicating your position and getting feedback from Receiver until you reach a natural break in your thoughts.

   b. Receiver: ask Sender questions about any part of Sender's message that you are not quite clear on, or you are curious about his or her underlying assumptions, or you wonder how she or he got to that position. If Sender makes any generalizations, ask Sender to identify how, why, when, what, and where.

   c. Recorder: note whether or not Sender's questions are successful efforts to clarify, subtle efforts to distract Sender, or efforts to confront or change Sender's mind.

6. Switch roles until all have had the opportunity to practice each role. Discuss your observations and what you learned in each role.

7. Report your observations, conclusions, and questions to the rest of the class.

# Exercise 2

**Purposes:**  *Refine listening skills*
                *Construct arguments*
                *Examine multiple points of view*

## DIRECTIONS

Brainstorm a sizeable number of issues that directly concern members of the entire class. Do not be shy. If an issue concerns you, it will most likely concern others. List the issues on the board so everyone can see them.

Once you have identified many issues, pare the list down to just those issues about which the group is equally divided: half are pro and half are con. Then:

1. Form dyads so that each dyad consists of a person who is pro and one who is con on the same issue.

2. Each person in the dyad should state his or her position on the issue and identify supporting reasons.

3. Each person then should change her or his position on the issue. The person who was "pro" now assumes the "con" position and vice versa. Present as persuasively as possible the reasons given by the other person.

When you have completed the exercise, describe what it was like for you to argue the opposite side of the issue. Were you able to do so convincingly? What did you learn by participating in this exercise? Did you change your opinion or perspective on the issue? Why?

# Exercise 3

**Purpose:** *Assess the acceptability of premises*

## DIRECTIONS

Brainstorm statements about the relationship between diet and health using these examples:

- ▼ Eating a diet high in fat and cholesterol contributes to plaque deposits in the arteries.
- ▼ Compliance with a carefully controlled diet contributes to fewer complications for diabetic clients.
- ▼ A diet high in calcium will prevent elderly men and women from developing osteoporosis.
- ▼ Cruciferous vegetables have antineoplastic properties that help prevent cancers of the gastrointestinal tract.

Select the statement about which you are most interested. Go to the library and look for all the reports you can find about the diet and its effects. What evidence is given to support the conclusion? Is the evidence based on research findings? On authority? How many reports did you find? Is the evidence sufficient? Is the evidence acceptable? Why or why not? Is further research needed? Report your findings to the class.

# Exercise 4

**Purpose:** *Evaluate premises*

## DIRECTIONS

Read the following statements and determine if the premises support the conclusion:

- ▼ Brett is a better nurse than Nancy because he is always prompt and neat in his appearance.
- ▼ Mr. George is more informed about his illness because he is a college graduate.
- ▼ Mr. Tan will like to eat fried rice and egg rolls because he is Asian.
- ▼ Mrs. Gonzales will need help getting around because she is elderly.
- ▼ Tyrone is so intelligent. He is so articulate and good-looking.
- ▼ Mrs. Rose is a better mother than Mrs. Tannen because she keeps her house so clean and tidy.

If the premises do not support the conclusion, restate each argument and provide better reasons to support the conclusion.

## Exercise 5

**Purpose:** *Evaluate arguments based on criteria*

### DIRECTIONS

Evaluate the following arguments using the criteria shown in the box on p. 257. Restate them to create strong arguments. Be creative!

1. The asbestos you were exposed to in your home will not hurt you. Government officials have overplayed the harm associated with asbestos. My dad worked as a plumber for many years and was exposed to far greater amounts of it than you have been exposed to. He is still living and doing fine. You will be okay. Do not worry.

2. Did you know that excess amounts of vitamin A can be toxic? I thought it was a good practice to take extra vitamins to stay strong and healthy. I read in the newspaper about a person who had all kinds of health problems and had to be hospitalized because of excess intake of vitamin A.

3. Workplace violence is increasing. Nurses should take precautions to protect themselves against clients who try to slap, punch, stab, or rape them. All nurses should be trained in violence prevention and self-defense and required to carry a deterrent such as mace. Delicia, the emergency room nurse, was severely injured when a client high on cocaine kicked her in the abdomen.

4. Participating in group counseling sessions has many positive benefits. Besides enriching your life and making new friends, it helps you gain personal insights into your behavior that you may not otherwise have discovered. You also can try out new behaviors in a safe environment knowing you have the support of friends. Here is my card; be sure to call when you are ready to join us.

## Exercise 6

**Purpose:** *Evaluate arguments using the fallacy approach*

### DIRECTIONS

Evaluate the following arguments and determine if they contain an error in reasoning. If erroneous, identify the fallacy in reasoning then restate it. Be creative!

1. Nurses should not become fractionalized, internally focused, or reactionary to change because these are not appropriate behaviors for nurses according to an editorial in September, 1994, issue of *The American Nurse,* the official publication of the American Nurses Association.

2. Nurse are the most underappreciated and underpaid group of health care providers. Why should nurses continue to work in a system that devalues their efforts? It is time nurses unionize along with millions of other Americans who have found appreciation, equity, and parity through the collective bargaining process.

3. In hospitals where nurses can routinely exercise their professional judgment, the implications for quality and client care outcomes are positive. If you disagree, you should state your reasons; otherwise, you will have to acknowledge the accuracy of my statement.

4. Senator Sims is responsible for bringing diverse groups together to support child care issues. He does it by diverting attention away from the substantive issues and focusing on trivial ones. He is crafty and devious.

5. Chaos would result if women were in charge of hospitals. Men are better managers than women. Everyone knows that.

6. Did you hear about the two children who were admitted for lead poisoning? I bet some paint manufacturers continue to add lead to paint even though it is illegal.

7. Everyone should always tell the truth—no matter what the circumstances are.

8. Something needs to be done! Either the federal or state government should pass legislation curbing workplace violence.

9. Yesterday Margie went ice skating and became chilled. Today she has an upper respiratory infection. You just know that becoming chilled contributed to her illness.

10. If the United States Congress passes strict handgun control legislation, then only crooks will have handguns and law-abiding citizens will be defenseless and vulnerable. Violence will get worse, and emergency rooms will become overburdened and chaotic.

## Exercise 7

**Purpose:** *Reflect by writing in your journal*

### DIRECTIONS

Consider the following question in your journal:

1. What positions have I taken recently (on any issue)? What were my reasons? Were my premises true? Did I reason logically from them to arrive at my conclusion?

2. Why was that issue important? What significance did it have?

3. Regarding my interactions today: What arguments did I use or hear that did not meet a criterion for a good argument? Did I commit a fallacy of reasoning? How would I replay the interaction given an opportunity?

4. What sparked my curiosity today? yesterday?

# REFERENCES

Babcock, D.E., and Miller, M.A. (1994). *Client education: Theory and practice.* St Louis: Mosby.

Borg, W.R., and Gall, M.D. (1989). *Educational research: An introduction* (5th ed.). New York: Longman.

Browne, M.N., and Keeley, S.M. (1994). *Asking the right questions* (4th ed.). Englewood Cliffs, N.J.: Prentice Hall.

————. (1986). *Asking the right questions* (2nd ed.). Englewood Cliffs, N.J.: Prentice Hall.

Chaffee, J. (1994). *Thinking critically* (4th ed.). Boston: Houghton Mifflin.

Copi, I.M., and Cohen, C. (1994). *Introduction to logic* (9th ed.). New York: Macmillan.

Corell, J. (1984). Ethnicity and cancer prevention in a tri-ethnic urban community. *Journal of the National Medical Association, 76*(10), 1013-1019.

Engel, S.M. (1994). *With good reason: An introduction to informal fallacies* (5th ed.). New York: St. Martin's Press.

Giger, J.N., and Davidhizar, R.E. (1995). *Transcultural nursing* (2nd ed.). St Louis: Mosby.

Green, I. (1938). Rules for freshmen. In *Golden Cords Yearbook.* Lincoln, Neb.: Union College.

Hales, D. (1994). *An invitation to health* (6th ed.). Redwood City, Calif.: Benjamin/Cummings.

Hughes, W. (1992). *Critical thinking.* Lewiston, N.Y.: Broadview Press.

Implant debate lucrative. (1995, March 24). *The Denver Post,* p. 25A.

Kelley, D. (1994). *The art of reasoning.* New York: W.W. Norton and Co.

Kim, J.C.S. (1994). *Introduction to logic* (rev. ed.). New York: McGraw-Hill.

Missimer, C.A. (1990). *Good arguments: An introduction to critical thinking* (2nd ed.). Englewood Cliffs, N.J.: Prentice Hall.

Moore, B.N., and Parker, R. (1992). *Critical thinking* (3rd ed.). Mountain View, Calif.: Mayfield.

Neufeldt, V. (1991). *Webster's new world dictionary* (3rd ed.). New York: Webster's New World.

Ruggiero, V.R. (1991). *The art of thinking* (3rd ed.). New York: Harper Collins.

Satir, V. (1967). *Conjoint family therapy* (rev. ed.). Palo Alto, Calif.: Science and Behavior Books.

Wassman, R., and Rinsky, L.A. (1993). *Effective reading in a changing world.* Englewood Cliffs, N.J.: Prentice Hall.

# *Persuading and Articulating*

Chapter **10**

## OVERVIEW

Chapter 10 discusses the process of persuading others to consider your point of view and articulating your position. The chapter begins by explaining how to build on communication (see Chapter 9), because communication allows us to share insights and find common ground in our interactions with others. Theoretical views of persuasion are then considered. Articulating your position from the perspective of preparing your thoughts and materials, organizing your message, and choosing your methods of delivery also are covered. Feedback is an important component throughout all of these processes because as human beings we grow when we interact with each other.

## COMMUNICATION VARIABLES

Whenever people communicate, they send and receive messages at several levels. Some of these levels are obvious to an observer, and others are less visible but no less important. The words each sender uses to convey meaning to the receiver gives evidence of the amount of thought he or she put into the message. The sender's vocabulary tells something about his or her educational level and his or her sensitivity to the receiver.

The context of communication also matters. Circumstances in which communications occur, such as in a busy unit, a private office, or a public rally, affect what the communicating partners convey and receive. Each of these contexts also affects the outcome. The comparative height of the communicating partners, their body posture (such as leaning forward or turning away), the distance between them, and the positioning of their arms all convey messages. They shape the message's meaning and impact on the communicating partners. The relationship between the communicators in terms of trust, intent, and power are very important. These factors affect both the process and the outcomes. Some questions to consider include: Who listens to whom? Do we have a history together? What do we have in common? What have each of us done to increase or decrease trust between us? Is either one of us vulnerable to the other (subordinate/supervisor)? Not only are these variables important, but also the *perception* of the communicating partners is extremely important. It is common for the person in the more favored position not to notice it or to discount its importance (Bohan, 1992).

Culture is a variable that is just beginning to be acknowledged as a powerful factor in communication. Some questions to consider include: What are the general norms, values, and world view to which the communicating partners subscribe? Are they similar? Are meanings sufficiently shared to allow us to communicate? What evidence do we have to support our conclusion that we can, indeed, communicate effectively about the issue at hand? For example, what does a head shake (up and down) with a smile mean? I agree with you? I acknowledge your opinion? I am being courteous? I acknowledge your authority? I acknowledge your right to speak your opinion? When the interacting other looks and acts as you do, it is easy to make some very outlandish assumptions such as: that others grasp what you intend to convey, you grasp what others intend to convey, and you and the interacting other both derived the same meaning from the utterances of a third person. To test this out, listen carefully at the next meeting you attend. Ask if you may summarize or paraphrase what you just heard, or what you think the purpose of the meeting is, or what the assignments are. Watch what happens. All of the above issues are important to keep in mind when you attempt to communicate with anyone about anything.

Persuasion is a human communication during which one person or group attempts to influence another to change attitudes, thoughts, and behavior (Rappsilber, 1982). What does persuasion have to do with nursing? Nurses who want to help people become healthier are persuaders. When you attempt to get clients to take better care of themselves, take actions that will speed their recovery, prevent relapse, or achieve health care goals, you are persuading.

When you join a committee to simplify, strengthen, or write new policies and procedures or to streamline the functions of personnel, or when you attempt to manage conflict, or share new knowledge with colleagues, you are adopting the role of persuader. When you attend a committee meeting at your facility or a public meeting at which an important issue is being discussed, and you prepare to discuss the issue before you go, you are persuading.

When you attempt to get peers in your group to do their fair share of the work or get the instructor to change a teaching strategy or give an example, you are functioning as a persuader. Whenever you are acting as a change agent, teacher, resource person, collaborator, or advocate, you are using persuasion.

## PERSUASION THEORIES

### Theoretical Approaches

Littlejohn and Jambusch (1987) identified four approaches to studying persuasion. They are transmissional, behavioristic, interactional, and transactional.

The transmissional approach stresses the sending and receiving of messages and emphasizes persuasion as a one-way manipulation of the person to be persuaded. The manipulator achieves this through skillful use of conventions of human behavior; that is, he or she engages strong psychological principles to personal gain. This approach would be used by those who are in a position of power such as administrators (Belenky, Clinchy, Goldberger, and Tarrule, 1986) and those who believe that changes can be evoked without the persuadee's conscious cooperation.

The behavioristic approach focuses on the response to the message. Does the stimulus (persuasive message) produce the desired responses? What do people do, feel, or think in response to this particular message transmitted in that particular package?

The behavioristic approach concentrates on effects, or measurable, observable behaviors. It makes use of well-known behavioral principles such as: behaviors that have been reinforced in the past are more likely to be repeated than behaviors with no responses or behaviors with negative consequences. Adherents of the behavioral perspective concentrate on behavior outcomes as the key to understanding persuasion. The advantage of the behavioristic approach lies in the specific measurable behavioral changes that result from a particular message delivered in a particular way.

The interactional perspective is the model with which most nurses are familiar today. It emphasizes reciprocity. It was the model presented in Chapter 9: The sender encodes and puts forth a message to the receiver, who takes in the message and decodes it. The receiver then becomes the sender by giving feedback to the original sender (see Fig. 9-1).

The transactional approach focuses on the give and take of the communicating partners. It attempts to account for the motivation of the person who will attempt to modify his or her behavior. The person may "shop" for a message that is appealing, a persuader who presents a message in an appealing manner, or a person who is an attractive or inspirational persuader (i.e., has charisma). The persuadee actively participates in the persuasion. If the persuader is to succeed, he or she must listen to the persuadee to learn what he or she wants to be persuaded to do, think or feel differently. Further, the persuader must be open to the persuadee's hunches about which influencing strategies will be most influential to the persuadee. The foci of the transactional approach are common ground and mutual actions. This model emphasizes that persuasion is an exchange of messages and that giving and receiving on both sides of the persuasion transaction are necessary for success. This approach emphasizes the relationship of the nurse with the interacting other as client (Fig. 10-1).

## Social Psychology

Ajzen (1991) examined the history of persuasive communication in social psychology. He emphasized source, receiver, channel, and message factors.

***Source Factors.***   A number of writers identify the sender of the persuasive message as the source. Source factors are observed or inferred characteristics of the communicator such as the communicator's appearance. The communicator's age, grooming, gender, body, and breath odors are examples of source factors. Behavioral factors are the communicator's posture, stride, eye contact, physical closeness, body language (e.g., confident, respectful, open), credibility, and attractiveness.

***Receiver Factors.***   The ability of the receiver to process the message is related to internal factors such as familiarity with the issues, age, gender, status, intelligence,

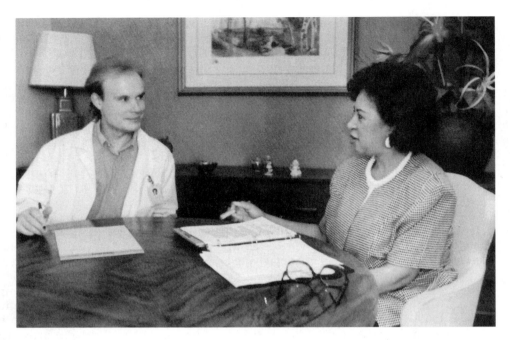

**Fig. 10-1** Persuasion involves mutual listening and respect between the nurse and the interacting other.

From Wise Y: Leading and managing in nursing, St Louis, 1995, Mosby.

educational preparation, preexisting beliefs, attitudes, and involvement of the receiver. These all influence the success of the persuasive transaction. The myth of the passive receiver that dominated much of the research on persuasion in the past is no longer considered accurate (Ajzen, 1991). Motivation to process a message and elaborate on its implications is dependent on the receiver's willingness to be involved. Motivation comes from the receiver's enduring values and whether or not the receiver perceives the work of involvement to lead to desirable consequences such as improved health or improved self-esteem. The determination and desire of the receiver to recover or change is extremely important.

The bond between the source and the receiver is an extremely important variable (Hasemeier, 1994). An example of the power of this relationship is meaningful support; for example, when nurses carry both the client and family through their darkest times of discouragement with expressions such as "I have faith in you. You can make it."

***Channel Factors.***     The channel through which the message is sent and received greatly affects the clarity of the message and how fully it is received. Situational factors can aid or interfere with the message. Noise, other external distractions, and internal distractions all affect the power of the message. For example, a client in severe pain or anxiety has trouble hearing the message.

For some individuals one-to-one and face-to-face communication is the most effective way to persuade. Others may gain most from a multimedia production. A written message has the advantage of being available for further study and digestion. If the multimedia production is captured on videotape, it too can be redigested at a later time, when the receiver is in a more receptive mode. Both of these channels allow the receiver to share the experience with important others.

***Message Factors.***   The message itself affects the receiver. Is the message one-sided? Does it agree with what the receiver already believes? Is it fair-minded and two-sided? Does the message appeal to reason or emotion? Is the message likely to evoke amusement or fear? Is the tempo of the message lively? Is it too long to sustain the attention of the receiver?

## Attribution Theory

Attribution theory refers to the receiver's beliefs about his or her ability to influence the outcome of involvement in the persuasive process. When an individual tends to find external explanations for success or failure, that person is giving evidence of having an external locus of control. A person who has worked hard and succeeded is likely to have a more internal locus of control. Success influences locus of control, and vice versa. Cultural groups vary in their orientation to locus of control. It is important for you to learn your client's orientation and make use of it in planning your intervention. For example, a nursing student was all set to teach a man how to clean his colostomy, when he noticed that the client was not paying attention. The student had the good sense to ask, "How do you expect to manage this when you go home?" The answer was "My wife will do it for me. She spoils me." The client in this example had an external locus of control; that is, he placed the responsibility of his care on someone else—his wife.

## Expectancy Theory

Expectations are very important to results. Both the persuader and persuadee have expectations. Raudenbush (1984) synthesized the findings of 18 experiments that measured the effects on pupil IQ when the teachers of those pupils believed that the students had differing IQs. The students responded to unconscious cues from the teachers, and their IQs drifted in the direction of their teachers' expectations. These studies have been replicated in other fields including industry, and the results support the conclusion: your expectations matter; what you expect is what you get. As a nursing student you should note your friends' and relatives' expectations carefully. Spend more time with relatives who expect you to succeed and avoid those who do not. You have a responsibility to choose your friends carefully. Surround yourself with friends who expect you to succeed. You should practice reality-based, hopeful optimism when you relate to clients. Let the client know that you expect him or her to succeed, giving evidence that is convincing. For example, consider the older client who was sure she could not learn to handle a piece of equipment that was necessary to her discharge. The nurse and client had the following dialogue:

**Client:**   I'm sure that I can't learn to use this equipment. I haven't been in school for 60 years!

**Nurse:**   That's a long time! I can see why you have some big doubts. Tell me what kind of place you live in.

**Client:**   (Describes an average house with a stove, a refrigerator, a vacuum cleaner, etc.)

**Nurse:**   Do you drive a car? Have you bought any new appliances lately? (Quizzes client about any opportunities for learning.)

**Client:**   (Describes a new appliance.)

**Nurse:**   Was it hard to learn?

**Client:**   Oh, no. I just took my time and . . .

**Nurse:**   Well, this equipment is no more complicated than that!

### Dissonance Theory

An important aspect of people's self-esteem is their feelings of internal consistency; that is, their thoughts are congruent with one another and that their beliefs, thoughts, and behaviors are consistent. One of the reasons people resist change is that they keep tension to a minimum by holding beliefs that promote this internal consistency.

People experience tension or discomfort when a deeply held value or belief is challenged by a psychologically inconsistent belief or behavior (Festinger, 1957). To make use of this theory, you would need to uncover the conflicting beliefs and values that interfere with change and then create strategies to lower the negative forces and reinforce the positive forces. For example, if you attempted to get yourself or a peer to quit smoking, you might start with a pro and con list (see the Pro and Con List for Smoking Cessation box on p. 285).

Discuss ways to unbalance the resistance at this point. How could you or the client make the pros outweigh the cons? What pros can you think of to add to the pro list? Are there any cons that you could weaken?

Establishing a set (or mood of optimistic expectancy) is an important early step in the persuasion process. Spend time convincing the client of the importance and interest of the material about to be presented. Maintain curiosity. Find out what motivates the client and use that feedback in planning your persuasion strategies.

## APPLICATION OF PERSUASION THEORIES

Examples of applying theories relevant to persuasion were given in the previous pages. The following are other applications and examples of persuasion while applying the nursing process.

**Pro and Con List for Smoking Cessation**

**PROS**

If I make the change I:
- ▼ decrease my risk of lung cancer
- ▼ smell better to others
- ▼ enjoy the smell and taste of food
- ▼ increase my self-esteem
- ▼ gain more energy
- ▼ become a better model for health

**CONS**

If I do not change I:
- ▼ avoid the risk of failure
- ▼ avoid the pain and discomfort of withdrawal
- ▼ avoid change
- ▼ enjoy the periodic "lift"
- ▼ have a quick and easy relaxation technique
- ▼ have a good excuse for a "break"
- ▼ do not have to find something else to do with myself

## Assessment

Find out what the client knows and does not know. Consider as many beliefs as possible. What are the current myths that the client believes? How narrow is the client's perspective? Is it possible that you could bring up other perspectives that the client has not considered? Where is the client's locus of control? Does the client believe that he or she can change? What motivates the client? Does she or he believe that the benefits outweigh the trouble of changing?

## Analysis

Look for points of agreement, especially aims. If you cannot agree on ends, recognize the importance of the problem or issue that you decide to raise. If the interacting other has already made a commitment to another solution or has endorsed it, consider remaining neutral until the solution does not work. Face all significant objections and look at them with courage. Learn the advantages and disadvantages of all major options. Does the persuadee understand the whole picture?

## Plan

Establish set, tone, and mood. Be enthusiastic and confident. Your energy and confidence may inspire others. Avoid being overbearing, but state your intent and your credentials. People are more easily swayed by those who appear credible. Give evidence of your academic credibility and life experiences that make you credible to this audience. For example, a social worker, whenever she spoke to welfare mothers, started by telling them that she had five children, and that when her husband was in medical school, they were eligible for food stamps and housing assistance. Endorsements from trusted people in the community also help.

If you cannot agree on ends, point out the advantages and disadvantages of other points of view as well as your own. Perhaps all you can agree on is the importance of the issue. Prepare to answer all significant objections, especially if you do your persuading on paper. Recognize the importance of timing. Choose a time when the interacting other is free to give you his or her full attention. Use a time when no other pressing concerns are competing for your attention. Make sure your body language matches your words. If you cannot find someone to give you feedback, videotape yourself and study the tape. Appeal to the logic of the client: use the client's vocabulary when building your case.

## Implementation

Do what you planned to do, but stay open to feedback. Show respect for your interacting other. Listen with undivided attention. Take the client's concerns seriously. Treat the client like a person, not just a recipient of your wisdom. You may learn much from the client. Talk *with* the client. Use full eye contact with the client before going on to other issues. Introduce yourself. Respect the client's privacy. Make sure she or he does not mind discussing your topic in those surroundings. Do not use jargon that may make your instructions unintelligible. Use more than one channel to convey your message (e.g., one-to-one, memo, picture, cartoon, poster, videotape). Make your message complete and specific. Claim responsibility for your work by signing it.

## Evaluation

Keep looking for feedback. Make sure the receiver is receiving what you intend to send. Watch the client's body language. Have him or her paraphrase the message you hoped to convey. Ask the client what part of the message seems possible or true, and what part seems impossible or untrue, or contrary to experience. Ask the client to show or tell you how he or she might implement the change. If the client is unwilling to change the whole thing, find out if the client is willing to accept or try any part of the recommended plan. Try to build in some periodic feedback from the client to continue the change process. Note that changes in attitude often precede changes in behavior. Count that as a step.

## ARTICULATING YOUR POSITION ·

Now that we have discussed theories and strategies of persuasion, let us consider communication from the perspective of articulating your position in the clearest manner possible.

### Preparation

***Purpose.***   The first question to ask and answer is what are your motives? Are you searching for truth? Do you wish to promote better understanding? Do you have economic or political motives? Why articulate your position? To improve the health behaviors of clients? To improve their recovery rate? To create a system that is more supportive to your own and clients' health? To support ANA's and NLN's agenda of creating a more equitable health delivery system?

What are your values? How do your values influence what you articulate? Nurses are clearly not motivated by money alone. What motivates you? What does service to others mean to you? What is your intent? Are you presenting your thoughts to be challenged and do you welcome opposing views or problems that you have not considered? Do you want to show a particular group what a good thinker you are? Do you wish to make yourself more visible in the organization? Are you dealing with an issue that is of grave importance to you?

To clarify the outcomes of your presentation is important. What do you hope the listeners will gain? A better understanding of your point of view? A change of opinion closer to your own? More information with which they can consider your position? Willingness to consider a different plan of action than the one they proposed? A different plan of action than the one they now use?

***Audience Analysis.***   After you confront yourself and your own agenda, you should analyze your audience. If you wish to communicate with an individual, you must begin by establishing rapport. Rapport is essential to opening lines of communication with the other person. A friendly, warm demeanor usually helps. Eye contact can be important, depending on the culture of the person you wish to influence. Maintaining a comfortable geographic space also can be used to open communication, (e.g., pulling up a chair and getting on an equal level).

The first section of Chapter 9 is devoted to listening. This is a key component in one-to-one communication. After carefully listening to your client, family, colleague, or administrator, you should use all that you learned about this person in preparing your reasons. Use the metaphors that you heard when that interacting other was speaking. Look for benefits to that person to agree with your arguments or to follow your advice. Thinking out your reasons and jotting down the points you want to make are good ways to organize your thoughts. For some people, internal rehearsal is effective.

For example, getting a teenager to stop smoking would require effective persuasion. You would have to assess and build on her knowledge of anatomy and pathophysiology and use words that she could comprehend. Showing her pictures of diseased lungs might be an important accompaniment to your explanation of how the various tars damage the lungs. If she is very conscious of her appearance and uses perfume, she may be motivated to quite smoking if you point out the connection between smoking, wrinkles in the skin, odors, and the inability of her own nose to detect them. Knowledge alone may not be adequate to help her change. You and she may need to set up a behavioral change program together. This would include further investigation into what motivates her. The skills you learned in counseling would be important to be effective in such a situation. The feedback you receive from your interacting other gives you clues on how to proceed.

Another example of a nurse reasoning with medical staff follows. She was present when the staff was considering surgery on an extremely elderly and debilitated person. She stated her objections to the surgery based on the client's age, physical condition, chances of gaining a better quality of life, or even surviving the surgery, and the client's statements about being "ready to go." She also pointed out the feelings of futility that the medical staff must feel in conducting such an expensive procedure that brings no satisfaction or feelings of success. She organized her thoughts, spoke clearly, and listed each of her reasons in a courteous but strong tone of voice. She looked into their eyes and spoke with conviction. She did not succeed in changing their minds that particular time, but she felt good about herself and the quality of her communication. In subsequent interactions, she detected a more respectful attitude from those who were involved in the discussion. She joined the ethics committee and over time, she helped shape more holistic decisions about surgery.

When you plan to speak to a group, what generalizations can you make about your audience? What characteristics can you predict or discern that would impinge on their reception of your message? Are you speaking to peers, subordinates, or administrators? When addressing teenagers you would need to use a much different approach than when you speak to retirees. Are you speaking to fitness buffs? Are members of your audience hearing or vision impaired? Is the audience relatively homogeneous in composition, or is the group comprised of widely diverse individuals? Individuals with a particular disease such as multiple sclerosis, arthritis, or diabetes may be very well informed no matter what their formal educational level is.

What is the educational level of most of the audience? What are their reading and media preferences? Would they find your use of technical words awe inspiring? Would they conclude that you are an authority and that your message is important? Or would they be confused by "big words" and stop listening? This is a particular risk if you are trying to reach women from deprived and abusive settings (Belenky, Clinchy, Goldberger, and Tarule, 1986).

One psychiatric nurse specialist said, "I personally have watched ethnic neighborhood workers tune out at meetings during which the professionals were using technical jargon. We were discussing important treatment protocols and problems in the political system that impinged on the subsystem in which we worked. Privately, the ethnic workers conceded that they brought knitting and did their nails because they believed the meetings were 'just a bunch of words with no meaning.'"

Your audience's socioeconomic characteristics also will give you clues to the appropriate level of conceptual sophistication. If the audience consisted of members of government grant or private funding committees, health care administrators, physicians, or other colleagues, you would inform yourself about their priorities. You must emphasize the connection between their objectives and the proposal you wish them to consider. Clinicians will find your presentation more weighty if you include facts that are easily observed in their setting. Items such as statistics and reputable sources of information also will add worth to your argument. Critical thinkers will look for the holes in your reasoning. Many would be favorably impressed at the breadth of your thinking if you presented selected opposing views and counterarguments. One of the judgments you must make is to decide how many opposing views to present. You want to reach a balance between conveying the metacommunication that you have done your homework and thought about all of the angles, yet not weaken your position by giving opponents more ammunition than they had prepared themselves.

If you are dealing with an audience less sophisticated in critical thinking, you should consider other tactics. If you hope to change the nutritional patterns of welfare recipients, for example, focus on the value and preparation of foods known as excess commodities.

If members of the audience are from other cultures, you may need to consult literature on portions of that culture's belief system that are relevant to your purpose. Choices of topic, examples, and the way the material should be prepared may all be affected by the culture's view of the topic under consideration.

For example, when a nurse explained the various available methods of birth control to Asian women, the nurse had to be aware that if any men came in during the discussion (the presentation took place in one of their homes), the session had to end. It was important for the women to see and touch the birth control paraphernalia to enhance communication, but all paraphernalia had to disappear instantly if any men approached. The nurse did not understand all of the cultural taboos, but she understood enough to respect and comply with them.

Searching for appropriate audiovisuals and testing their effectiveness is a time-consuming process that should be started as early in the preparatory phase as possible. Such materials should be chosen with careful attention to your audience. You want materials that are convincing, arousing, respectful of their expertise, and clear. The next section includes more information on the selection and use of audiovisual aids.

We also must note the expectations of the audience. What do they want to know or hear? What have they heard before? Are the people you wish to address here because they *want* to hear your point of view? Are they listening to you because they believe it is the courteous thing to do? What is their intent? Do they realize that open communication fosters a better and more effective working climate?

Do they already value you as an authority? Do they respect you as a careful thinker? If not, then your first priority is to create a set conducive to their hearing you and your point. Show them that you can think carefully and that your message is a product of that process.

If your presentation involves persuading people to change their behavior, you need to provide inspiration and persuasion to get them to change. Changing our behavior is work. It is easier to stay the same. Inspiration can help us find the motivation to start that process and to continue it. Inspiration is most effective when it is connected to an important mutual goal (Johnson and Eagly, 1989).

***Self Analysis.*** In addition to assessing your audience and their wants and expectations, you should assess yourself (Kaufman and Raphael, 1991). Are you preparing to speak to people who think like you do, or do they think quite differently? Are you field dependent, preparing to speak to people who are field independent? Or are you field independent, preparing to speak to people who are field dependent? You may need help from a colleague whose learning style is more like your audience to refine your approach and your examples. Your choice of points and examples will be based on conclusions you reached from thinking about the previously mentioned phenomena. In translating your knowledge into a frame of reference that suits this audience, you may find it useful to ask: what analogies and real life examples will be meaningful to them? This is essential if you wish to convince individuals in positions of power.

## Organization

***Ordering Your Ideas.*** The organization of your talk should be appropriate to your message. A number of intellectual processes for building knowledge, argument, and other aspects of thinking are treated throughout this text. One way to sequence ideas in a logical progression is to examine cause and effect. Chronological order is very useful for describing events that have historical relationships to one another. Geographical positions may be useful when discussing populations, ecological systems, or the map of the workstations (current or recommended) within a building. Moving gradually from the simple to the complex is another effective method. Describing the problem and the possible solutions is another useful way to organize your thinking. Chapter 3 points out how important it is to show the connection between your assumptions and your conclusions. It is equally important to highlight the connection between your assumptions and reality. Presenting opposing views and arguing against them or counterpointing them with your own observations is another.

When you present information that you suspect is totally new to the audience, you must find tactful ways to help them comprehend it. An effective method is to develop a familiar context in which to present the new concepts. You can translate the new information by using analogies that are familiar to the audience. You also can use personal stories that include the new information. You have read many such examples throughout this text.

Ideas should be grouped to make them easier to grasp and remember. Few listeners can hold simultaneously more than seven thoughts in their minds at once (Poon, Fozard, Cermak, Arenberg, and Thompson, 1980). These thoughts include both those that you intend to convey and the connotations that are evoked in each listener's mind by your presentation. Three groups of three are easier to remember and less formidable to the listener than nine separate ideas. You also can make use of memory principles by organizing the ideas into comprehensible and associated groups. This also will make it easier for the audience to grasp and remember the flow of your argument. An illustration of this technique has been used in organizing this section of this text. Although several ideas have been addressed, they have been organized into three basic categories: preparation, organization, and delivery.

One way to capture the audience's attention is to start with statistics that are particularly meaningful to the group. Statistics also help to create the impression that you are well informed on the topic at hand. Telling a story about yourself can be fun or even arresting because when you share a human experience, you give the audience a sense of who you are as the speaker. The story is most meaningful when it relates to the topic. Telling stories about yourself is particularly important if you are dealing with a speaker/audience trust issue: "Why should we listen to you? You have all that money, and you do not know what a life of hardship really is. What do you know about our lifestyle and our problems? How could you possibly know what we need? What are you really up to?" Story telling is particularly helpful when your sociocultural or educational background is quite different from that of your audience.

***Audiovisual Aids.*** Other senses besides the auditory channel must be considered. The rare orator who can capture an audience's attention for an extended period usually does so by creating visual imagery (i.e., painting pictures with words). Most speakers rely on audiovisual aids. You should time audiovisuals throughout your presentation to accomplish several objectives. Frequently a picture conveys an idea much more clearly than words.

A graph can help to clarify the meaning of statistics (Fig. 10-2). You can leave the graph, cartoon, or other display on the screen for the audience to absorb. Think about

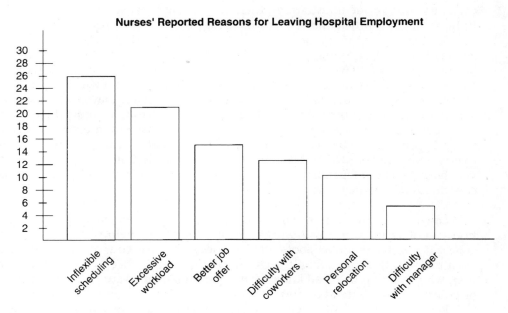

**Fig. 10-2** A graph helps clarify the meaning of statistics.
From Schroeder: Improving quality performance, St Louis, 1994, Mosby.

the length of time your words are heard by your audience. Words are much more short-lived than visuals. Even if your argument is very sound and well thought out, a crucial member of your audience may not be listening during the few moments you present the key point of your argument. A good idea is to present your main ideas more than once and through more than one sensory channel. The key points may be presented in the form of cue words or cartoons.

For example, consider a group of home health nurses who wanted to persuade legislators to increase Medicare benefits to cover the cost of ostomy dressings. In addition to presenting some short personal stories of their own observations, they included very graphic slides of makeshift dressings that clients had used and the badly damaged wounds that had resulted from such efforts. The legislators were horrified at what they saw, and, indeed, they did change the law to include the cost of dressings.

## Delivery Style

***Appearance.***    Your appearance helps establish an atmosphere before you begin to speak. Whether you want to believe it or not, the first impression is indeed very powerful. Your clothing and your stride when you approach the podium or take control of the meeting all create a mind-set in the audience that will enhance or detract from the power of your message. Your appearance should be that of a well-educated and sophisticated professional who is worthy of the audience's undivided attention (Fig. 10-3).

Within those parameters, your appearance should be suitable to the topic and your audience. If your point is to persuade your audience to do more physical exercise with some demonstrations, then a becoming sweat suit might be appropriate. If the audience is little children and you are a woman, wear a pant suit or a long, full skirt so that you can sit comfortably on low chairs or participate in the activities that are mandatory for young, restless children. A dark suit would be suitable for a business audience. If your audience is older, you also will be received more easily when you present a conservative appearance. A woman with a wild hairdo or a man wearing a ponytail when talking to a conservative audience may create insurmountable barriers. On the other hand, if the audience is a group of individuals with low socioeconomic status, a very sophisticated and expensive outfit can impact negatively. If you want to be heard, and you want to promote critical thinking, be sensitive to your audience. A field-dependent thinker may automatically adjust for these variables. A field-independent thinker may fail to consider them or need to make a conscious effort to take into account their importance.

***Language.***    Language should be appropriate to the audience. Use the information you acquired when you assessed your audience to help you choose your language. If you have doubts about the knowledge base of your audience and do not want to insult them, you might begin by saying "I would like to review the information, which you probably all know, that is particularly relevant to the topic (position or point of view) I intend to present."

Remember the positive effects of enthusiasm. Your own natural gestures and body movements add to your presentation (Babcock and Miller, 1994). Distracting phrases and mannerisms, however, can diminish the impact of your message.

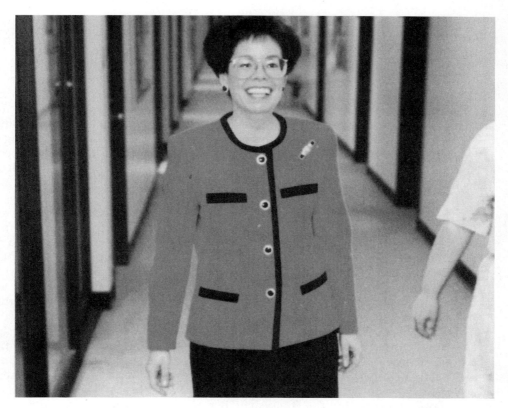

**Fig. 10-3** Your appearance should be that of a professional worthy of full attention.
From Wise Y: Leading and managing in nursing, St Louis, 1995, Mosby.

The pace of the speech must be geared to those whom you wish to reach. If the members of your audience are older, you should use a low, slow, and loud voice. Members from large urban areas, particularly on the Northeast Coast, would probably enjoy a pace that is much brisker than individuals from a rural community or from the South. If your accent is very different from that of your audience, you may need to enunciate carefully.

Individuals very familiar with the issue will be able to comprehend the point of your presentation much more quickly than people to whom the information is very new. Think of yourself when you read an article on new medical discoveries. Not only can you comprehend it better than your clients, but you also can make some educated guesses about the accuracy of the reports.

Your voice should be clear, loud enough to be heard, and conversational in tone. A monotone is usually a sign of anxiety. If you concentrate on how important the topic is and how much the audience will benefit from perceiving your point of view, your natural enthusiasm will modulate your voice. If you have a high, soft voice we strongly urge you to become familiar with a loudspeaker, to the point at which it becomes a friend and communication enhancer. Try to eliminate speech patterns that are distracting. Do not laugh off your words, particularly when you are speaking over a microphone. The laugh diminishes the weight of your message.

*Eye Contact.* Eye contact is very important in our culture for reasons very similar to those you learned when you studied assertiveness. When you maintain eye contact, you increase your authenticity, sincerity, and authority. Pick out a few friendly faces on each side of the room and talk to them. Members of the audience characteristically respond to this kind of attention in a very warm, encouraging way. Eye contact also allows you to determine when the audience has not grasped the message you intend to convey. At that point you can slow down, repeat, or ask what seems to be the trouble.

*Rehearsing Your Thoughts.* Practice cannot be overemphasized. It is a very effective device for easing anxiety. Practice is as important for the neophyte as it is for the experienced speaker. Practice should be done with feedback. It may be done in front of a mirror. This is particularly important if you are easily intimidated, or if you will present your points to listeners who think differently than you do. Rehearsal with an audiocassette recorder is useful in general and mandatory for anyone with a soft voice. If you speak too softly or mumble, you rob your thoughts of their importance. Listeners will think, "She or he is not very convincing."

Ruth Strang made excellent use of the microphone. She was one of the first educators to write about "personnel relations" (the euphemism for mental health) in the school. She was a wonderful teacher at Columbia University's Teachers College in the 1950s. She held her audience spellbound while she "conversed" with a 200-member audience in a large auditorium. One of her students describes the experience: "She was a very old lady then, but she could share her precious insights into life and teaching while sitting there in a comfortable chair with just a microphone. I remember being fascinated by the informal atmosphere she managed to create without draining her energy."

Practice your presentation with trusted friends or relatives who will give you honest and helpful feedback. Young children and adolescents also can be very frank. Role-play with your friends; have them challenge your thinking and practice dealing with their feedback.

*Dealing with Anxiety.* Feeling anxious when you speak publicly is a normal experience. We still experience some feelings of anxiety before we begin any important transaction, particularly if our audience is new to us, or if we suspect everyone will not agree with us. One way of coping with tension is to reframe the experience. Note the "butterflies" and have them fly in formation (Babcock and Zak-Dance, 1981). Redefine your anxiety as a raised epinephrine level and excess energy (Babcock and Miller, 1994). Find ways to use up your excess energy. Arrive at the speaking site very early and arrange the furniture to suit your needs. Greet members of the audience when they enter.

Before your speech, use familiar ways to calm yourself such as breathing deeply, praying, chewing gum, or sucking on clear candy (remove either before speaking), and employing comforting magic. Fantasy also is helpful. Imagine yourself giving a very poised and well-presented argument, and then imagine smiling while the audience nods approvingly after each important point (Dobson, 1988).

Many individuals find positive affirmations or "self-talk" useful in a variety of situations (Fishel, 1988). Try the following phrases: "This is an important issue. They must be aware of this side of the argument. They need to know this for the well-being of our clients." Such phrases may help you assume a positive attitude.

It is important that you *talk from notes,* rather than read from a paper. One reason to avoid reading your argument is the negative effect it has on you as the speaker. When you look at a piece of paper instead of the audience, you may lose touch with your listeners and not notice their nonverbal feedback. You may fail to notice when they are interested, puzzled, or getting restless. If you notice the latter, you may find it wise to change your approach.

If you are nervous, you may speed up your language. When you have complete sentences in front of you, you may be tempted to talk faster. Notes that are incomplete clues instead of sentences help your presentation. You can see the cues briefly, so your eye contact with the audience is maximized and you do not end up looking like you are bobbing for apples. When you look at the next line and reconstruct what to say, you automatically pause. During your pause, the audience has time to absorb what you just said. It thus allows them time to reflect on the idea and to associate it with experiences with which they are familiar. Notes that stimulate recall also allow you to be more spontaneous. A fresh example may occur to you during the reconstruction process. It may be stimulated by feedback you receive from your audience, even while you speak. This helps keep the presentation more lively and avoids the feeling that your point of view is "canned."

## Delivery Method: Exposition

After preparing and organizing your thoughts, you must decide upon your method of message delivery. The formal presentation is a very common method. Exposition may be defined as setting forth facts, ideas, and detailed explanation; it is writing or speaking that sets forth or explains (Neufeldt, 1991).

## Delivery Method: Discussion

Suppose your main reason for meeting with a group is not to persuade them of something but to share information. Perhaps your main objective is to promote critical thinking in your audience. Perhaps you are struggling to solve a difficult problem or to obtain a more comprehensive understanding of an issue. For example, should the state board of nursing no longer require or track mandatory continuing education? Discussion may be the best way to discover all of the important aspects of the issue (Fig. 10-4).

Discussion may be defined as a two-way verbal interaction. It involves talking, listening, asking questions, and answering questions. Discussion implies an egalitarian approach to transacting. An assumption underlying this method is that the audience has some knowledge and experience in the area under scrutiny, and that their

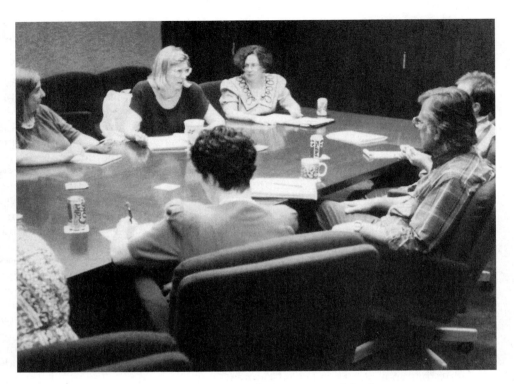

**Fig. 10-4**   Discussion helps obtain a more comprehensive grasp of the issue.
From Wise Y: Leading and managing in nursing, St Louis, 1995, Mosby.

thinking, knowledge, opinions, conclusions, and views of the issue are valuable input. You are more likely to succeed in persuading the audience to your point of view when they are actively involved in addressing the issue with you.

Discussion is useful when your main objective is to get closer to the truth or to obtain a more comprehensive grasp of the issue. "Basic to effective critical thinking is the ability to make connections, to bring to bear on an issue, a question, or a problem all the factors or influences that attend it" (Hanford, 1994, p.7). Discussion can be used to gather data before, during, or after your formal presentation.

If you lead the discussion, you may find it helpful to think through and write out a number of questions. Questions can serve many purposes in the process of persuasion: to find out what the others already believe, to detect the power and breadth of your opposition, to stimulate interest in divergent points of view, to explore ideas with your colleagues, and to discern whether or not others grasped the main points of your position. You can use the information you gain to guide the rest of the discussion.

***Initiating the Discussion.***    One of your first tasks is to get the discussion started. It is often helpful to review the purpose of the meeting with the group. Sometimes a summary of past discussions or areas of agreement and disagreement helps. Another task is to keep the group on target. All of us think by associating one idea with another, but associations are likely to vary with each individual. You must keep alert to the topic at hand and direct others. Summarizing periodically is important. At the closing of the session you may do it yourself or you may ask another to summarize. Chapter 9 is devoted to evaluating arguments. Use these listening and evaluating skills when you proceed with the discussion.

**Guiding the Discussion.**   As with any method of discourse, there are problems associated with the discussion strategy. We give up some of the control. Others share some of the leadership. At times this may mean that the others diverge to a very different path than we had in mind. At that point we must make a decision about whether or not to attempt to refocus the group or to go with the energy of the group. Is the new path in some way relevant to the goal you hope to reach? In your opinion, does the new path have merit? Is your main goal more likely to be reached by pursuing this path? Does this path show promise of leading to an important truth that you had not considered? Is the digression timely? Your attempt to refocus under such circumstances also might be an attempt on your part to avoid an issue that you find uncomfortable to address, or you may be semiconsciously trying to steer the group away from an insight that will highlight the flaws in your argument. One of your obligations as a critical thinker is to address that possibility.

**Participating in a Discussion.**   How do your tasks differ when you are a participant in a discussion and not the leader? Study the agenda carefully and determine the purpose of the meeting. If you have been given a specific slot of time on the agenda, write out your message with documentation in case anyone expresses an interest, or in case someone usurps your time. In addition, have an outline with your most important points highlighted so that you can easily find them. You may introduce an idea when it fits with another's perception, or you may bring it up when a lull occurs.

## Delivery Method: Team Presentation

Team presentation exists when two or more presenters with different preparations, abilities, and skills cooperate and share with one another the responsibilities for planning and presenting the argument or position. This exemplifies the collaborative function of the nurse (Fig. 10-5).

In team presentations, different types of individuals combine their strengths to make their view of the issue more potent. For example, consider the two nurses who agreed with one another on the need for changing from primary care to managed care on their unit. The first nurse, a very logical and structured thinker, gave a very scholarly, logical presentation that was obviously the work of a critical thinker. Her partner subsequently evoked a lively discussion among the other participants about the consequences of the change in the workplace in the real world of today's changing times.

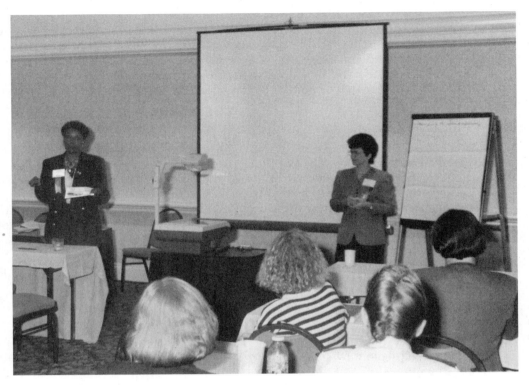

**Fig. 10-5**  Team presentations exemplify collaboration.
From Nursing Quality Connection (Special Conference Report, Supplement to 4[3] Nov/Dec 1994), St Louis, Mosby.

They both participated with the group in receiving and sharing ideas on how to implement the change.

### Delivery Methods:  Other

Other delivery methods involve more physical participation from the audience. Other methods are demonstration, simulated environment, and role playing.

***Demonstration.***    Demonstration may be defined as an activity that describes or illustrates by experiment or practical application; during demonstration one displays, operates, and explains (Neufeldt, 1991). You are most likely to use the demonstration method when you decide that it will be the most persuasive strategy. It may be that the decision makers are people who have little exposure to a particular procedure, yet they are the ones whose decision will affect the use of the procedure, such as implementing a no COR (cardiopulmonary resuscitation) policy.

***Simulated Environment.***   Suppose you decide that your audience is more likely to get your point if they experience some measure of the actual situation as it impinges on the real life of individuals? The simulated environment may be defined as an artificial situation that is designed to evoke in the participant the same coping responses that are likely to occur in the real situation. The simulated environment provides the participant with an opportunity to practice under low-risk conditions, the dilemma for which a crucial decision must be made.

Earlier in this chapter we presented the task of persuading welfare mothers to make better use of food commodities. The best setting for conducting such a presentation would probably be in a kitchen. Your effectiveness in changing behavior would be enhanced if you included the family cooks in the development of recipes and tested them then and there. During World War II, efforts were made to help homemakers use foods to substitute for ingredients that were in short supply (e.g., butter, eggs, and sugar). Women who were involved in group discussions and helped create the recipes were using them years later. Women who were given demonstrations and ready-made recipes tended not to incorporate those recipes into their cooking.

***Role Playing.***   Role playing may be defined as assuming the characteristics and expected behaviors of an assigned individual. The individual may be yourself in an anticipated position, or the player may take the position of another to better understand that other individual or role. This technique also is useful in assisting an individual to consider attitudes, beliefs, and thoughts that were heretofore incompatible with that individual's self-perception.

Jurors sometimes employ these methods to help themselves decide more wisely about the circumstances of a crime and the logical or realistic possibilities, or the probable sequence of events. These strategies are quite useful in helping the participants develop a more accurate frame of reference through which to judge a particular dilemma. When there is no easy answer, participants can learn how to cope more successfully with their own feelings. They also can anticipate more realistic options, as well as the consequences of those options. You also must be able to convince the participants that logic and discourse alone will not allow them to gain a comprehensive understanding of the issue under investigation. They must believe that investing in such an activity will deepen their understanding of important aspects of the situation.

## Selecting the Right Method

When planning your method of communication, select one to suit your style, your intent, the audience, and the reality of the situation in which your transactions will occur. Consideration also should be given to the situation in which the new information or point of view will be used.

A thoughtful and logical sequence is necessary to whatever method you use. Field trips provide participants with the opportunity to think about your ideas in context. Attitude adjustments are facilitated by discussion and participatory activities such as games, role playing, and simulated environments. These methods of unconscious influence and personal confrontation are helpful for assisting participants to modify their values. One such approach is to have them enact simulations or role-play situations that confront the attitudes they currently hold. "Teaching people to become critical thinkers does not mean simply equipping them with certain intellectual tools; it involves their personal transformation and its commensurate impact on the quality of their lives and those around them" (Chaffee, 1994, pp. 24-25).

Your delivery method should suit the participants' thinking style. If the participants cannot read, a strategy that involves reading or writing would be ineffective. If a substantial number of participants are kinesthetic thinkers, then at least one of the strategies should provide an opportunity for "hands-on" experience. Use as many senses as possible such as hearing, seeing, touching, and smelling. Some speakers prefer to talk from their slides or from transparencies with cue words or cartoons.

To assume that your audience received what you intended to convey is easy; do not deceive yourself with that assumption. To elicit feedback is important. An interesting example of differing perceptions occurred during the Al Gore Jr. versus Ross Perot debate before the 1993 elections. Two people, a father and grown daughter, watched the debate because both listeners took their constitutional privilege to vote seriously. Both people were intelligent and had a similar level of education, and both valued critical thinking. They watched the same program, but their perceptions diverged. The father said, "Perot won!" The daughter said, "Gore walked all over Perot!" To elicit feedback conduct a discussion or survey, ask for written responses, or invite the members of your audience to write down other thoughts they did not have time to say. Keep in mind that many human beings believe that what they believe is true.

## WRITTEN EXPOSITION

Articulating your position in writing is another option. You have been writing academic papers throughout your college and high school career. When you prepare to write your position paper, you should think about many of the same variables that you consider for oral presentation. All of the critical thinking skills you have been developing throughout your professional development will be useful in your preparations. All of the concepts and skills you learned in your course on writing the research paper are applicable to articulating your position. The information in Chapters 6 and 7 of this text should help you organize your paper.

### State Your Purpose

When you write, you should make your underlying assumptions and premises explicit. You must consider your motive in writing your ideas, values, and intent. You must make your objectives clear to the reader. The reader will want to know where you are coming from, so she or he can follow where you are going and how you intend to get there.

## Assess the Target Population

Analysis of your audience will help you decide how to write the paper for the same reasons that it will help you decide how to speak. The literacy level of your readership is very important. If your readership is less sophisticated in abstract thinking and vocabulary level, you must adjust your writing style. Shorter sentences; studied use of common words; and inclusions of cartoons, sketches, and photographs all facilitate the readability of a document. Examples from the lived experiences of your readership also will facilitate their comprehension of your message (Babcock and Miller, 1994).

## Be Clear and Explicit

When you write, you cannot accompany your message with body language, facial expressions, or vocal intonations. You cannot get immediate feedback from your audience to guide you in adjusting your communication strategies during your presentation. You have the advantage, however, of being able to write and rewrite until your words convey exactly what you mean in the clearest, most thoughtful, and most readable manner. You can and should ask at least two people to edit your paper. One reader should have expertise in the topic of your paper, and the other should have a different background or have a background similar to your target audience. The second person will pick up words that need definition and ask for assumptions you failed to specify. Count the number and length of words used in your sentences. It is a measure of the "fog index" you may create; that is, the sentences may be technically correct but unintelligible due to the use of big words or strange vocabulary.

## Organize Your Thoughts

Getting your message on paper is a personal experience. Many authorities suggest preparing an outline and then filling it in. An experienced writer explains, "Organization comes first. Get the organization set in your mind and then write. If you just start, you may come up with a jumble of 14 different parts and not know how to put them together." Another equally experienced writer writes as ideas and relevant insights come to her. She allows the organization to flow out of her ideas later in the process. Once she gets the organization, she uses it, unless a better one comes along later. Still others talk their way through a paper. If you are a talker, you may find it effective to tell an audiocassette recorder your thoughts on the way to work, class, or on a lengthy drive. You may find a quiet, repetitive activity such as walking or lap swimming helps you move into a meditative state. While in that state you may find it easier to create analogies and/or organize your thoughts. If you have an unreliable memory, keep a small notebook with you, so you can capture insights before you lose them. Your journal can serve this purpose.

Make your ideas orderly. One idea should flow into another. Make use of all you have learned in this book about preserving the logic of your arguments and sticking to the issues that are pertinent to your purpose. Say what you want to say as simply and clearly as possible. Try to avoid using the same word repeatedly in the same or nearby sentences. Varying your sentence length adds interest, whereas, using run-on sentences confuses and irritates the reader.

## Edit Carefully

The polish with which you present your written position will affect your reader as much as your physical grooming affects your listener when you present your position verbally. Proper use of English enhances the acceptance of your work and the attitude of the reader toward your message. Poor grammar and careless construction of sentences is distracting to the reader and generally obstructs your purpose. It is crucial to the image you create as a scholar and to the positive reception of your thoughts. A colleague reported, "When I wrote this paper, I asked my husband (who wrote 35 technical papers) to critique it for me. He edited it and then said, 'Correct the errors and then I'll read it for content. The errors are distracting.'" Another teacher said, "If I find a certain number of errors, I hand the paper back. I won't finish reading it." If you are writing for a particular teacher, administrator, or publisher, pay attention to what your intended reader wants in the way of exposition. Ask to see samples of papers he, she, or they consider quality writing. Some busy executives want a proposal no longer than one or two pages. If this is the case, you may present an abbreviated abstract with a lengthier document attached or easily available. Your abstract in such a situation should refer to the situation or problem you address and a summary of your proposal for change.

If your instructor is interested in fully developing your idea, take his or her stated and written guidelines very seriously. Do not be afraid to consult with the instructor or supervisor. Give him or her a draft of your best effort and ask, "Is this what you want?"

## Heed Rules of Style

Various publications have their own style rules. If you want your writing to be published, you raise your chances of having it accepted if you make it fit the subjects, style, and length of typical publication articles. In a sense, your writing must be tailor-made for the publisher. You can discover this by reading the target periodicals and looking for publication guidelines in the document. Some periodicals like *Publication Manual of the American Psychological Association* (APA) have very specific requirements. Editors of *Readers Digest,* for example, include in each issue a list of criteria for each section of the magazine along with limits on word count. The publication company Mosby–Year Book, Inc., has a general style manual as well as additional instructions on how to prepare a manuscript electronically. You may write to your intended publisher and request guidelines. The APA publishes a manual that contains valuable information on the correct expression of ideas. We strongly recommend that you get yourself an appropriate reference if you have trouble with any of the following recommendations and helpful hints. Other respected manuals are available. *The Chicago Manual of Style* is an excellent reference book for publishing. *The Elements of Style* is an excellent reference for undergraduate academic writing. *The Associated Press Stylebook and Libel Manual* is a helpful reference for journal and newspaper writing.

## Obey Rules of Grammar

This section addresses some of the most common mistakes in grammar that nursing students at the baccalaureate level make.

Use parallel construction. If you have a list make sure that each member of the list matches. For example, if one of your verbs ends in *ing*, be sure all of the other verbs in the list do too; for example, list*ing*, emphasiz*ing*, show*ing*, and throw*ing*.

If you write a bulleted list, be sure each bulleted phrase is expressed with the same type of language and construction. Each bulleted phrase begins with a dot resembling a bullet or a triangle. They are usually not complete sentences, but they convey a series of important ideas in the most economical language possible without compromising clarity. The following is an example of a bulleted list of punctuation marks:

▼  .  =  end of a complete thought that contains a subject and predicate
▼  ;  =  end of a complete thought followed by another related complete thought
▼  :  =  beginning of a series. All of the verbs in a series should match
▼  ,  =  one of a series. All of the items in the series should match

One of the most common grammatical errors nursing students make is failing to make pronouns agree in number: "A *person* (singular) does what *they* (plural) think is right." The most common reason for mismatching the words is to avoid the pronoun *him* or *her,* or *his* or *her.* This usage is frequently heard in conversation, but it is incorrect and should not appear in a paper that will reflect your ability to think and communicate effectively. Exercise 2 at the end of this chapter contains a sample of that type of error.

Many students appear unaware of the number of drafts they can expect to write to produce a scholarly paper. Today there is less excuse for grammatical and spelling errors. You can purchase word processing software with spell checking and grammar checking capability. Such programs also will count the number of words you employ and estimate your paper's readability level. Such capability also is available on the word processors in college laboratories.

While evaluating resources for students, a teacher made a trip to the computer laboratory on campus. He asked the lab assistants (students) about the software package titled "Grammatik" on the computers. They told the teacher that the program was "no good," because it stopped at every other sentence saying "passive voice." Many students of science and related fields have learned to use the passive voice. Until recently the passive voice was encouraged in an attempt to avoid the appearance of egocentrism and to give the appearance of objectivity. What it actually does is lead to dangling participles. Some authorities now recognize that authors who use the passive voice fail to be clear and concise in their writing (*Publication Manual,* 1994). Writers using passive voice tend to write with many dangling participles and fail to claim their own work and opinions. We recommend that you claim your thoughts in the clearest and most concise manner possible. An example of passive voice and active voice follow:

In writing this book, it is hoped that it will fill a gap in the critical thinking literature and be useful to nurses.

The above sentence is written in the passive voice. It also avoids the author's use of "I" or "we," which in the past was considered bad form. The preferred way now is to make clear whose observations are being conveyed (*Publication manual,* 1994). A more forthright way to write the above thought is,

> We wrote this book on critical thinking to fill a gap in the nursing literature.

The above sentence is written in the active voice, which is more direct and vigorous than the passive.

## SUMMARY

In summary, each method of discourse has advantages and disadvantages. Each is more suitable for various types of changes you hope to induce in your audience, the argument you wish to defend, or the truth that you are seeking. Research confirms what critical thinkers have always known: using a variety of strategies greatly enhances the amount of communication that you achieve (Claxton and Murell, 1987) and promotes critical thinking in the person or groups with whom you engage. A variety of methods helps us to communicate, assess, persuade, and approach the truth. Feedback is essential to an accurate evaluation of what was in fact communicated. To write an effective position paper, you will proceed through intellectual processes very similar to those you employ when preparing an oral presentation. The advice Dale Carnegie (1980) learned from a politician is just as relevant to an oral presentation as it is to a written paper: Tell them what you intend to tell them; tell them; tell them what you have told them.

# EXERCISES

▼

## Exercise 1

**Purpose:** *Apply persuasion theories to real nurse–interacting other experiences*

### DIRECTIONS

1. Think about the four types of persuasive approaches that are outlined in this chapter. Describe four situations in which you acted as the nurse and functioned from the perspective of the

   a. Transmission mode (persuader acts; persuadee increases compliance)

   b. Behavioral mode (persuader provides stimulus; persuadee changes in desired direction; persuader reinforces desired change)

   c. Interactional mode (persuader is modified by feedback from persuadee)

   d. Transactional mode (mutual goals; persuadee indicates a desire for help with change; persuader uses knowledge from persuadee to help plan change)

## Exercise 2

**Purpose:** *Raise awareness of common grammatical errors*

### DIRECTIONS

Identify the errors in agreement in the following example and correct them:

1. A *person* cannot benefit from examples that are unfamiliar to *them*.

2. The *client* does not automatically believe or agree with *their* doctor.

3. It is rather difficult to persuade some*one* to change *their mind* unless you have contact with *them*.

## Exercise 3

**Purpose:** *Develop further skill in conveying your thoughts through exposition*

### DIRECTIONS

Write a position paper on a current nursing issue of your choosing.

1. Submit the topic to the instructor for approval during the selected week of the semester.

2. Address the following components:

a. statement of the issue

b. statement of your reasons and evidence to support your position

c. conclusion(s)

## Exercise 4

**Purpose:** *Practice speaking thoughtfully and articulately*

### DIRECTIONS

Make a speech of persuasion concerning your issue.

1. Sign up to present your issue in class.

2. See the instructor for the sign-up sheet.

3. See the schedule for available dates.

## Exercise 5

**Purpose:** *Promote critical thinking about written and verbal communication*

### DIRECTIONS

Write in your journal about your own process of collecting and ordering your thoughts.

## Exercise 6

**Purpose:** *Promote reflective thinking*

### DIRECTIONS

Go back and read and reflect on the entire journal you have kept as you have progressed through this book. Evaluate your critical thinking abilities. Reflect on the following:

- ▼ In what areas do you feel skilled?
- ▼ In what areas do you need more depth?
- ▼ Can you see a difference in the type, amount, and depth of your thinking from the beginning to the end of this book?
- ▼ How has this content in critical thinking helped you in your professional life?
- ▼ How has it helped you in your personal life and the choices you have made?

# REFERENCES

Ajzen, I. (1991). Persuasive communication theory in social psychology: A historical perspective. In M.J. Manfredo (Ed.), *Influencing human behavior: Theory and application* (pp. 1-27). Champaign, Ill.: Sagamore.

*The Associated Press Stylebook and Libel Manual* (30th ed.). (1995). New York: Associated Press.

Babcock, D.E., and Miller, M.A. (1994). *Client education: Theory and practice.* St Louis: Mosby.

Babcock, D.E., and Zak-Dance, C. (1981). Developing skills as a public speaker. *AORN Journal, 33*(5), 994-1000.

Belenky, M.F., Clinchy, B.M., Goldberger, N.R., and Tarule, J.J. (1986). *Women's ways of knowing: The development of self, voice and mind.* New York: Basic Books.

Bohan, J.S. (1992). *Replacing women in psychology: Readings toward a more inclusive history.* Dubuque, Iowa: Kendall/Hunt Publishing Co.

Carnegie, D. (1962). *The quick and easy way to effective speaking* (2nd ed.). New York: Dale Carnegie and Associates.

Chaffee, J. (1994). Teaching for critical thinking. *Educational Visions, 9*(2), 6-7.

Claxton, C.S., and Murrell, P.H. (1987). *Learning styles: Implications for improving education practices* (ASHE-ERIC Higher Education Report No. 4). Washington, D.C.: Association for the Study of Higher Education.

Dobson, K.S. (Ed.). (1988). *Handbook of cognitive-behavioral therapies.* New York: Gilford Press.

Festinger, L.S. (1957). *A theory of cognitive dissonance.* Evanston, Ill.: Peterson.

Fishel, R. (1988). *Time for joy: Daily affirmations.* Deerfield Beach, Fla.: Health Communications, Inc.

Hanford, G. (1994). The danger of fragmentation. *American Visions, 9*(2), 6-7.

Hasemeier, C.S. (1994). The nursing life: Best friends. *American Journal of Nursing, 94*(10), 27-28.

Johnson, B.T., and Eagly, A.H. (1989). The effect of involvement on persuasion: A metaanalysis. *Psychological Bulletin, 106*(2), 290-314.

Kaufman, G., and Raphael, L. (1991). *Dynamics of power: Fighting shame and building self-esteem* (2nd ed.). Rochester, Vt.: Schenkman.

Littlejohn, S.W., and Jambusch, D.M. (1987). *Persuasive transactions.* Glenview, Ill.: Scott, Foresman and Co.

Neufeldt, V. (Ed.). (1991). *Webster's new world dictionary* (3rd ed.). New York: Webster's New World.

Poon, L.W., Fozard, J.L., Cermak, L.S., Arenberg, D., and Thompson, L.W. (Eds.). (1980). *New directions in memory and aging.* Proceedings of the George A. Talland Memorial Conference. Hillsdale, N.J.: Lawrence Erlbaum Associates.

*Publication manual of the American Psychological Association* (4th ed.). (1994). Washington, D.C.: Author.

Rappsilber, C. (1982). Persuasion as a mechanism for change. In J. Lancaster and W. Lancaster (Eds.), *The nurse as change agent* (pp. 132-145). St Louis: Mosby.

Raudenbush, S.W. (1984). Magnitude of teacher expectancy, effects on pupil IQ as a function of the credibility of expectancy induction: A synthesis of findings from 18 experiments. *Journal of Educational Psychology, 76,* 85-97.

Strunk, W. Jr., and White, E.B. (1979). *The elements of style* (3rd ed.). New York: Macmillan.

*The Chicago manual of style: The essential guide for writers, editors, and publishers* (14th ed.). (1993). Chicago: The University of Chicago Press.

# Learner Assessment Tool

## Appendix A

### LEARNING NEEDS ASSESSMENT TOOL
### CRITICAL THINKING STUDENT LEARNING PROFILE

Name _____

Course _____

### Student Expectations

1. I expect to learn the following about critical thinking:

2. I am interested in learning more about critical thinking because:

3. To me, critical thinking in nursing means:

### Previous Experiences

4. I have had a course in: _____ logic

_____ statistics

_____ speech

_____ debate

5. I have had the following experiences related to this course (other than the courses noted):

6. I believe that I know the following about critical thinking: _____ a little

_____ a moderate amount

_____ a lot

## School and Work Time Commitments

7. I am taking _____ semester hours this semester.

8. I am employed _____ hours per week this semester.

## Family/Other Responsibilities

9. Age(s) of/relationship(s) to the children for whom I care:

10. Others for whom I have or share responsibility:

11. Community responsibilities that I have (list):

12. Other commitments and pressing responsibilities that I have this semester are (describe):

## Learning Style/Needs

13. I learn best in the following ways:

14. Instructor behaviors that help me learn:

15. Instructor behaviors that inhibit my learning:

16. To help me participate and be successful in this course, the instructor should know:

# Example of Quantitative Research Report

Appendix B

_____

## EVALUATION OF THE SAFETY AND EFFICACY OF TOPICAL NITROGLYCERIN OINTMENT TO FACILITATE VENOUS CANNULATION

Patricia Griffith • Barbara James • Ann Cropp

*The purpose of this study was to determine the safety and efficacy of 2% nitroglycerin ointment to facilitate venous cannulation. In a double-blind experimental design, 80 adult subjects were randomly assigned to receive a 2% nitroglycerin ointment or a placebo ointment prior to cannulation. Variables measured before and after ointment application included heart rate, electrocardiogram, vein size, and presence of headache. No statistically significant differences were found in vein size or adverse effects following nitroglycerin ointment application.*

Venipuncture is an integral part of performing diagnostic procedures and administering therapy during a patient's hospitalization. Many techniques to facilitate venipuncture are advocated, such as tourniquet application, use of heat, dangling of the extremity, and tapping the vein. Recently, the topical application of nitroglycerin ointment has been advocated to dilate veins and facilitate venous access (Enich and Hindever, 1991; Wong, 1987). Minimal data exist to support this recommendation. A major concern with this practice is the potential for systemic absorption of nitroglycerin and the development of significant side effects related to the vasodilating properties of nitroglycerin.

Since the 1950s, nitroglycerin ointment has been used to treat angina when oral nitrates do not control chest pain. Topical application of nitroglycerin (2%) ointment is frequently prescribed to achieve systemic vasodilation and preload reduction. Side effects such as postural hypotension, headache, flushing, and reflex tachycardia may occur with therapeutic doses of 22.5 mg every 6 hours (McEvoy, 1989). Hemodynamic effects occur 15 to 60 minutes after ointment application and last 2 to 8 hours when therapeutic levels are >0.5 ng/mL. No major side effects of subtherapeutic doses have been reported.

From Griffith P, James B, and Cropp A: Nurs Res 43(4):203-206, 1994.

Plasma concentration data are unavailable after 2% nitroglycerin ointment is applied to the dorsal surface of the hand. It is thought that this absorption is site dependent, with peripheral sites leading to fewer hemodynamic effects (Deans and Hartshorn, 1986; Hansen, Woods, and Wills, 1979). In general, skin permeability, surface area of the ointment, thickness of the layer applied, and the concentration gradient all influence nitroglycerin plasma concentrations (Curry, et al., 1984).

The ability of nitroglycerin ointment to facilitate venous access has been examined in adult and pediatric patients. Three out of seven studies have reported improved venous access after topical application of nitroglycerin (Hecker, Lewis, and Stanley, 1983; Parakh and Patwaori, 1983; Roberge, et al., 1987). Generalization of these findings to other situations is not possible due to methodological problems with the studies. While current professional literature recommends applying topical nitroglycerin ointment to facilitate venous cannulation, the purpose of this study was to determine the safety and efficacy of topical nitroglycerin ointment application to facilitate venous cannulation.

## Method

*Sample:* Eligibility criteria included absence of cardiovascular disease, no current cardiac medications, a systolic blood pressure greater than 100mm Hg, and no previous allergies to medications. Subjects included 50 females and 30 males. Forty subjects received topical nitroglycerin ointment, and 40 received placebo ointment. Subjects ranged in age from 21 to 69 years, with a mean age of 41.3 (SEM ± 1.3) years. Forty subjects were normal volunteers, and 40 subjects, who had interstitial lung disease, were admitted for diagnostic bronchoscopy.

The study was approved by the institution's Investigational Review Board (IRB). Written informed consent was obtained from each subject. Data collection was conducted in an 18-bed pulmonary medical unit, part of a 54-bed federal research hospital.

*Instruments:* Blood pressures were recorded with a Sentrol automatic blood pressure monitor/printer, Model 400 (Bard Biomedical Division, Lombard, IL). The accuracy of the cuff pressure measurement displayed on digital readout correlated with a pressure standard ± 1% full scale. The zero pressure was computer corrected prior to each cuff inflation. Heart rate and rhythm were measured in the first 20 subjects using the Hewlett-Packard cardiac monitor, Model HP78334A (Waltham, MA). This monitor had a heart rate range of 15 to 300 beats/min = 0.15v to 3v. The accuracy was ± 5 beats/min with a resolution of 16 beats/min.

A visual analogue scale (VAS) was used to measure changes in subjective complaints of headache pain intensity. This is a valid and reliable paper-and-pencil test to assess clinical pain (Kramer, Atkinson, and Isnelzi, 1981; Lee and Kieckhefer, 1989; McGuire, 1984; Ohnhaus and Adle, 1975). The two extremes of the 100-mm VAS were "no headache" and "worse headache." Subjects were asked to draw a verticle line through the 100-mm horizontal scale to indicate the severity of their headache.

ECG calipers (Ciba, Philadelphia, PA), commonly used for fine measurements of electrocardiograms (ECG), were used to measure vein diameter. The numerical reading of the caliper measurement was determined by having a second investigator place the caliper against a millimeter ruler.

Plasma nitroglycerin samples were analyzed by trained personnel using a mass spectrometer (Model 5988A, Hewlett-Packard, Atlanta, GA) following manufacturer's specifications. Mass range is 10 to 1000 atomic mass unit (amu), with an accuracy of ± 0.13 amu.

*Procedure:* Subjects were randomly assigned to one of two groups prior to the venous cannulation procedure. One group received 2% nitroglycerin ointment (15 mg), and the other received a placebo ointment with the same lanolin base. A computer-generated randomization procedure was used, with the code held by the pharmacy. All persons directly involved in data collection were blind to the group assignment.

Subjects were placed in a comfortable, supine position. Both arms were examined to identify the best vein for cannulation. The criteria used for selecting the best vein were palpability, size and condition of the vein. The same investigator identified the best vein in all subjects.

An automated blood pressure monitor was applied to the arm not selected for IV cannulation. Before ointment application, blood pressure was measured every 5 minutes for 15 minutes, after ointment application, every 5 minutes for 30 minutes, and then every 15 minutes for another 30 minutes. Headache was measured with the VAS before ointment application and 15, 30, 45, and 60 minutes and 2, 4, and 8 hours after ointment application.

The study arm had a soft latex penrose tourniquet applied approximately 6 inches above the vein to be cannulated. The vein was identified, and one point of the ECG calipers was placed on one side of the vein and the other point placed on the opposite side of the vein. A second investigator then quantified all caliper vein measurements against the millimeter ruler.

The tourniquet was released and one inch of ointment (placebo or nitroglycerin) was applied to a 1 × 2 inch area over the selected vein using a template to confine the ointment. An occlusive dressing was then applied over the ointment and template. After 15 minutes, the remaining ointment was removed by a second investigator, lightly wiping once with a dry gauze sponge. The tourniquet was then reapplied and vein size remeasured as previously described. The skin over the selected vein was aseptically cleansed and allowed to dry for 30 seconds. The vein was then cannulated with a 21-gauge butterfly needle using a standard intravenous insertion technique. Blood samples were obtained as ordered for therapeutic purposes, the tourniquet was released, and the needle was either removed or attached to intravenous tubing for fluid administration. The same investigator performed all caliper vein measurements and venous cannulation in all subjects. This investigator was considered an expert in venous cannulation.

In addition to the above procedures, systemic nitroglycerin levels, cardiac rhythm, and heart rate were monitored in the first 20 subjects. A heparin lock was placed in the nonstudy arm prior to the start of the study for nitroglycerin blood samples. Blood samples were collected in precooled heparinized vacutainer tubes prior to ointment application and at 15 and 30 minutes after ointment application. Samples were immediately placed on ice and then centrifuged at 2400 rpm at 4°C for 5 minutes. The plasma was then transferred to siliconized glass tubes and frozen at −17°C. Frozen samples were sent for analysis (National Medical Services, Inc, Willow Grove,

PA). Nitroglycerin metabolites were determined by mass spectrometry (Model 5988A, Hewlett-Packard). Analysis of metabolites was determined by capillary gas chromatography and electron capture detection as recommended by Jaeger, Lutz, Michaelis, and Salama (1987).

A cardiac monitor was applied using standard technique. Cardiac rhythm strips (6 sec) were obtained every 5 minutes for 15 minutes before ointment application; and every 5 minutes for 30 minutes after ointment application. Heart rate and rhythm were later determined by the same experienced critical care nurse using standard ECG diagnostic criteria (Conover, 1992).

## Results

No statistical difference between groups was found for systolic or diastolic blood pressures over time. The systolic blood pressure pre-nitroglycerin-ointment application was $119 \pm 1.7$ ($M \pm SEM$) mm Hg, while the postmeasurement was $120 \pm 1.9$ mm Hg. Diastolic blood pressure pre-nitroglycerin-ointment application was $76.7 \pm 1.5$ mm Hg, and the postmeasurement was $76.1 \pm 1.6$ mm Hg. The systolic blood pressure pre- and post-placebo-ointment application was the same $122.4 \pm 2.0$ and $122.4 \pm 2.0$ mm Hg. The diastolic blood pressure before placebo application was $75.6 \pm 1.5$. It was $75.8 \pm 1.8$ mm Hg after application.

Both groups reported headaches. Ten subjects who received nitroglycerin ointment and 13 who received placebo ointment developed a headache within 8 hours of ointment application. The majority of VAS scores were below 5 mm. Scores > 5 mm primarily occurred 2 to 4 hours after ointment application.

Plasma nitroglycerin levels obtained in the first 20 subjects revealed no significant detectable drug levels. Plasma levels pre-nitroglycerine-ointment application were $0.01 \pm 0.01$ ng/mL and postapplications were $0.02 \pm 0.02$ ng/mL.

No significant changes in heart rates or cardiac rhythms occurred during or after the application of nitroglycerin or placebo ointment. The heart rate pre-nitroglycerin-ointment application was $74.0 \pm 1.4$ ($M \pm SEM$) beats/min, while the post measurement was $74.0 \pm 1.4$ beats/min. Heart rate pre-placebo-ointment application was $73.0 \pm 1.5$ beats/min, while the postmeasurement was $71.0 \pm 1.5$ beats/min.

Mean vein size increased after the application of both placebo and nitroglycerin ointment. Vein size pre- and post-placebo ointment was $6.9 \pm 0.33$ and $7.7 \pm 0.44$ mm, respectively. Vein size pre- and post-placebo-ointment was $6.6 \pm 0.3$ and $7.4 \pm 0.3$ mm, respectively. Significant differences in vein size were found before and after ointment application ($F_{2,154} = 3.18$, $p < .05$) but not between the nitroglycerin and placebo groups ($F_{1,154} = 0.96$, $p = .33$) Scheff's Multiple Comparison Test revealed a significant difference between the pretreatment vein size of the nitroglycerin and placebo groups ($p < .05$), as well as the posttreatment values ($p < .05$). Controlling for pretreatment vein size with analysis of covariance, no difference was found in posttreatment vein size. Venous cannulation was successful in all subjects with one attempt.

Erythema at the site of ointment application occurred in 8 subjects, 7 of whom received nitroglycerin and 1 who received placebo ointment. This erythema consisted of a fine, circumscribed rash ranging in size from $10 \times 20$ mm to $45 \times 100$ mms. The rash was observed 15 to 20 minutes after ointment application, resolving within 15 to 45 minutes. Eight subjects in the study were receiving therapeutic doses of steroids; however, none of these subjects developed erythema.

## Discussion

This study evaluated the safety and efficacy of topical nitroglycerin ointment application to facilitate venous cannulation. This is the first study to report plasma drug levels in evaluating this technique. Despite the finding that topical application of 2% nitroglycerin ointment was safe to use, vein size did not increase significantly.

The results with regard to safety in a highly controlled experimental design are similar to the findings of previous studies (Hecker, et al., 1983; Lohman, Moller, Brynitz, and Bryerrum, 1984; Manifold, et al., 1986; Maynard and Oh, W., 1989; Parakh and Patwaori, 1983; Roberge et al., 1987; Vaksman, Rey, Breviere, Smadja, and Dupuis, 1987). Because nitroglycerin may cause serious problems such as hypotension and headache, plasma drug levels were measured to determine systemic absorption. Results found in this study (0.5 ng/mL) were well below therapeutic nitroglycerin plasma levels (Jordan et al., 1986).

Only three previous studies measured blood pressure and pulse rate (Lohman, et al., 1984; Maynard and Oh, 1989: Roberge et al., 1987). These studies reported no significant hemodynamic changes after nitroglycerin administration, similar to the findings in the current study.

Headache, which was reported in both groups before and after the application of ointment, was higher in the control group. This underscores the importance of using placebo study designs in clinical trials. Evaluation of headache in previous studies was based on verbal complaints by subjects. Only one incidence of headache was reported (Parakh and Patwaori, 1983).

Several factors could have caused the erythema at the site of ointment application. These include the nitroglycerine, the occlusive dressing, or the lanolin base of the ointments. It is unlikely that the latter two factors caused the erythema since both the placebo and the nitroglycerin group had the same occlusive dressing and the lanolin base ointment. Findings from only previous study identified erythema associated with topical nitroglycerin (Maynard and Oh, 1989). However, anecdotal reports frequently describe skin irritation at the site of ointment application (Deans and Hartshorn, 1986; Hansen, et al., 1979; Hansen and Woods, 1980).

The efficacy of nitroglycerin ointment to aid venous access has been studied in both adult and pediatric populations in a variety of clinical settings, including emergency rooms, preanesthesia, chemotherapy clinics, nurseries, and in normal volunteers. Of the seven studies reported, five claimed that nitroglycerin increased vein size or caused vasodilation (Hecker, et al., 1983; Lohman, et al., 1984; Manifold, et al., 1986, Parakh and Patwaori, 1983; Roberge, et al., 1987). Methods for evaluating vein size, however, were poorly described and/or subjective, using visual estimates or vein size. A precise, objective measurement tool was used in this study. Other methodologic problems in previous studies included poor control of extraneous variables, small sample sizes, and no evaluation of systemic response to topical nitroglycerin. These problems may invalidate many of these studies' findings.

It is unclear what caused the measurable increase in vein size found in both groups of this study. Because vein size was measured before and after ointment application, the reapplication of the tourniquet may have trapped more blood the second time. Another explanation could be the positioning of the subjects during data collection, with arms resting below chest level on the bed for 15 minutes prior to the post-ointment-application measurement. This quiet, dependent position may have increased blood pooling in the extremity. No additional aids were used to increase vein size, such as tapping the vein, heat application, fist clenching, or extreme arm dependency.

Another important aspect of efficacy is the ability to cannulate the vein successfully. Two of the three previous studies reported that the degree of difficulty of cannulation was less when nitroglycerin ointment was applied (Hecker, et al., 1983; Parakh and Patwaori, 1983; Vaksman, et al., 1987). Of the three studies that evaluated cannulation success, one study found no difference (Manifold, et al., 1986), one found increased success (Roberge, et al., 1987), and one found decreased cannulation success after nitroglycerin ointment application (Maynard and Oh, 1989). Because of the lack of cannulation failures in the placebo group of this study, it is not possible to evaluate the efficacy of nitroglycerin ointment to facilitate venous cannulation.

Despite the frequent mention of aids to facilitate venous cannulation, there are no studies to document their efficacy. Future studies should evaluate the efficacy of heat application, arm dependency, fist clenching, and tapping of the vein to improve vein palpability and successful cannulation. Due to the increasing numbers of the patients with poor venous access from chronic illness, prolonged intravenous therapy, and administration of intravenous irritants, future studies should focus on patients with extremely poor venous access.

# REFERENCES

Conover, M. B. (1992). *Understanding electrocardiography: Arrhythmias and 12 lead ECG.* St Louis: Mosby.

Curry, S. H., Kwon, H. R., Perrin, J. H., Culp, J. R., Pepine, C. J., Yu, W. C., and Stevens, J. L. (1984). Plasma nitroglycerin concentrations and menodynamic effects of sublingual, ointment and controlled-release forms of nitroglycerin. *Clincial Pharmacology and Therapeutics, 36,* 765-772.

Deans, K., and Hartshorn, J. (1986). Cardiovascular pharmacology. *Journal of Cardiovascular Nursing, 1,* 81-86.

Enich, N., and Hindever, G. (1991, February). Performing venipuncture in elderly patients. *Nursing, 91,* 32C, D, H.

Hansen, M., and Woods, S. (1980). Nitroglycerin ointment: Where and how to apply it. *American Journal of Nursing, 80,* 1122-1124.

Hansen, M., Woods, S., and Willis, K. (1979). Relative effectiveness of nitroglycerin ointment according to site of application. *Heart and Lung: The Journal of Critical Care, 7* 16-720.

Hecker, J. F., Lewis, G. B., and Stanley, H. (1983). Nitroglycerin ointment as an aid to venipuncture. *Lancet, 2,* 332-333.

Jaeger, H., Lutz, D., Michaelis, K., and Salama, Z. B. (1987). Determination of nitrates in plasma. *Drugs, 33,* 9-22.

Jordan, R. A., Seth, L., Casebolt, P., Hayes, M. J., Wilen, M. M., and Franciosa, J. (1986). Rapidly developing tolerance to transdermal nitroglycerin in congestive failure. *Annals of Internal Medicine, 104,* 295-298.

Kramer, E., Atkinson, J., and Isnelzi, R. (1981). Patient preference does not confound pain measurement. *Pain, 10,* 241-248.

Lee, K., and Kieckhefer, G. (1989). Technical notes measuring human responses using visual analog scales. *Western Journal of Nursing Research, 1,* 130-132.

Lohman, M., Moller, P., Brynitz, S., and Byerrum, O. (1984). Nitroglycerin ointment as aid to venipuncture. *Lancet, 6,* 1416-1417.

Manifold, I. H., Cole, R., Mackintosh, M., Smith, W., Champion, A. E., and Hancock, B. E. (1986). A double blind trial of nitroglycerin vasodilator ointment in patients undergoing chemotherapy. *European Journal of Surgical Oncology, 12,* 67-68.

Maynard, E., and Oh, W. (1989). Topical nitroglycerin ointment as an aid to insertion of peripheral venous catheters in neonates. *Journal of Pediatrics, 3,* 474-476.

McEvoy, G. (Ed.). (1989). *American Hospital Formulary Service,* Bethesda, Md.: American Society of Hospital Pharmacists.

McGuire, D. B. (1984). The measurement of clinical pain. *Nursing Research, 33,* 152-156.

Nitroglycerin ointment: An aid to cannulation (1987). *American Journal of Nursing, 12,* 1656.

Ohnahaus, E., and Adle, K. (1975). Methodological problems in the measurement of pain: A comparison between the verbal rating scale and the visual analogue scale. *Pain, 1,* 379-384.

Parakh, S. C., and Patwaori, A. (1983). Experience with Nitrobid (2% Nitroglycerin) ointment as an aid to venipuncture. *British Journal of Anesthesia, 5,* 822.

Roberge, R., Kelly, M., Evans, T., Hobbs, E., Sayre, M., and Cottington, E. (1987). Facilitating intravenous access through local application of nitroglycerin ointment. *Annals of Emergency Medicine, 5,* 546-549.

Vaksman, G., Rey, C., Breviere, G. M., Smadja, D., and Dupuis, C. (1987). Nitroglycerin ointment as aid to venous cannulation in children. *Journal of Pediatrics, 3,* 89-91.

Wong, D. L. (1987). Venipuncture made easy and less painful. *American Journal of Nursing, 11,* 1403.

# Example of Qualitative Research Report

Appendix C

## A HEIDEGGERIAN HERMENEUTICAL ANALYSIS OF SURVIVORS OF INCEST

Lori L. Kondora

*The phenomenological study described in this paper examined the lived experience of adult women survivors of childhood incest. Self-identified incest survivors (N=5) participated in non-structured, audiotaped interviews. Subsequent transcripts were analyzed by a team of researchers using Heideggerian phenomenology to identify common meanings and themes in the texts. The major findings of the study suggested two constitutive patterns of lived experience among incest survivors: "Remembering As a Coming of What Has Been" and "Care: Reconstituting a Sense of Me."*

*(Keywords: abuse; sexual exploitation; women's issues; violence)*

Incest was traditionally thought to be rare, but it is now acknowledged to be reaching epidemic proportions. Current statistics suggest that about one in four females is sexually abused by the time she reaches 18 years of age with about 75 percent of the perpetrators being family members (Finkelhor, Hotaling, Lewis, and Smith, 1990). Incest is defined as sexual relations of any kind perpetrated by a biologically or nonbiologically related individual functioning in the role of a family member. The critical element of this definition is the role relation as opposed to genetic relation. It is both the biological and "pseudo" family from which the child justifiably expects sexual distance and protection.

In adulthood, many victims of childhood incest have chosen to call themselves survivors (Kelly, 1988). The notion of survival implies that these women have persevered. Children who are victims of incest often are forced or coerced into secrecy and silence. It is not unusual for a woman to lose contact with the memory of incestuous abuse until adulthood when a trigger event occurs (Briere, 1989). Many adult women survivors are choosing to tell their stories and break the long-standing silence thereby

From Kondora LL: Image J Nurs Sch 25(1):11-16, 1993.

gaining a sense of self-respect (Brady, 1981; Wisechild, 1988). Telling one's story can be a liberating experience and can provide opportunities for healing if the story is received by an engaged and knowledgeable listener (Bass and Davis, 1988).

Nurses are in a unique position to listen to these stories because our practice takes us into schools, public clinics, emergency rooms, industries, hospitals, communities, counseling centers and private practices. We provide intimate bodily care to women, and accompany them through birth and death as well as the crises of illness and injury. We are present during their moments of greatest sorrow, pain and joy. We are frequently in contact with survivors of incest, yet so few of us are sensitive and knowledgeable about their lived experience. We talk very little about incest in our nursing literature, curricula, research, theory development and practice. Striving to understand the meanings of incest to its survivors through study, self-reflection and dialogue can break the silence of our profession and transform our practice to be genuinely available to women who are struggling to heal from childhood incest.

## Literature Review

Typically incest survivors are studied according to what group of impairments they present (Browne and Finkelhor, 1986). The adult after effects of childhood incest can be quite diverse and range from little life disruption (Herman, Russell, and Trocki, 1986) to devastating psychiatric and/or physical illnesses (Beck and vanderKolk, 1987). Most survivors experience after effects that fall somewhere in the middle (Briere, 1989). The most widely recognized health consequence of incest is depression (Bagley and Ramsey, 1985; Briere and Runtz, 1988; Butler, 1978; Courtois, 1988; Finkelhor, 1979; Gil, 1988; Lowery, 1987; Peters, 1988; Sedney and Brooks, 1984). Other after effects frequently identified include sexual dysfunction, revictimization, anxiety and low self-esteem (Briere and Runtz, 1988; Brunngraber, 1986; Burgess and Holmstrom, 1978; Carson, Council, and Volk, 1988; Edwards and Donaldson, 1989; Feinauer, 1988; Gorcey, Santiago, and McCall-Perez, 1986; Herman and Hirschman, 1981; Kroll, 1988; Lowery, 1987; Sedney and Brooks, 1984; Stein, Golding, Siegel, Burnam, and Sorenson, 1988). Other after effects identified with less frequency include dissociative reactions (Briere and Runtz, 1988), addictive disorders (Peters, 1988; Stein, et al., 1988), sexual promiscuity (Brunngraber, 1986; deYoung, 1982), self-injurious behavior (deYoung, 1982; Kroll, 1988; Lowery, 1987), eating disorders (Bulik, Sullivan, and Rorty, 1989), somatization (Briere and Runtz, 1988), hallucinations (Ellenson, 1985; Feinauer, 1988), recurrent nightmares or terrors, flashbacks and amnesia related to childhood (Brunngraber, 1986; Edwards and Donaldson, 1989; Ellenson, 1986), and parenting problems (Goodwin, McCarthy, and Divasto, 1981). In addition to emotional and psychological effects there can be a host of physical sequelae including pelvic inflammatory disorder, bladder infections, chronic pain, hemorrhoids, headaches and chronic sore throat, most of which are felt to be directly related to the abuse experience (Bass and Davis, 1988; Brunngraber, 1986; Courtois, 1988; Gil, 1988; Walker, Katon, Harrop-Griffiths, Holm, Russo, and Hickok, 1988).

Child victims become adult survivors because they used creative survival strategies while the abuse was occurring. One such strategy, that of dissociation, is thought to be implicated in later memory impairment (Putnam, 1985). The impairment is usually in the form of complete or partial amnesia regarding the abuse experiences. However, the gap in memory may encompass entire chronological periods of childhood (Blake-White and Kline, 1985; Gelinas, 1983; Herman, 1986). Blocking or burying the details, sensations and feelings surrounding incest is a natural coping response to the severe pain of these traumatic experiences. But later they can recur in the form of flashbacks, nightmares, intrusive memories, panic attacks, anxiety and dysphoria (Blake-White and Kline, 1985; Horowitz, 1976). Many incest survivors do not have access to their incest histories until some trigger event allows remembrance, such as giving birth, returning to the childhood home, sexual assault or death of a loved one (Briere, 1989).

The overwhelming investigatory focus on post-incest symptomatology has left a gap in our knowledge about what it means on a day-to-day basis to be a survivor of childhood incest. Many autobiographical accounts in the popular press describe incest survivorship (Bass and Thornton, 1983; Brady, 1979; Donaforte, 1982; Morris, 1982; Sisk and Hoffman, 1987; Wisechild, 1987). However, nurses need phenomenologically based studies to reveal the personal journeys of survivors and help us understand their difficulties, their endurance, and their healing. Such was the purpose of the research reported here.

## Method

The methodology used in this study was ontological hermeneutics, which is a phenomenological approach based on the philosophical world view of Martin Heidegger (1927/1962). The method of Heideggerian hermeneutics seeks to uncover shared meanings through understanding rather than prediction and explanation. Everyday practical activities become part of our life stories, and this everydayness is the focus of hermeneutics (Woolfold, Sass, and Messer, 1988). Therefore, to understand a given culture (in this instance, the culture of adult women survivors of childhood incest) one must seek common, everyday, shared meanings (Benner and Wrubel, 1989). These common, everyday meanings provide an inside-out view of everyday experiences and become visible through instructured conversation.

Participants were recruited through the posting of notices in bookstores and university classroom buildings. Volunteers responding to the notices were fully informed about the study and their eligibility was established. Exclusionary criteria ruled out the participation of any women who were currently experiencing suicidal ideation, had experienced suicidal ideation and/or difficulty functioning within the last year, and/or had been hospitalized for acute emotional difficulties within the last year. Part of the process of obtaining informed consent was to assure each participant of confidentiality.

All five participants were recruited from a midwestern city and ranged in age from 26 to 48. Most were college educated, white and employed. Most of the participants were involved in partnered relationships, two of which were lesbian.

Participants were interviewed individually at a mutually agreed upon location. Four of the interviews took place in the homes of participants and one at the participant's place of employment. In an attempt to increase rapport, I typically brought food and/or coffee or tea to share during our conversation. Prior to each interview, the participant and I would spend about one hour conversing about topics of a general nature. The interviews themselves lasted about 90 minutes and were audiotaped. Consistent with the method introduced into nursing by Benner (1984), the interviews were unstructured and open-ended; therefore, no questionnaire or agenda was followed. Participants were asked to respond to the question "What does it mean to you to be a survivor of childhood incest?" The purpose of such a question was to call forth experiences that had meaning to the participant. Most of the participants required little prompting; it was common for participants to talk for up to one hour without need of further questions. When prompting was required, it consisted of "Tell me more about that," or "What did that mean to you?" There were periods of silence in some of the interviews lasting up to five minutes, four of the five women cried off and on throughout the interview and all five laughed occasionally.

Data obtained from the transcribed interviews were analyzed by the author and a research team according to the seven stage hermeneutical approach described by Diekelmann, Allen, and Tanner (1989). Initially, all five of the transcribed interviews were read by research team members to obtain an overall feel for the interviews. Weekly meetings were held thereafter where individual written interpretations of each interview were discussed. Any disagreements or contradictions in interpretations of team members were clarified by returning to the original interview text. The goal of the discussions was group consensus on interpretations, relational themes and patterns. Relying largely on the team's findings and discussions, the author then composed the final report. At this point in the analysis, two of the participants were contacted to read and validate the team's findings. Each of the participants agreed that the patterns, themes and analyses suggested by the research team were meaningful and consistent with their experience as survivors of childhood incest. This multistage process of analysis and expert consensual validation, in which participants are considered to be the experts, have been suggested as bias control strategies when conducting hermeneutical research (Benner, 1984; Diekelmann, Allen, and Tanner, 1989).

The analysis procedure described above was rigorously adhered to in order that the results would accurately reflect the meanings of the participants. Adequacy of interpretive research was achieved through several different measures described by Hall and Stevens (1991), including credibility, coherence, rapport, complexity, consensus, honesty and mutuality and reflexivity. Liberal use of quotes from participants will be used in this paper which will allow the reader to validate and establish adequacy of the study.

## Findings and Discussion

What was sought in the analysis was shared meanings and themes that were common in the texts. The highest level of hermeneutical analysis is a constitutive pattern, which is a shared meaning that is characteristic of all texts and expresses a relationship among themes. What follows is a description of the two constitutive patterns of lived experiences that emerged from these incest survivors' texts. The constitutive patterns were "Remembering As a Coming of What Has Been" and "Care: Reconstituting a Sense of Me."

### Remembering As a Coming of What Has Been

Remembering emerged as a central pattern in the analysis with each participant sharing numerous stories about it. The women took different paths to remembering. Some never lost contact with the memories of abuse, while others were recovering memories for the first time in adulthood. The stories remembered by incest survivors reflect what Heidegger termed a "coming of what has been" (1947/1971, p. 10). This "coming of what has been" is understood to be a commemorative thinking back. That is, we always have our memories, but we may not have access to them at certain times; therefore, the "coming" is an opening to experience "what has been." Participants in this study live this "coming of what has been" through allowing their past to inform their present and create new possibilities for themselves. This opening to remembrance is of central importance to incest survivors. The opening to remembrance is sometimes prompted by a traumatic even as this woman described:

> I had no memories whatsoever, then my daughter died . . . her death is what finally hit me behind the knees, up until that point, I had been so closed off from myself . . . I don't feel like it's ever been the same.

The process of remembering for these survivors of incest was very painful. Participants in this study told of feeling stalked by unwelcome remembrances of painful incest-related memories, as this woman described:

> I think that I'll probably go to my grave and the day before I die, one more thing will happen to let me know that incest is still a part of my life.

The pervasiveness of the memories was prominent in the womens's stories. As one woman shared:

> It is just these strange little pieces, they all seem to relate somehow to my incest . . . it permeates my thoughts so much, it's never gone, it's always there, I never expect it to leave.

All of the participants told stories of the return, during intimacy, of unwelcome and unpleasant memories of abuse which created many challenges. Hugging a friend, being touched on the shoulder or being sexual could call forth incest memories for survivors. One participant described olfactory, tactile and visual rememberings that intruded upon her when she was being sexually touched by a lover:

> . . . It made me remember things . . . all of a sudden the smells come back and the sights and the feelings . . . gag me

Another woman spoke of the intrusions that her remembrances caused during intimate moments:

> Sometimes my lover would do things that would just haunt me and all of a sudden it was like, I was really on the defensive, get away from me right now and my mood would change . . . it made me remember things . . . and then my lover feels like this bad person because of the memories of my Dad that came back . . . it's hard.

Likewise, what seemed like everyday events to most people, served as painful reminders of past abuse to many of these women. For instance, one woman was revisited by the same painful memory every time she suffered from an upper respiratory infection. As she described it:

> My Dad would hold my nose and put his mouth over my mouth so he could stick his tongue in my mouth, then he wouldn't let me breathe . . . I still get real depressed when I have a cold . . .

In addition to these painful reminders, many stories were told of the possibilities that emerged after recovering the memories of abuse. By allowing oneself to experience what has been, new possibilities and opportunities were created for the present. The possibility that was created for these women through the coming of remembrance was described by this woman:

> Before getting in touch with memories, I never went to bed with anyone that I didn't feel raped . . . finally, I feel like I have a real sexual relationship . . . this feels like an authentic relationship, and that we have a celebration of love, we have an expression of our passion for each other.

Remembering gives meaning to their daily lives through connections that the women make between their pasts and their presents. This woman described how remembering has given her life meaning and created new future possibilities for her:

> Certainly all of those years that I was experiencing all of the effects, but didn't know what they were, I just felt like I was living this huge lie, but since getting in touch with memories [of incest] I get to be real, I don't feel all bottled up inside . . . and that feels just wonderful—to be honest. That's one of the goodies.

Another participant told of her experience upon reaching her opening to remembrance:

> I just knew something awful was wrong. I had felt for a long time in my life that somehow if my life was a pie, there was a piece missing . . . I feel I am finally a whole pie.

Both of these participants had lost contact with memories of their abuse until adulthood. It was only after recovering those memories that they were able to create meaning regarding their feelings and feel as if the "missing piece" had been discovered. This woman described how the realization of incest memories influenced her life:

> It's like this double-edged sword you know, on one side there is bitterness and on the other side there is compassion and growth and understanding. I don't think I got a lot of bitterness, but I do think it [incest] has given me a way to treat other people more gently.

Childhood experiences are to assist us as we learn to dwell in the world. For these women, however, the childhood experiences of incest were unchosen and unwelcome. Remembering is constitutive of human life. We are always remembering, it shapes and is shaped by our experience. Memory and remembering are taken for granted because of their pervasiveness. We cannot get clear of remembering, it is always already (Casey, 1987). Adult women survivors of childhood incest experience a centrality of remembering such that their past is always illuminated in front of them.

### Care: Reconstituting a Sense of Me

Caring emerged as a central pattern in these stories. Participants talked of the lack of care they had experienced as children and how this affected their sense of self. Women talked of feeling worthless and weak as children. One participant described living in a "soup of neglect" in which she was seldom able to experience nurturance, guidance or protection from a caring adult. As children, the women described feeling different from those around them. This differentness was apparent to them as they compared their reality to that of those around them and were left feeling as if they had missed out on something. The presence of incest in their lives constricted many childhood possibilities. This woman described what she missed:

> It [incest] prevented me from learning so many skills and things that kids learn . . . for example, I don't know how to ice skate or swim . . . you don't have a lot of adult skills . . . like problem solving . . . there was no way to learn them because you carried so much fear that trying new things was just not something you did as a child.

When caring acts were experienced, they were very meaningful and often prompted women to care for themselves. Through this caring for self, women were able to reconstitute a sense of themselves and regain a reciprocity in caring, in which they began to gain self-acceptance and feel a sense of personal empowerment. This woman reflected on being a child, nine years old, with virtually no self-esteem. Her own parents showed no interest in her education and her grades were indicative of that. Then, a friend's parents began to care:

> As soon as I met my first girlfriend, my life really started to change. I was a really bad student, and being with her and her parents, ah, I could be nothing but a student that should be improving her grades. I jumped to an A-B student, I learned how to study.

It was her friend's parents concern and interest in her that prompted her to care for herself. The simple fact that her friend's parents asked her "How were your grades?" and then listened to her response inspired her to improve them. Prior to receiving this care from her girlfriend's parents, this woman was unable to care for herself. It was only after experiencing care, that this participant recognized herself as being worthy of love, nurturance and attention.

Another woman described a caring act she experienced as an adult that created the possibility for her to care for herself. She told a lengthy story in which she was without financial resources and unable to provide for herself and her children. A woman from her church community offered to give her money, food and child care until the participant could get back on her feet. She described this incident that created the possibility for her to care for herself:

> There was this woman in the church . . . she kept caring about me . . . it was really strange to have her care for me because I didn't care much for myself and neither did my family . . . I finally had to understand that there were people that cared about me, maybe there had to be something of redeeming value somewhere in me.

As nurses we can care by concentrating on positive meanings and strengths rather than losses and deficits stemming from incest trauma. Through concentration on positive meanings and strengths, the relationship between nurse and incest survivor will no longer need to focus on the language of pathology and symptoms, but on stories that celebrate the human spirit.

What stands out about these particular stories, is that these women talked of feeling as if they had actually been chosen as being worthy of care from others. They had not received that kind of invested, engaged, reciprocal caring from family members. Receiving this care from others set up the possibility for them to care for themselves and to construct a new sense of themselves.

Part of the reclaiming of self is in the retelling of the story. There is transformative power in telling the story of incest, not the details of the abuse, but the story as it is lived. The act of telling one's story is thought to be therapeutic and empowering in and of itself (Diekelmann, 1991; Mishler, 1986; Polkinghorne, 1988). When a survivor tells her story and it is received by a caring, engaged listener, a healing dialogue is set into motion. These women shared what telling was like for them:

> I appreciate the opportunities to talk about the amount of work this is . . . I am also aware that it is healing, it helps me on my journey.

> It feels good to talk about this . . . each time I talk about these things I get farther away from it [incest] but also closer, closer to myself.

One woman said to me, "no one wants to hear this." We must maintain a place in our practice for listening to stories. This listening is not a simple skill that everyone can do, but a complex and engaged hearing. This type of hearing does not seek to guide nor direct; the engaged listener accompanies the storyteller on the journey, walking alongside the teller. Perhaps, engaged listening can best be described as a type of presence in which the listener actually becomes a part of the story.

Many of the women in this study talked of feeling as if they had missed out on important childhood experiences because they were traumatized by abuse. Many participants had to unlearn (not re-learn) childhood behaviors in their adult years. This learning how to live anew in adulthood was an important part of the claiming of personal power and strength that characterizes these women's redefinition of self:

> When you begin this healing work, it's like leaving one planet, going to another where the language, the culture, the dress, everything's different and having to learn all of that again. It's like starting from square one.

Each participant talked of long and arduous journeys that she had undertaken to reach the point where positive meanings were possible. This woman who previously viewed herself as weak, figuratively expressed the fervor of her self-care:

> That I am strong, that I can absolutely do anything that I want to. There is a part of me that I recaptured through this healing that I love. In a sense, it's a crude part, but it's basically, ah, if you try to hurt me, I will kill you. It is that absolute, that inner strength.

Another woman describes her connection with herself that came only after getting in touch with memories of previous abuse:

I am not sure I would be so in touch with myself had I not had to go through this process. I think most people pass over that, if they don't have something happen to really feel themselves, all the way to their toes. It's sort of like setting fire to yourself to see if you have any feeling.

Paradoxically, caring was missing from the childhood memories of these women, but it is what finally enabled them to care for themselves. Positive meanings began to emerge following the recognition of self-worth. Each of these women participated in a personal transformation that occurred in response to caring.

## Conclusion

Women in this study live the coming of memories on a day-to-day basis for a lifetime. As nurses, we must be aware of the pervasiveness of incest remembering and consider the potential influence that remembering can have on the life of an incest survivor. We must be open to bearing witness to these stories, painful as they may be, because in the telling, healing and transformation occur. What can potentially happen is a transformation of nurses through understanding the meanings of incest to its survivors. If we, as nurses, remain open to all possibilities and allow these womens' stories to speak to us, we will hear transformation, healing, surviving, and resiliency.

After taking part in these conversations and bearing witness to this reconstitution of self, I have come to rejoice in the tenacity and resoluteness of the human spirit. Each of the participants has reconstituted a sense of self through her ability to survive and perservere. These positive meanings and this strength can be the focus of our interaction with survivors.

# REFERENCES

Bagley, C., and Ramsey, R. (1985, February). *Disrupted childhood and vulnerability to sexual assault: Long term sequels with implications for counseling.* Paper presented at the Conference on Counseling the Sexual Abuse Survivor. Winnipeg, Canada.

Bass, E., and Davis, L. (1988). *The courage to heal: A guide for women survivors of child sexual abuse.* New York: Harper and Row.

Bass, E., and Thornton, L. (Eds.). (1983). *I never told anyone: Writings by women survivors of child sexual abuse.* New York: Harper and Row.

Beck, J., and vanderKolk, B. (1987). Reports of childhood incest and current behavior of chronically hospitalized psychotic women. *American Journal of Psychiatry, 144,* 1474–1476.

Benner, P. (1985). Quality of life: A phenomenological perspective on explanation, prediction and understanding in nursing scirnce. *Advances in Nursing Science, 8,* 1–14.

————. (1984). *From novice to expert: Excellence and power in clinical nursing practice.* Menlo Park, Calif.: Addison-Wesley.

Benner, P., and Wrubel, J. (1989). *The primacy of caring.* Menlo Park, Calif.: Addison-Wesley.

Blake-White, J., and Kline, C. (1985). Treating the dissociative process in adult victims of childhood incest. *Social Casework: The Journal of Contemporary Social Work, 66,* 394–402.

Brady, K. (1979). *Father's days: A true story of incest.* New York: Dell.

Briere, J. (1989). *Therapy for adults molested as children: Beyond survival.* New York: Springer.

Briere, J., and Runtz, M. (1988). Symptomatology associated with childhood sexual victimization in a non clinical adult sample. *Child abuse and neglect, 12,* 51–59.

Browne, A., and Finkelhor, D. (1986). Impact of child sexual abuse: A review of the research. *Psychological Bulletin, 99,* 21–27.

Brunngraber, L. (1986). Father-daughter incest: Immediate and long-term effects of sexual abuse. *Advances in Nursing Science, 8,* 15–35.

Bulik, C., Sullivan, P., and Rorty, M. (1989). Childhood sexual abuse in women with bulimia. *Journal of Clinical Psychiatry, 50,* 460–464.

Burgess, A., and Holmstrom, L. (1978). Recovery from rape and prior life stress. *Research in Nursing and Health, 1,* 165–174.

Butler, S. (1978). Conspiracy of silence: The trauma of incest. New York: Bantam Books.

Carson D., Council, J., and Volk, M. (1988). Temperament, adjustment and alcoholism in adult female incest victims. *Violece and Victims, 3,* 205–216.

Casey, E. (1987). *Remembering: A phenomenological study.* Bloomington, Ind.: Indiana University Press.

Courtois, C. (1988). *Healing the incest wound: Adult survivors in therapy.* New York: W.W. Norton and Co.

deYoung, M. (1982). Self-injurious behavior in incest victims: A research note. *Child Welfare, 61,* 577–584.

Diekelmann, N. (1991). The emancipatory power of the narrative. In *Curriculum revolution: Community building and activism* (41–62). New York: The National League for Nursing Press.

Diekelmann, N., Allen, D., and Tanner, C. (1989). *The NLN criteria for appraisal of baccaluareate programs: A critical hermeneutic analysis.* New York: The National League for Nursing Press. Pub No. 15-2253.

Donaforte, L. (1982). *I remembered myself: The journal of a survivor of childhood sexual abuse.* Ukiah, Calif.: Self-published.

Edwards, P., and Donaldson, M. (1989). Assessment of symptoms in adult survivors of incest: A factor analytic study of the responses to a childhood incest questionaire. *Child Abuse and Neglect, 13,* 101–110.

Ellenson, G. (1986). Disturbances of perception in adult female incest survivors. *Social Casework: The Journal of Contemporary Social Work, 67,* 149–159.

Ellenson, G. (1985). Detecting a history of incest: A predictive syndrome. *Social Casework: The Journal of Contemporary Social Work, 66,* 525–532.

Feinauer, L. (1988). Relationship of long-term effects of childhood sexual abuse to identity of the offender: Family, friend or stranger. *Women and Therapy, 7,* 89–107.

Finkelhor, D. (1979). *Sexually victimized children.* New York: The Free Press.

Finkelhor, D., Hotaling, G., Lewis, I., and Smith, C. (1990). Sexual abuse in a national survey of adult men and women: Prevalence, characteristics and risk factors. *Child Abuse and Neglect, 14,* 19–28.

Gelinas, D. (1983). The persisting negative effects of incest. *Psychiatry, 40,* 312–332.

Gil, E. (1988). *Treatment of adult survivors of childhood incest.* Walnut Creek, Calif.: Launch Press.

Goodwin, J., McCarthy, T., and Divasto, P. (1981). Prior incest in mothers of abused children. *Child Abuse and Neglect, 5,* 87–96.

Gorcey, M., Santiago, J., and McCall-Perez, F. (1986). Psychological consequences for women sexually abused in childhood. *Social Psychiatry, 21,* 129–133.

Hall, J., and Stevens, P. (1991). Rigor in feminist research. *Advances in Nursing Science, 13,* 16–29.

Heidegger, M. (1947/1971). *Poetry, language, thought.* (A. Hofstadter, Trans.). New York: Harper and Row.

Heidegger, M. (1927/1962). *Being and time.* (J. Macquarrie and E. Robinson, Trans.). New York: Harper and Row.

Herman, J. (1986). Histories of violence in an outpatient population: An exploratory study. *American Journal of Orthopsychiatry, 56,* 137–141.

Herman, J., and Hirschman, L. (1981). *Father-daughter incest.* Cambridge, Mass.: Harvard University Press.

Herman, J., Russel, D., and Trocki, K. (1986). Long-term effects of incestuous abuse in childhood. *American Journal of Psychiatry, 143,* 1293–1296.

Horowitz, M. (1976). *Stress response syndromes.* New York: Jason Aronson.

Kelly, L. (1988). *Surviving sexual violence.* Minneapolis, Minn.: University of Minnesota Press.

Kroll, J. (1988). *The challenge of the borderline patient: Competency in diagnosis and treatment.* New York: W.W. Norton and Co.

Lowery, M. (1987). Adult survivors of childhood incest. *Journal of Psychosocial Nursing and Mental Health Services, 25,* 27–31.

Mishler, E. (1986). *Research interviewing: Context and narrative.* Cambridge, Mass.: Harvard University Press.

Morris, M. (1982). *If I should die before I wake.* New York: Dell.

Peters, S. (1988). Child sexual abuse and later psychological problems. In G. Wyatt and G. Powell (Eds.). *Lasting effects of child sexual abuse.* Beverly Hills, Calif.: Sage.

Polkinghorne, D. (1988). *Narrative knowing and the human sciences.* Albany, N.Y.: State University of New York Press.

Putnam, F. (1985). Dissociation as a response to extreme trauma. In R. Kluft (Ed.). *Childhood antecedents of multiple personality* (66–97). Washington, D.C.: American Psychiatric Press.

Sedney, M., and Brooks, B. (1984). Factors associated with a history of childhood sexual experiences in a non-clinical female population. *Journal of the Academy of Child Psychiatry, 23,* 215–218.

Sisk, S., and Hoffman, C. (1987). *Inside scars: Incest recovery as told by a survivor and her therapist.* Gainsville, Fla.: Pandora Press.

Stein, J., Golding, J., Siegel, J., Burnam, M., and Sorenson, S. (1988). Long-term psychological sequelae of child sexual abuse: The Los Angeles epidemiologic catchment area study. In G. Wyatt and G. Powell (Eds.), *Lasting effects of child sexual abuse* (135–156). Newbury Park, Calif.: Sage.

Walker, E., Katon, W., Harrop-Griffiths, J., Holm, L., Russo, J., and Hickok, L. (1988). Relationship of chronic pelivic pain to psychiatric diagnoses and childhood sexual abuse. *American Journal of Psychiatry, 145,* 75–80.

Wisechild, L. (1988). *The obsidian mirror: An adult healing from incest.* Seattle, Wash.: Seal Press.

Woolfolk, R., Sass, L., and Messer, S. (1988). Introduction to hermeneutics. In S. Messer, L. Sass and R. Woolfolk (Eds.). *Hermeneutics and psychological theory: Interpretive perspectives on personality, psychotherapy, and psychopathology* (2–26). New Brunswick, N.J.: Rutgers University Press.

# Guidelines for Writing an Issue Paper

## Appendix D

## ISSUE SELECTION

A suitable issue for this paper may be social, political, educational, environmental, cultural, economic, or psychological in nature and related in some way to nursing and health care. Think about what concerns you most about your world, nursing, and health care. Select an issue that you would like to examine in greater depth. Your frame of reference should be professional and may be neighborhood, city, state, national, or international in scope.

Remember that an issue is a matter about which intelligent, informed people disagree. An issue often generates strong emotional responses among people who hold different points of view.

Confirm the acceptability of your selected issue with the instructor. *Do this no later than* _____ (date).

## ISSUE CLARIFICATION

1. Express your issue in writing. By externalizing it, you can further examine, clarify, and refine your wording. Express the issue in the "Is . . . ?" "Does . . . ?" or "Should . . . ?" form. See Chapter 8 for examples.

2. Distinguish between the central issue and peripheral issues.

3. Present your issue in class. Listen to the feedback provided by your colleagues. They will help you clarify your thinking and further focus your issue. Notify the instructor when you are ready to present your issue. *Do this no later than* _____ (date).

## ISSUE DEVELOPMENT

1. Define the key terms and concepts.

2. Describe the context of your issue.

3. Identify your assumptions. What are you taking for granted?

## REASONS AND CONCLUSION

1. To resolve the issue means to choose a conclusion, belief, or point of view that you believe to be the most reasonable in response to your issue.

2. Construct your reasons and determine how you will present them to lead to your conclusion.

3. Support your reasons with relevant data, evidence, experience, and other information as appropriate.

4. What do your reasons value? What are your priorities?

5. Acknowledge alternative points of view and prepare a defense for each anticipated objection.

## IMPLICATIONS

Discuss the implications of your position. What positive and negative consequences might result? Are the consequences of your position acceptable? To whom? Who or what is affected?

## REFERENCE LIST

A reference list is required. Use the American Psychological Association format.

## GRADING

This issue paper is _____ % of your final grade for the course. It should be type-written.  It will be graded as follows:

| | |
|---|---|
| Issue clarification | 10% |
| Issue development | 20% |
| Reasons and conclusion | 40% |
| Implications | 20% |
| Style, readability, clarity, spelling, punctuation | 10% |
| Total | 100% |

Due date for written paper _____


Due date for oral presentation in class _____

# Index